Diversity and Aging Among Immigrant Seniors in Canada

Changing Faces and Greying Temples

Editors

Douglas Durst

Michael MacLean

DETSELIG
ENTERPRISES LTD

Detselig Enterprises Ltd.
Calgary, Alberta

Library and Archives Canada Cataloguing in Publication Data

Diversity and aging among immigrant seniors in Canada : changing faces
   and greying temples / edited by Douglas Durst and Michael MacLean

Includes bibliographical references.
   ISBN 978-1-55059-407-2

1. Older immigrants – Canada. 2. Minority older people – Canada
 I. Durst, Douglas II MacLean, Michael J., 1947-

HQ1064.C2D59 2010   305.26086'9120971   C2010-905042-8

DETSELIG
ENTERPRISES LTD

Detselig Enterprises Ltd.
210, 1220 Kensington Road NW
Calgary, Alberta
T2N 3P5

Phone: 403-283-0900   Fax: 403-283-6947
email: temeron@telusplanet.net
www.temerondetselig.com

We acknowledge the support of the Government of Canada through the Canada
Books Program for our publishing program.

We acknowledge the support of the Alberta Foundation for the Arts for our publishing program.

Alberta
Foundation
for the Arts

978-1-55059-407-2   SAN 113-0234   Printed in Canada

Contents

Acknowledgements

Working on this volume has been a "labor of love" mainly because of the importance of the topic and the contributions from the many current researchers. Thank you to all the contributors for their timely and relevant chapters and their superb work in meeting deadlines and quick responses to our "pesky" questions. It has been a real pleasure working with such high calibre of colleagues.

Our sincere gratitude goes to the Metropolis Canada and especially the Prairie Metropolis Centre for their encouragement and financial support to see the completion of this project. Their continued and consistent support for research and, just as importantly, dissemination of knowledge on Canada's immigration, is gratefully recognized. Thank you to Dr. Baha Abu-Laban for his initial support and Drs. Linda Ogilvie and Tracey Derwing, Co-Directors of the Prairie Metropolis Centre, for their on-going encouragement.

We thank Karen Martens Zimmerly and Alaina Harrison for assistance in proof reading and editing. Thank you to the Faculty of Social Work and the Social Policy Research Unit, University of Regina, for their "support in kind."

On the production side, we thank Ted Giles, for editing, production and design. We thank James Dangerous for his cover design.

Reading the chapters, we are touched by the stories of those individuals who left their homelands to come to Canada. We are moved by their personal commitment to their new home and how they have shaped Canada's past, present and future.

Douglas Durst and Michael MacLean

Preface

When considering immigrants, many people assume that immigrants are "young" but senior immigrants are not new in Canada. Throughout the history of Canada, our foreign-born members have aged in Canada and made important and significant contributions to our country. It is surprising to many people to learn that the prairie provinces of western Canada have the highest percentages of foreign born seniors; they emigrated from Europe many decades ago. However, in recent years, the faces of our senior population have been changing. With changes in source countries, our senior population is beginning to reflect the diversity in demographics of the nation as a whole. With increasing ethnic diversity among our aging population come some new challenges and opportunities. Some of these seniors immigrated as adults and aged in Canada and others aged in their homelands prior to family unification. All of them bring diversity and contribute in all aspects of Canadian society whether it is social, economic, political or spiritual. Little attention has been given to this demographic, social change. We know so little about them and the challenges they face. This edited volume attempts to address this lack in knowledge and makes an important contribution for policy and program planning. Readers in social policy, social gerontology, social work, public health/administration and community development will be informed and challenged by the discussions proposed by scholars from across Canada. Many of the chapters provide specific and concrete recommendations for practitioners and policy planners. Some of the contributors come from a social gerontological background with an emphasis on aging while others have a research background on immigration or ethnicity. It is exciting to see these two important backgrounds come together and teach us what they know. There are numerous chapters addressing gender concerns from a feminist perspective and structural issues with a critical analysis. The book is interdisciplinary with contributions from economics, nursing, medicine, sociology, social work and psychology. Its diversity across theoretical perspectives and disciplines is its strength.

The book is divided into major sections. The first section is meant to have chapters that are broader in focus to include issues pertaining to most immigrant seniors. It is offers a foundation and a context for the topic of aging and immigration. In the second section, the chapters are more focused on various ethnic groups but with important implications for the broader population. The book concludes with a chapter by the editors that attempts to link the major themes and leads the reader into future topics of discussion and research.

The volume will be of interest to a matrix of readers. First, there are those who are primarily interested in immigrants, cultural diversity or ethnicity and, second, those interested in the field of gerontology, aging and seniors. These two themes can then be intersected with three readerships: service providers who practice or deliver programs and services in either communities (seniors or immigrants); social and health policy developers in either themes (seniors or immigrants) and; academics and researchers who research and teach in either theme (seniors or immigrants). The volume is a useful resource for practitioners, policy researchers, academics and students.

The introductory chapter gives an overview of the topic and includes a brief history of immigration, classes of immigration and refugees, and current demographics of immigrant seniors. It also introduces concepts of aging and a summary of current issues.

Herbert C. Northcott and Jennifer L. Northcott provide a review of recent literature examining the integration of immigrant seniors in Canada. This chapter examines various issues relating to the economic, health, social, linguistic and cultural integration of immigrant seniors in Canada. Key priorities regarding the integration needs of immigrant seniors are identified and recommendations made.

Lynn McDonald argues that an enduring complaint about research on aging is its atheoretical nature, so it comes as no surprise that theorizing ethnicity and aging is minimal. Most theory is still caught at the intersection of gerontological theories and general theories of ethnicity. Specifically, in multicultural countries like Canada, most of the focus has been on inequality by examining the additive disadvantage of being old and belonging to an ethnic group. In this chapter, the author reviews assimilation and modernization theories through to age stratification and ethnic stratification and the construction ethnicity. She concludes with an examination of the life course as a cultural construct that may have promise for theorizing about ethnicity.

Sharon Koehn, Charmaine Spencer and Eunju Hwang outline the legal, social, and health implications of the immigration laws and policies related to sponsorship of elderly relatives under the Family Class immigration category. Examples are drawn from original case studies of the South Asian and Chinese immigrant populations in British Columbia.

Referring to both the literature and their own research among immigrant older people and their families, Jean-Pierre Lavoie, Nancy Guberman, and Shari Brotman explore cultural versus structural debates regarding differences in care patterns among immigrant and non-immigrant families, including the role of methodology in the maintenance of confusion about the respective role of cultural/structural factors. They review the dangers of overemphasizing the role of culture in intervention with immigrant seniors.

Hugh Grant and James Townsend present the economic issues facing immigrant seniors. They tell the reader that elderly immigrants are more likely to live with economic families that are earning less than the LICO; the differences are more pronounced for men (12.5% for immigrants versus 8.0% for native born) than for women (20.1% for immigrants versus 17.6% for native born). These figures mask a number of worrying patterns; immigrants that arrived after the age of 30 or came from developing countries have much higher poverty rates than the native born. Regardless of immigrant status, individuals living alone experience rates of poverty exceeding 30%.

The purpose of the chapter by Atsuko Matsuoka, Antionette Clarke and Darlene Murphy is to present an alternative intervention for addressing elder abuse and neglect of minority older women at risk. The alternative intervention presented here is based on restorative justice mediation and strengths-based critical social work. The authors apply the intervention model to two minority populations: Japanese and Caribbean seniors.

Recent research in end-of-life care shows there has been considerable work in this area in the past few years but that very little of this research considers end-of-life issues for immigrant seniors. Michael MacLean, Nuelle Novik, Kavita Ram and Allison Schmidt explore this limited research on immigrant seniors and use qualitative data from interviews with immigrant seniors to document some of the issues faced by these seniors and their families at this stage of life.

The face of residential care has been changing and issues confronting long term care facilities and personal care homes are explored by Douglas Durst. This chapter introduces the concepts of continuing care and types of long-term care facilities in Canada. Since there are a lot of myths and fears about long-term care, this chapter provides readers who are new to the field a foundation from which to understand the issues facing ethnic minority seniors and their families.

Edward Makwarimba, Miriam Stewart, Zhi Jones, and Knox Makumbe, Edward Shizha and Denise Spitzer present the investigated perceptions of support resources, and perspectives on support programs preferred by immigrant seniors from four different ethnic groups (i.e., former Yugoslavians, Spanish-speaking Latino, Chinese (Mandarin-speaking), and English-speaking Afro-Caribbean. They offer insights on how services and policies can be adapted and improved.

Social capital is an emerging concept in social policy and research arenas. According to Daniel Lai and Shirley Chau, no research has specifically examined the role of social capital on the health of elderly Chinese immigrants. Based on their findings from a multi-site study of a random sample of aging Chinese adults in Canada, their chapter examines the effect of social capital on health and well being of 1 537 elderly Chinese immigrants. The findings are useful in informing policy makers and health service providers the directions for enhancing health of elderly immigrants.

Elder abuse is a major problem with profound effects on the quality of life of older persons. In Canada, demographic shifts and the increased need for care provision make this issue particularly salient. Christine. A. Walsh and Shelina Hassanali discuss elder abuse of Chinese immigrant elders, exploring those cultural variables which make this experience similar to and different from elders of other ethnic backgrounds.

The experiences of the African immigrant are quite unique and editor, Douglas Durst, and Godknows Kumassah present the history of the immigration of Africans to Canada. They present research on immigrants and refugees, and the conceptual/theoretical perspective of the image of Africans in North America is examined with references to aging and seniors.

Siavash Jafari, Richard Mathias and Souzan Baharlou's ethnographic observations and qualitative study of elderly Iranian-Canadians reveal several cultural and religious factors as the barriers to successful acculturation and mental well-being. Poor integration in the main stream culture, improper communication, lack of English language skills, and strong cultural ties were among the main barriers to access to and use of mental health services.

Cheuk Fan Ng and Herbert C. Northcott examine the integration and adaptation of 161 elderly South Asian immigrants 60 or more years of age surveyed in Edmonton, Alberta in 2003. Comparisons are made between older immigrants who came to Canada recently and those who came less recently, and between females and males. This study focuses on three sets of factors relevant to immigrant integration: social and cultural factors, family and interpersonal relationships, and living arrangements.

Carlos Teixeira's interesting case study explores issues related to neighborhood change in Toronto's "Little Portugal." The author indicates that gentrification, steadily rising property taxes, and increasing housing maintenance costs are all major concerns that are forcing some Portuguese seniors to sell their properties.

In Louise Racine's chapter, the everyday struggle to reconcile paid work with caring activities of middle-aged Haitian Canadian women caregivers is described. More specifically, the extent to which women caregivers are torn between Haitian cultural traditions and the need to adapt to the Canadian market economy are examined. Second, the influence of immigration in redefining family dynamics of Haitian Canadian families is examined. Third, a detailed description of the lived experiences of two aged men caregivers is presented to illustrate the social and economic impact of caring among older immigrants.

Nuelle Novik's study draws upon three generations of elderly Ukrainian immigrant women to explore the factors impacting their lives. This qualitative study involved 20 women from 7 distinct families in Saskatchewan. The women told her that quality of life is all about relationships: marital, family and community.

Ann H. Kim considers the structural and cultural implications of various housing arrangements for Korean immigrant older adults. Using census data and interviews, she examines issues of access to housing, barriers to institutionalized housing, and the degree to which cultural prescriptions regarding family responsibilities to house aging parents have shifted for the Korean community.

Ben Kuo applies a bidirectional model of acculturation to examine the demographic, psychosocial, and health predictors of Canadian Acculturation and Chinese Identification, respectively, in a sample of 213 elderly Chinese Canadian immigrants. Interestingly, he finds that the identification to either Chinese or Canadian orientations is not related and the two identifications are primarily independent of each other.

Gurnam Sanghera provides a personal and reflective discussion on the perspectives of elderly Punjabi in Canada. He provides some interesting background to their cultural perspectives on growing old and living in their new land. His chapter nicely summarizes the humanity and companssion called for in many of the previous chapters.

In the final chapter, editors Douglas Durst and Michael MacLean attempt to weave the discussion and link the various themes into concluding comments. They identify critical issues and offers some suggestions for further research and debate.

The volume uses Canada Census data so a number of definitions should be explained. When the term "foreign-born population" is used, it includes permanent residents and citizens who were born outside of Canada and excludes persons born outside Canada who are Canadian citizens by birth. The term "visible minorities" is defined by the federal *Employment Equity Act* as "persons, other than Aboriginal peoples, who are non-Caucasian in race or non-white in color." The Act specifies the following groups as visible minorities: Chinese, South Asians (eg., Indian, Pakistani), Blacks, Arabs, West Asians (eg. Iranian, Afghan), Filipinos, Southeast Asians (eg., Vietnamese, Cambodian), Latin Americans, Japanese, Koreans and other visible minority groups, such as Pacific Islanders.

The editors have avoided the term "race" to describe differences between groups, populations and cultures because it has no bearing physically. Biologically, it does not exist and its frequent use perpetuates this myth that there are significant physiological differences between groups. However, it does have social and political contexts and we prefer "racialization" to describe the often false assumptions, beliefs and attitudes towards people who appear differently. Some of our contributors have used the word "race" and when the word "race" appears in this volume, it is in a social and "racialized" context.

The astute reader will find mistakes in this text. There will be missed editorial corrections, poor choice of words and weak sentence structure. The mistakes are ours and we seek the reader's patience and indulgence.

We hope that this text adds and builds our body of knowledge and understandings of these special people. It is only the beginning and not the last word. The readers' feedback and comments are always welcomed.

Douglas Durst and Michael MacLean
Editors
October, 2010

Part 1

Foundation: Setting the Stage

1

Elderly Immigrants in Canada: Changing Faces and Greying Temples

Douglas Durst, (University of Regina)

The phrase, "Canada is a nation of immigrants," has been repeated so frequently that it has become a cliché; however, this fact has shaped and formed every aspect of Canada. Since Samuel de Champlain brought the first settlers to Port Royal in 1605, newcomers have crossed the Atlantic Ocean, and now the Pacific, to make this northern land their permanent home.[1] For the most part, the First Nations peoples welcomed the newcomers but with tragic and devastating long term impacts. Throughout most of Canadian history, 16-20% of the population has been foreign-born. As these newcomers lived and worked, they also aged and eventually died in their new land. They aged in their homes and communities that they built themselves and with a steady stream of young immigrants, the aging of the older immigrants went unnoticed.

In recent years, two interesting demographic trends have been silently progressing. First, the Canadian population has been aging as the post war baby-boomers approach their senior years. Second, with greater choice, couples are having fewer children resulting in a population growth that is based upon immigration. These trends combine to form a new group of aging immigrants that seems to have evaded notice (Durst, 2005).

For those studying aging, the gerontologists have been slow to recognize ethnicity or culture as a relevant issue in the psycho/social process of aging. For many studying diversity, culture and ethnicity, social researchers have failed to recognize aging as a relevant variable. As recently as 1980, the public policy report called *A Profile of Canada's Older Population* neglected ethnicity as a subject matter. Although social science researchers have always been interested in ethnicity and aging, little consideration has been given to the combined impact of these two intersecting variables. These developments have created a new field in social gerontology called **Ethno-gerontology**: the study of the influence of ethnicity, national origin and culture on individual and population aging (Chappell, Gee, McDonald & Stones, 2003). In recent decades, the source countries of immigrants have changed from European to Asian regions

15

resulting in a significant increase in visible minorities. Elderly Canadians no longer appear the same. The senior populations are no longer homogeneous and have diversity in religion, values and customs.

Defining "Senior": It Looks Different the Closer One Gets!

Aging and attitudes towards aging are culturally specific and change over time (McPherson, 2004). The connotations towards terms such as elder, old, and senior vary from highly regarded and respected to disdained and mocked. In western society, the gifts and gags associated with aging demonstrate a discriminatory "agism" not present in other cultures. With western emphasis on youth, elderly are often dismissed. About 100 years ago, Chancellor Otto von Bismark of Germany noted that the average life expectancy of his citizens was a mere 65 years of age. Feeling that a person did well to live that long, he implemented his retirement and pension programs for citizens aged 65 years. Over time, life expectancy has increased and yet his benchmark did not change. Anyone 65 years of age or older is considered in a broad nebulous category as "senior." In China and other Asian countries with its youthful demographics, men are expected to retire at 60 years of age and women at 55 years.

Curiously, "old age" is frequently considered as a single stage of life – infant, child, youth, young adult, mature adult and old age. A retired individual is "a retired senior" regardless of whether he is 65 or 95 years of age, representing a 30-year lifespan. It could be considered as similar to combining a 5-year-old child as part of the same life stage as a 35-year-old adult. Or, it would be similar to placing a 20-year-old adult and a 50-year-old together. The issues facing each age are very different and do not allow for simple comparisons. In order to address this problem, the "seniors" category is subdivided into three stages of aging: the young-old (65 to 75/80), the old-old (75/80 to 90) and the very-old or frail-old (over 90) (Suzman and Riley, 1985).

Figure 1

Stages of Seniors' Aging

- Young-Old (65 to 75/80)

- Old-Old (75/80 to 90)

- Frail-Old (90 plus)

In spite of these categories, chronological age is a weak criterion for clustering or classifying individuals. It does not allow for individual and cultural diversity in economic, health and social capacities and deficiencies. For example, in Vietnam most women are expected to retire at 55 years of age and men at 60 years of age. With 50% of the population less than 25 years of age and the country having serious unemployment issues, "seniors" are expected to retire, giving their employment opportunities to younger persons with families. In many cultures including most Asian, elders are viewed with respect and as possessing special wisdom that begins before 65 years of age (Sung, 2001). In spite of the limitations of using chronological age, these age categories do allow statistical clustering and the application and analysis of census data.

As any parent will know, a child's growth and development are most dramatic in the first 5 years of life. Other than these first years, the physical and mental changes during the last thirty years of life are more significant than at any other period. The three groups differ in important and significant ways but they all experience loss. Over time, persons experience financial loss (income, savings, increasing health costs), physical loss (strength, hearing, seeing, mobility), emotional loss (family, friends, death, isolation, loneliness) and mental loss (memory, cognitive, emotional control). The young-old often remain active, and normally, enjoy full and rewarding roles and activities. For some, this stage can be extremely expressive and creative. They are more like the "middle-aged" but with more time and sometimes more disposable money! The old-old experience increasing loss but can enjoy fulfilling lives with environmental and social supports. The very old are often physically and mentally impaired and need extensive supports sometimes from formal institutions (Schaie & Willis, 1998). They are often referred to as the "frail elderly" and these are the individuals who enter long-term care, regardless of their chronological age.

Canada's Immigration Policies: Historical Racism

This section provides a brief background on Canada's immigration with an emphasis on its implications for minorities. It critically examines the policies from its racist undertones and assumptions.[2]

The first immigrants to permanently settle in Canada were Europeans who began to arrive in this country at the beginning of the seventeenth century (Dirks, 1995). During the next three centuries, Canada's population, comprised mainly of European immigrants, grew slowly. In 1763, the European population in the new colony of Canada stood at approximately sixty thousand. By Confederation in 1867, the number had reached approximately three million and was comprised mainly of British and French settlers (Dirks, 1995). At the beginning of the twentieth century, the population had only reached five million according to the 1901 Census (Verbeeten, 2007). However, by the 1950s, Canada's population had grown to more than thirteen million, and with marked change in its ethnic composition. Up until then, only Europeans or white Americans were almost exclusively allowed into Canada (Dirks, 1995). The only exception, in terms of the presence of other ethnic groups, were the free and fugitive Black slaves from the United States, and Chinese immigrant laborers (Knowles, 1997).

In 1783, 3 000 free Blacks from among the British loyalists of the American Revolution were the first significant influx of refugees to settle in the colony of Nova Scotia (Knowles, 1997; Kelley & Trebilcock, 1998). The free Blacks, who expected that they would be dealt with on the same terms as white Loyalists in their new home, were faced with a scourge of racism and a host of other obstacles with regard to land grants and provisions. "Bitterly disappointed in their hopes of finding equality and a good life in Nova Scotia, nearly 1 200 of them sailed in 1792 for Sierra Leone to start afresh on the west coast of Africa" (Knowles, 1997, p. 24 -25).

The first Chinese immigrants arrived in Canada from California in 1858 at the beginning of the Fraser River gold rush in the colony of British Columbia (Li, 1998; Knowles, 1997; Kelley & Trebilcock, 1998). By 1859, more Chinese immigrants arrived directly from Hong Kong on chartered ships. The largest numbers began arriving in the 1880s, after Andrew Onderdonk, an American builder, was awarded the contract to construct the section of the Canadian Pacific Railway from the Pacific Ocean through the Rocky Mountains (Knowles, 1997). Between 1881 and 1884, an estimated 15 701 Chinese men entered British Columbia, primarily to participate in the dangerous construction of that historic stretch of railway (Knowles, 1997, p. 50). They were treated with contempt and hostility (Lo & Wang, 2004) and in 1885, the Canadian government passed an act restricting and regulating Chinese immigration (Knowles, 1997). It came in the form of a Head Tax of $50 for every Chinese person from entering Canada and in 1903 it was raised to an astronomical $500, approximately two years of wages for a Chinese laborer (Fernando, 2006; Li, 1998). Despite the Head Tax, Chinese immigrants continued to trickle to Canada. In 1923, the Canadian Parliament passed the *Chinese Immigration Act* excluding all but a few Chinese immigrants and effectively ceasing immigration until 1947 when this Act was repealed (Fernando, 2006).

By the 1950s, 84.6% of immigrants living in Canada were European by birth (Dirks, 1995, p. 9). Between Confederation and the mid-twentieth century, Canada's immigration policy consistently favored people from northern and western Europe as well as from the United States (Dirks, 1995, p. 9). In spite of this preference, by 1900, government immigration officials and railroad company land agents began to accept applicants from eastern and southern Europe to meet the need for farmers to develop the vast Canadian West (Dirks, 1995, p. 9; Knowles, 1997, p. 61-78).

Before the 1970s, the ideas and thinking that shaped the formulation of immigration policy in terms of the types and numbers of people to be admitted as immigrants revolved around three factors: (1) the preferred ethnicity of immigrants, (2) Canada's "absorptive capacity" as measured by a variety of vague criteria, and (3) the economy's presumed labor market requirements (Dirks, 1995; Knowles, 1997; Kelley & Trebilcock, 1998). In 1947, the Prime Minister, Mackenzie King, in a landmark statement on immigration he read to the House of Commons, reiterated these ideas of racism and discrimination. In that statement he defended Canada's right to discriminate, stating that "the racial and national balance of immigration would be regulated so as not to alter the fundamental character of the Canadian population" (Dirks, 1995, p. 10; Knowles, 1997, p. 131). The contents of his statement became the guidelines that influenced the thinking of policy makers and officials for the next two decades (Dirks, 1995, p. 10).

By preferred ethnicity, Canada's immigration policy sought to limit its selection or choice of immigrants to those from the United Kingdom, northern and western Europe, and the United States (Dirks, 1995; Knowles, 1997; Kelley & Trebilcock, 1998). A more liberal immigration policy was adopted during the post-World War II period. After the war, Canada's economy was booming, creating a demand for both skilled and unskilled workers. However, immigration was still restricted mainly to immigrants from continental Europe (Knowles, 1997, p. 124). As a result of pressure and demand from the Canadian general public for Canada to admit World War II refugees and displaced persons from United Nations' International Refugee Organization (IRO) camps in Europe, the Canadian government was compelled to adopt a more humanitarian immigration policy. Nearly a quarter of a million European refugees immigrated to Canada between 1946 and 1962 (Knowles, 1997, p. 124-144; Kelley & Trebilcock, 1998, p. 337). Ethnic origin was still central to the screening of these refugees and displaced persons. Acting on instructions from Ottawa, the Canadian immigration officials routinely rejected Jewish applicants and also took into account the persons political and ideological views that were considered incompatible with that of Canada (Knowles, 1997, p. 132-133).

By 1962, the wave of criticism from the Canadian public, especially the discriminatory nature of Canada's immigration policy, resulted in significant changes (Kelley & Trebilcock, 1998, p. 345). In the centennial year of 1967, the Minister of Citizenship and Immigration in John Diefenbaker's government tabled new regulations in the House that "eliminated racial discrimination as a major feature of Canada's immigration policy" (Knowles, 1997, p. 151). Although this was a major and historic initiative on the part of the government, there were two factors that forced the government to take this action. First, racist policies were being attacked within Canada and the world over. During this period, there were international interest groups, churches, organized labor, and many liberal-minded Canadians criticizing Canada's racially discriminatory immigration policy. This was also the period when South Africa was under condemnation for its apartheid policies and Australia under scrutiny for maintaining policies that favored white immigrants. As such, Canada could not afford to ignore the charges of racism in the "government's practices and programs" (Dirks, 1995, p. 10). The other factor concerned the international impact of Canada's discriminatory immigration policies. The policies were hampering its operations at the United Nations and the multi-ethnic

Commonwealth. At this time the stronghold of Britain and other European empires, as colonial powers, was waning and independent nations in Asia, Africa, and the Caribbean were emerging. Canada needed to develop positive relations with these new governments that could not be possible with an immigration policy that "in practice excluded nonwhites" (Dirks, 1995, p. 10; Knowles, 1997, p. 152). In 1967, Canada implemented the "points system" that rated immigrant applicants on skills, language, education and other criteria rather than ethnicity or political/social background (Verbeeten, 2007). The policy shifted immigrant priorities from agricultural and rural basis to urban, post-industrialized economy (Verbeeten, 2007).

In theory, racial discrimination in Canada's immigration policy was removed and any independent immigrant, regardless of ethnicity, appearance, or nationality, had equal chance to be considered suitable for admission into Canada. However, in practice, the changes had little significant difference for certain ethnic groups in terms of gaining admission into Canada (Jakubowski, 1997).

The impacts of the evolving policy did change the "face" of Canadians with increasing numbers of visible minorities who did not quietly melt into mainstream society. Not only did these newcomers look different, they brought new cultures reflecting differing beliefs, values and customs. Canadians began to define their country as a "multicultural society" with a "mosaic of cultures" under one nation. Although the mosaic ideology is viewed as a goal, it is understood by many as illusive and unobtainable (Kallen, 2008).[3] Canada remains the only nation in the world that has an official *Canadian Multicultural Act* (1988) designed to promote diversity within the national framework. Although meant to be inclusive, the Act and its resulting policies have not eliminated the tensions between and within groups (Rimok & Rouzier, 2008). Acknowledging that over time ethnic immigrants change, perhaps the description of "flux" is more accurate than "mosaic."

Immigrating to Canada: Class of Immigrants

The study of "immigrants" is complex and becomes even more confusing when considering aging. It is not easy to determine who is an "immigrant." For example, researchers often aggregate refugees and immigrants together and ignore the different classes of both immigrants (Family, Economic, Other) and refugees (Assisted, Sponsored, Asylum). Often those persons under economic classes immigrated when they were young or young adults. For example, the universities and health care fields have recruited individuals who have diverse backgrounds. Many of the individuals hired in the expansion of the universities in the 70s are at or near retirement and enter the seniors group. They have raised their families here and Canada is now "home" even though they may have thought about returning to their country of origin when they first arrived in Canada. They do not return to their homeland and make significant impacts in our communities. Their situations can be very different than the elderly who recently arrived in Canada. Under the Family Class, immediate families sponsored their parents and/or grandparents. Many from regions such as Asia do not speak English or French and are socially and economically dependent upon their children. They can be very isolated. These individuals will be older and have different social and health needs than business immigrants in the Economic Class. These family sponsored elderly will require different policies and programs. As immigrants age, Canada is experiencing an increase in the old-old immigrant group from two sources. Many immigrants and refugees aged in Canada and others immigrated as a "senior," having experienced most of their aging in their country of origin.

Citizenship and Immigration Canada provide six main categories of newcomers, and each category impacts differently on issues pertaining to integration, settlement and labor participation. There are also implications for aging and later years in life. In 2009, Canada admitted 25 179 newcomers, about 6 900 (2.7%) were over 65 years of age (Canada 2009).

Skilled Workers and Professionals have education, work experience, knowledge of English or French and other abilities that will assist them in integrating and adjusting to living and working in Canada. There were 95 962 admitted under this category in 2009. Normally, they quickly adapt and enter productive employment. As they age, they are normally acculturated and readily access services.

Canada has three classes of **Business Immigrants: Investors, Entrepreneurs and Self-employed Persons.** The program attempts to attract experienced business individuals who will support and build the Canadian economy. Business immigrants are expected to make a $400 000 investment or to own and manage a business in Canada. It is a successful way to buy oneself into Canada. In 2009, only 14 704 persons entered Canada under this program, a drop from 19 924 in 1997. As they age, they may keep their business active and participate in the economy well into their later years. After such an empowered and active life, they may have adjustment issues as they retire and become frail.

Canadian citizens or permanent residents can sponsor a spouse, common-law partner, dependent child or parent/grandparent under the **Family Class** or **Family Sponsorship Program.** The sponsoring relative assumes financial responsibility of the newcomer and must provide for him/her. In 2009, 65 200 family members entered Canada. Some of these newcomers such as elderly parents do not enter paid employment but may support their children through child care, enabling families to have multiple incomes. Having aged in their homeland, they may not speak English or French and have serious issues in social inclusion often suffering from loneliness and isolation.

With collaboration with individual provinces, the federal government implemented a Provincial Nominee Program a few years ago. In 2009, 11 801 workers with 18 577 family members entered Canada under this program. Manitoba was the first to sign an agreement with CIC and has been very successful in applying this so-called "fast track." Another goal of the program is the reunification of family members who may or may not participate in the labor market. Some of those family members may be elderly and the issues are similar to the Family Class of immigrants.

The federal government's **Temporary Foreign Worker Program** permits foreign workers entry into Canada to work for a specified period of time. Employers need to demonstrate that they were unable to find local employees and that the entry of the foreign workers will not harm the existing Canadian labor market. Since their working visas are time limited, these immigrants seldom comprise the senior immigrant population. During 2009, 178 478 temporary workers entered Canada.

With a history of humanitarian traditions and international obligations, Canada admitted 2 846 refugees in 2009 under the **Refugee Class**. Refugees seek protection from persecution, violence and/or torture in their homeland. They can be sponsored by government agencies, private organizations or individuals. If they arrive in Canada and claim refugee status, one of three tribunals adjudicates the claim as defined by international conventions. This group of immigrants is often in poor health – sometimes both physically and mentally. They may have been subjected to extreme violence and severely traumatized. They frequently have few skills and are poorly educated. Potential employers should be aware that there can be serious issues when hiring persons from this group. It pays to work closely with the sponsoring group to esnure success.

Figure 2

Categories of Immigrants to Canada

- Skilled Workers and Professionals
- Investors, Entrepreneurs and Self-employed Persons
- Family Sponsored
- Provincial Nominees
- Temporary Workers
- Refugees

Considering what immigrants offer and what they need, one can see how diverse so-called "immigrants" are and it is important to avoid "lumping" them together. For example, one can imagine the differences between two senior immigrants/refugees from Hong Kong. The former Governor General of Canada, the Right Honorable Adrienne Clarkson, immigrated as a "refugee" child during the Second World War. She grew up in Canada and experienced Canadian society throughout her entire life. She is very different than a "granny" who immigrated under the family reunification program at the age of 70 years old. It is important that researchers, policy analysts and programmers do not aggregate these differences and make false assumptions and generalizations.

The issues, pertaining to visible minorities, further complicate an already complex situation. For example, many European immigrants may be considered "mainstream," visible minority or invisible minority and therefore, generalizations may be false or misleading. Interestingly, the province of Saskatchewan has the largest percentage of foreign-born immigrant population over the age of 75 years. Fifty-three percent of Saskatchewans over 75 population is foreign-born from Germany, Ukraine, Norway, Hungary, and Poland. The large migration to the west in the 1920s has left its impact. Newfoundland and Labrador has the least percentage of over 75 as foreign-born at only 2% (Canada, 2005).

Gerontological research on minority groups has generally applied three conceptual frameworks: levelling theory, buffer theory and multiple jeopardy theory (Novak, 2006).[4] Researchers have suggested that there is a "levelling" and converging of indicators as people age. The disparity in the quality of life indicators between ethnic seniors and the dominant group diminishes as they age because of such variables as strong family connections and supports. If an ethnic minority person who is middle-aged has a low income, their income changes little as they move into retirement and from employment income and onto income support programs; hence a levelling between groups (Novak, 1997; Novak & Campbell, 2006).

Buffering theory argues that ethnicity protects and buffers the impact of aging and the loss of roles. The buffer may come in the form of family supports and cultural connections that support the aging elder. Ethnic seniors are more likely to live with their adult children and therefore they will receive social, emotional and physical support and engagement with the family. Being involved in cultural organizations or activities keeps the elder active and engaged, reducing loneliness and isolation. In these ways, the ethnic senior is buffered from the impacts of aging by his/her ethnicity (Novak & Campbell, 2006).

In multiple jeopardy, researchers use variables such as age, sex, income, education, disability, and ethnicity to classify individuals. Broadly speaking, each of these variables can be compared to mainstream society and since older immigrants or visible minorities have poorer health and lower incomes than the mainstream group, they experience the multiple "jeopardy" of their "status." Not all immigrants are "visible minorities" and many of the elderly immigrants can be considered part of the mainstream society. In addition, because women live longer, the percentage of women increases over time. So the "jeopardy" of age, sex, visible minority, ethnicity, language, health, income, and so on, compound to disadvantage the individual. If a cross section of the sample is studied, it neglects the change over time that the group experiences. If the group starts out poor in both wealth and health, then the group will remain so later in life. If multiple jeopardy factors affect only the lower class visible minority then it is only social class rather than ethnic status that creates the multiple jeopardy (Novak, 1997; Novak & Campbell, 2006). This theoretical approach has limitations.

However, levelling, buffer and the multiple jeopardy theories miss the diversity within minority groups and they also miss the effects of earlier life. For example, refugees and immigrants from Peoples Republic of China and Hong Kong come from very different cultures yet are frequently clustered together for statistical purposes. One could further complicate the demographics by adding ethnic Chinese who have come to Canada from Indonesia or Vietnam. Furthermore, recent immigrants and long term immigrants have different experiences and may not be comparable but are listed as "Chinese." In addition, some refugees, many of them from Central America, have experienced trauma and torture. This violence will influence them in subtle but important ways limiting the value of simple comparisons. The life experiences and subjective qualitative perspectives are major influences of integration, life satisfaction, mental health and emotional stability (Novak, 1997; Novak & Campbell, 2006). Changes are normal in one's life history and how the individual understands, interprets and responds to the aging process depends upon the individual and his/her situation. Hence, the life course perspective (or life-span development) offers a valuable framework in completing research on aging immigrants and refugees. Often, trauma that occurred decades ago resurfaces in frail elderly who are suffering from cognitive dysfunctions or emotional problems. Also, men and women experience the life course of aging differently and the impact of gender and social class is a critical variable in understanding aging in any culture or context (Chappell, Gee, McDonald & Stones, 2003; Novak & Campbell, 2006). The gendered life course offers a framework for considering these differences in work, retirement, health, social relationships and so on.

In recent years, there has been a growing interest in researching aging and ethnicity. Most of the published social research has focused on a single ethnic group and are generally categorized under Asian, Hispanic, African American and Native American (e.g., Olson, 2001). Ethnic-religious groups such as Jewish, Mormon or Amish have also been researched as well as special groups such as gays and lesbians, or rural elderly (e.g., Gelfand, 2003; Gelfand & Barresi, 1987; Olson, 2001). Often the contributors present a "case study" type of research that attempts to give an overview of the cultural group and its experiences in aging. Normally, they discuss topics such as health, income, housing and sometimes satisfaction. There is considerable Canadian research on Asian elderly, mainly Chinese (e.g., Lai, 2000; MacKinnon, Gien & Durst, 2001). There is little comparative research between mainstream society and ethnic groups or between ethnic groups. A few American studies cluster Asian, African

American (Black), Hispanic (Latino), and Native American and compare them under social determinants such as income, housing, health and so on (e.g., Gelfand, 2003; Manuel & Reid, 1982; Markides & Mindel, 1987). There is little conceptual literature that attempts to encompass the overall field of study. Although over 20 years old, the chapters on theoretical orientations by Rey, Lipman and Brosky (Manuel, 1982), are helpful as are Driedger and Chappell (1987), Gelfard (2003) and Ujimoto (1987). The danger of applying models and aggregating data from different groups is a form of reductionism and invites generalizations and assumptions, which may be false or misleading. For example, the role of family as an emotional and social support may look different between groups and within categories.

Recent research on inclusion and integration offers promising frameworks that are culturally sensitive and relevant to this population. Freiler's (2001) inclusion model was developed to research women in poverty and it can be appropriately used as a model for aging and ethnicity.

Social research on aging and ethnicity is complex. Issues on age categories, immigrant status, length of residency, age at immigration, ethnic background and history and familial relationships complicate the research and limit generalizations. Furthermore, language and cultural barriers and customs restrict access. Burton and Bengtson (1982) and Durst (1996) identify some of the stumbling blocks and barriers to researching aging and ethnicity.

Current Situation in Canada

According to the 2006 Census, 13.7% of Canada's population is over 65 years of age, representing an increase of 11.5% over the past five years. Correspondingly, the number of children under the age of 15 years has decreased to 17.7%, the lowest level ever. Since 2001, there has been an increase in immigration but it has not slowed the aging of Canada's population. Since 1966, the median age (the age that divides the population into two equal numbers) has steadily increased and is now at 39.5 years. There are now over 1.1 million Canadians over the age of 80. This means that 3.7% of the population falls into the category of "old" seniors. There are marked differences between provinces and territories with Nunavut at a low of 2.7% and Saskatchewan with a high of 15.4% senior populations (Canada, 2008). Alberta is a young province with 10.7% of its residents over 65 years of age.

Like most developed countries, Canada is experiencing an aging population due to an increasing life expectancy and a declining birth rate. However, comparing Canada to the developed G8 nations, it is one of the youngest as only the United States has lower percentage of seniors at 12.4% compared to Canada's 13.7%. The seniors' population is expected to continue to grow and Statistics Canada projects the percentage of seniors to reach 23% of all Canadians by 2041. The greatest growth will be in the old-old and very-old ranges. With a longer life expectancy, the senior population is predominantly female with 57% of the over 64 age group being women. The percentage increases to 60% for the old-old (75-84 years of age) and 70% for the very-old (over 85).

Table 1 presents the numbers and percentages of immigrants arriving in Canada in 2006. Under all classes, a total of 251 649 new immigrants and refugees in all ages arrived in 2006 with over 50.3% (n = 126 480) from Asian and the Pacific regions. Another 20.6% (n = 51 863) arrived from Africa and the Middle East. The pattern of those immigrants and refugees over the age of 65 years varies significantly from all ages. Only 6 911 of the newcomers were seniors representing 2.7% of the total immigrants. The percentages of Asian and Pacific to all seniors was a high of 67.3%, representing 4 651 seniors. There were 884 seniors arriving from Africa and the Middle East, representing 12.8% of all senior newcomers. Most of these immigrants are under the Family Class. Immigrants from the United States are consistent in all ages at 3.8-4.3%. The last column presents the percentage change in the past 10 years comparing patterns from 1997 to 2006. The total percentage of seniors has not varied in the 10-year period and has remained constant at 2.7% of all immigrants. However, amongst the senior immigrants, there has been a substantial increase from Asia and Pacific regions (7.9%) and a modest increase from Africa and the Middle East (2.3%). The number of senior immigrants from Europe and the United Kingdom

Table 1
Total and Percentages of Senior Immigration in the Year 2006

Source of Immigration	Total in 2006	%	65+	%	Percent of Total	10 year Change
Africa/Middle East	51 863	20.6	884	1.7	12.8	2.3
Asia and Pacific	126 480	50.3	4 651	3.7	67.3	7.9
South and Central America	24 306	9.7	353	1.5	5.1	-0.2
United States	10 943	4.3	265	2.4	3.8	-0.1
Europe/United Kingdom	37 946	15.1	756	2.0	10.9	-9.9
Not stated	111	0.0	2	1.8	0.9	
	251 649	100	6 911	2.7	101	0.0

dropped close to 10% over the ten year period. It seems clear that there are not large numbers of immigrant seniors arriving in Canada but the vast majority of them are Asian, under the family unification category. With increasing migration from these regions, the faces of Canada's seniors is changing.

Using Census 2006 data, Table 2 presents the percentages of foreign-born residents living in Canada by source region and age grouping. Foreign-born residents are also known as "the immigrant population" and they are defined in the 2006 Census as "persons who are, or who have been, landed immigrants in Canada."[5] The first column presents the percentages of all foreign-born residents (immigrants and refugees) identifying visible minorities and non-visible minorities.[6]

This table presents data collected in the Census 2006 under responses to "ethnic origin" (also known as ethnicity and ethnic ancestry). Over 200 different ethnic origins were reported in the 2006 Census and over five million identified themselves as a visible minority. Visible minorities represent 16.2% of the total population an increase

Table 2 Percentages of Foreign-Born as Visible Minorities by Source and Age				
	All Ages	**65+ Years**	**65-74**	**75+**
Total Foreign-Born	23.9	30.1	30.0	30.1
Visible Minorities	83.4	93.6	94.9	91.4
Not Visible Minorities	13.1	23.7	22.6	25.2
Asian				
Chinese	84.6	96.0	95.0	96.8
South Asian	85.6	98.6	97.7	99.0
Filipino	88.4	98.4	98.1	98.5
SE Asian	86.3	96.8	95.0	98.0
Korean	91.3	97.2	94.4	98.4
Japanese	43.2	27.1	19.5	34.1
Black	71.9	87.8	85.5	88.9
Latin American	89.8	95.3	93.9	96.0
Middle East				
Arab	88.3	92.1	99.2	94.1
West Asian	95.9	97.3	95.6	98.2

from 13.4% in 2001. Ethnic origin or ancestry is diffenerent than language, place of birth or citizenship. For example, an individual of Haitian ancestry may speak French, be born in Canada and have Canadian citizenship.

In the total population, 19.8% of Canada's permanent residents are foreign-born. Among visible minorities 83.4% are foreign-born compared to only 13.1% of non-visible minority persons (Caucasian and Aboriginal/First Nations). Amongst seniors, those percentages increase so that 30.1% of all seniors are foreign-born, higher than the national percentage for all Canadians (19.8%) and up from 16.9% in 1981. Although it is not surprising that the percentage of foreign-born population of visible minorities increases amongst the seniors to 93.6%, it seems surprising that it also increases among the non-visible minority population. Among the 75 years and older population of non-visible minorities, 25.2% are foreign-born.

There are some intriguing trends among the different ethnic groups. In most of the ethnic groups, the percentages of foreign-born residents increased between the young-old (65-74) and the old-old (75+). The overall percentages are lower for the group of Black, recognizing a long history of indigenous Black Canadians. Only the Japanese residents have a lower percentage of foreign-born seniors than the general population of Japanese (27.1% of seniors compared to 43.2% of all). Almost 83% of Japanese seniors (65-74) have been born in Canada, compared to less than 2-6% for other Asians. Most of these Japanese seniors were born in Canada in the years prior to the Second World War.

The Table presents four categories of visible minorities: Asian, Black, Latin American and Middle East. Among all ages, 57.3% are Asian with 21.7% Chinese and 20.9% South Asian including Indian and Pakistani are foreign-born. Only 10.3% of Blacks are foreign-born and a small percentage of 5.6% of Latin Americans are foreign-born.

Table 3 presents similar data but gives a comparison between groups of visible minorities and age. Of all visible minorities in Canada in all age groups, 57.3% are Asian (Chinese: 21.7% and South Asian: 20.9%). In the senior population of visible minorities (65 years plus), 71.7% are Asian. Senior Black Canadians represent 10.7% of all senior visible minorities and is close to the total representation at 10.3%. Latin Americans and Middle Eastern residents are a younger population with fewer seniors.

Immigration patterns from Asia show, in fact, that 9.1% (almost one in ten) seniors in Canada are a member of a visible minority which is a significant increase from 2001 (7.2%) and 1996 (6%). Asian seniors account for an amazing 6.9% of all seniors in Canada (Chinese: 3.2% and South Asian: 2.2%). These Asian seniors are concentrated in the major cities but are present throughout Canada.

Table 3 **Percentages of Foreign-born Visible Minorities by Age**					
Visible Minority	**All Ages**	**65+**	**65-74**	**75+**	**% of 65+**
Total – All VM					9.1
Asian	57.3	71.7	71.7	71.7	6.9
Chinese	21.7	33.8	31.6	37.5	3.2
South Asian – India	20.9	24.1	26.1	20.7	2.2
Filipino	7.2	7.0	7.1	6.8	0.6
Southeast Asian	4.1	3.7	3.6	4.0	0.4
Korean	2.7	2.2	2.4	1.9	0.2
Japanese	0.7	0.9	0.9	0.8	0.3
Black	10.3	10.7	11.4	9.4	1.1
Latin American	5.6	3.3	3.4	3.1	0.3
Middle East	7.5	5.2	5.6	4.6	0.5
Arab	4.4	3.1	3.3	2.7	0.3
West Asian	3.1	2.1	2.3	1.9	0.2

Table 4 provides the percentages of senior immigrants by continent. European immigrants represent 34% of the total immigrants in Canada and 63.7% of senior immigrants over 65 years of age. The immigrant population for the United States is also "greying" with 19.2% of its population over 65 years of age (4.0% of immigrant seniors). However, the growing population of Asian and Middle Eastern seniors is remarkable and now represents 22.8% of all immigrant seniors. Close to one in four immigrant seniors is from Asia/Middle East.

The assumption that "immigrants" are young is not supported. Canada has larger numbers of immigrants from diverse backgrounds and the senior population is mirroring the Canadian mosaic. By percentage, the youngest group is from Central and South American. Not surprisingly the African and South East Asia (Thailand, Laos, and Vietnam) are still fairly young. However since many South East Asians came to Canada as refugees during the Vietnam war, their senior population is expected to grow.

	Total	65+	% of Total Immigrants	% of Immigrant Seniors
Table 4 Senior Immigrants by Continent				
Total Immigrants	6 186 950	1 215 285	19.6	
United States	250 535	48 045	19.2	4.0
Central America	130 460	6 515	5.0	0.5
Caribbean	317 765	44 890	14.1	3.7
South American	150 710	23 325	9.3	1.9
Europe	2 278 345	773 770	34.0	63.7
Africa	374 565	32 600	8.7	2.7
Asia and Middle East	2 525 155	277 415	11.0	22.8
			101	99

The Canadian government provides two major income security programs for seniors that many immigrants can access. If they have been in Canada for 10 years, all immigrant seniors (over 65 years of age) are eligible for The Old Age Security program that provides a modest pension. If the senior immigrated at aged 62 then they could be eligible for benefits at aged 72 regardless if they have never been employed in Canada. If the senior has a low-income, he/she may be eligible for other benefits as early as age 60, providing he/she met the 10-year requirement.

Canada has international social security agreements with many countries to help people qualify for benefits from either country. An agreement may allow periods of contribution to the other country's social security system (or, in some cases, periods of residence abroad) to be added to periods of contribution to the Canada Pension Plan in order to meet minimum qualifying conditions. For example, these agreements would allow a citizen of Germany to access the Canada Pension Plan, including retirement, disability and survivor benefits in Canada. These agreements are with developed countries that have existing income programs for seniors and, although it is rare, there have been individuals who have immigrated specifically to "retire" in Canada. It may seem strange to retire in a country with snowy and cold winters, but for some immigrants it provides the opportunity to live near adult children in their children's new country. For others, it means escaping the crowded, congested and expensive lifestyle of European cities.

For those seniors who immigrated late in life under the Family Class, they may find that they are exclusively financially dependent upon their sponsoring family. Before leaving their homeland, they may have sold their businesses, homes or farms and moved to Canada to live under their children's care, often providing care for their grandchildren. These arrangements can be quite traumatic and stressful for once they held status and independence and, now they face loneliness and isolation (MacKinnon, Gien & Durst, 2001). In leaving their homeland, they give up their rich cultural heritage, community connections and life-long relationships, experiencing a "status discrepancy." Although living in comfortable spacious houses, they describe their children's home as a "golden prison."

Issues and Developing Needs

As the demographics shift there is a need to better understand and appreciate the diversity among the senior population. In all sectors of society, there is a need to improve understanding and appreciation of immigrant seniors. There is a need for further research and implications for policies and programs but researching ethnic aging requires careful planning and thought to ensure cultural relevancy (Durst, 1996). The Prairie Metropolis Centre, a Canadian Metropolis Site, recognized the paucity of research in this field and funded a Social Domain exploratory study. The study is holistic in the sense that it considers the senior immigrant as a total person with social, economic, physical, emotional and spiritual needs. Using both quantitative and qualitative data, it examined social and cultural factors, family and interpersonal relationships and living arrangements and conditions. Much of this edited volume is derived from this research.

Ethnic seniors must have decision-making powers regarding issues that affect them and need to be involved and represented at all level of organizations, government departments, and communities. As active participants, they will have a voice in policy, social, and program developments (CPHA, 1988). They are an emerging group that is empowered in ways that previous immigrants and especially visible minorities were not.

Immigrant seniors offer a potential resource to the larger Canadian society and methods should be developed to encourage volunteer service in agencies that provide services to ethnic groups. Sometimes volunteer service is "foreign" to some groups and efforts to develop volunteerism may be necessary. Many start by contributing to their ethnic community and expand their involvement to the larger community. Part of this process is the empowerment and also the acculturation skills to function in the mainstream community.

Information regarding services and programs must be accessible to ethnic seniors. Language barrier reduction in the service agencies must be improved through the use of interpreters, translation of materials, and employing multilingual staff. Language barriers have made services inaccessible by ethnic seniors and as a result, they frequently do not receive the assistance or the information they need or are entitled to receive.

Changes need to be made in major health and social services agencies so as to better serve ethnic seniors (Olson, 2001). Some of the service agencies do not meet their needs and are not culturally sensitive (Gelfand, 2003); however there are useful manuals and guidelines offering cross-cultural strategies and advice beginning to appear (See Elliot, 1999 and Fisher et al. 2000). Ironically, in most health and social agencies, the service providers, from the custodial and support employees through to the professional staff, are ethnically diverse and many are immigrants themselves. There is the need for an honest evaluation of the agencies' services. For example, one of the major issues for ethnic seniors is the inappropriate diet in long-term care facilities. Since many of these elderly are frail and immigrated under the Family Class, they have had little time to adjust to western life and foods. They often enter long term care in poor health and their final years are disappointing.

At times, there is a need for specialized services for special needs groups such as mental health, dementia, and end-of-life care (Butler, Lewis & Sunderland, 1998; Fisher, Ross & MacLean, 2000). Research on mental health and ethnic seniors is lacking, especially those who have suffered through past violence and trauma where the effects surface late in life.

There have been changing values in filial responsibility and more immigrant seniors wish to and are living independently. To achieve independent living, many need economic security and access to support services. They may need services such as home care, meals on wheels and day care/respite that are culturally appropriate.

Overall, the ethno-cultural seniors need to be recognized and valued for their diversity. They need to have more decision-making powers regarding policies, economics, health and social issues that affect them, and to have better knowledge about the services and programs that are available. Our diverse multicultural nation is facing new challenges with our aging population, making Canada an exciting place to live.

References

Biles, J., Burstein, M. & Frideres, J. (Eds.). (2008). *Immigration and integration in Canada in the twenty-first century.* Montreal, PQ: McGill-Queen's University Press.

Burton, Linda & Bengtson, Vern L. (1982). Research in elderly minority communities: Problems and potentials. in Ron C. Manuel. (Ed.). (1982). *Minority aging: Sociological and social psychological issues, pp. 215-222.* Westport CI: Greenwood Press..

Butler, Robert N., Lewis, Myrna I. & Sunderland, Trey, (1998). Aging and mental health: Positive psychosocial and biomedical approaches. Needham Heights, MA: Allyn and Bacon.

Canada. (2005). *http://www.statcan.ca/english/Pgdb/popula.htm#imm* or http://www12.statcan.ca/english/census01/products/standard/themes/

Chappell, Neena L., Gee, Ellen, McDonald, Lynn & Stones, Michael. (2003). *Aging in contemporary Canada.* Toronto, ON: Prentice Hall, Inc.

Canada (2010). http://www.cic.gc.ca/english/resouces/statistics/facts2009.

CPHA (Canadian Public Health Association). (1988). *Ethnicity and aging report: A National Workshop on Ethnicity and Aging 21-24 February 1988.* Ottawa: Ministry of State.

Dirks, G.E. (1995). Controversy and complexity: Canadian immigration policy during the 1980s. Montréal: McGill-Queen University Press.

Driedger, Leo & Chappell, Neena L. (1987). *Aging and ethnicity: Toward an interface.* Toronto, ON: Butterworths.

Durst, Douglas. (1996). *Multicultural research into healthy aging: Practical issues and wtrategies. in research into healthy aging: Challenges in changing times.* Conference Proceedings. Centre on Aging, Mt. St. Vincent University. Halifax, NS. Nov. 7-8.1996. pp. 143-157.

Durst, Douglas. (2005). *More snow on the roof: Canada's immigrant seniors. Immigration and the intersections of diversity.* Canadian Issues/Themes Canadien. Association for Canadian Studies. Spring 2005.pp. 34-37.

Cameron, Elspeth. (Ed.). *Multiculturalism & immigration in Canada: An Introductory Reader.* Toronto, ON: Canadian Scholars' Press.

Fernando, Shanti, (2006). *Race and the city: Chinese Canadian and Chinese American political mobilization.* Vancouver, BC: University of British Columbia Press.

Freiler, C. (2001). *What needs to change? Towards a vision of social inclusion for children, families and communities.* Draft Concept Paper. Toronto, ON: Laidlaw Foundation.

Fisher, Rory, Ross, Margaret M. & MacLean, Michael J. (2000). *A guide to end-of-life care for seniors.* University of Toronto: National Advisory Committee.

Elliot, Gail. (1999). *Cross-cultural awareness in an aging society. Effective strategies of communication and caring.* Hamilton, ON: Office of Gerontological Studies.

Gelfand, Donald E. (2003). *Aging and ethnicity: Knowledge and services.* 2nd Edition. New York, NY: Springer Publishing Company, Inc.

Gelfand, Donald E. & Barresi, Charles M. (Eds.). (1987). *Ethnic Dimensions of Aging.* New York, NY: Springer Publishing Company, Inc.

Kallen, Evelyn. (2004). Multiculturalism: Ideology, policy and reality. In Elspeth Cameron. (Ed.). *Multiculturalism and immigration in Canada: An introductory reader.* pp. 75-96. Toronto, ON: Canadian Scholars' Press.

Kelley, N. & Trebilcock, M.J. (1998). *The making of the mosaic: A history of Canadian immigration policy.* Toronto: University of Toronto Press.

Knowles, V. (1997). *Strangers at our gates: Canadian immigration and immigration policy, 1540-1997.* Toronto: Dundurn Press.

Kumassah, Godknows, (2008). *Giving voice: The lived experiences of African immigrants and refugees in the City of Regina.* M.S.W. Thesis. Faculty of Social Work. Regina: University of Regina.

Jakubowski, Lisa M. (1997). *Immigration and the legalization of racism.* Halifax, NS: Fernwood Publishing.

Lai, Daniel W.L. (2000). Depression among the elderly Chinese in Canada. *Canadian Journal on Aging. 19*(3), 409-429.

Li, Peter S. (1998). *The Chinese in Canada.* 2nd Edition. Toronto, ON: Oxford University Press.

Lo, Lucia & Wang, Lu. (2004). A political economy approach to understanding the economic incorporation of Chinese sub-ethnic groups. *Journal of International Migration and Integration. 5*(1). 107-140.

MacKinnon, M., Gien, L. & Durst, D. (2001). Silent pain: Social isolation of Chinese elders in Canada. in Iris Chi, Neena L. Chappell & James Lubeen (Eds.). *Elderly Chinese in Pacific Rim countries: Social support and integration. pp. 1-16.* Hong Kong: Hong Kong University Press.

Manuel, Ron C. (Ed.). (1982). *Minority aging: Sociological and social psychological issues.* Westport CI: Greenwood Press.

Manuel, Ron C. & Reid, John. (1982). A comparative demographic profile of the minority aged and nonminority Aged. In Ron C. Manuel. (Ed.). (1982). *Minority aging: Sociological and social psychological issues.* pp. 31-52.Westport CT: Greenwood Press.

Markides, Kyriakos S. & Mindel, Charles, H. (1987). *Aging and ethnicity.* Newbury Park, CA: Sage Publications, Inc.

McPherson, Barry D. (2004). *Aging as a social process, Canadian perspectives.* Fourth Edition. Don Mills, ON: Oxford University Press.

Novak, Mark. (1997). *Issues in aging: An introduction to gerontology.* New York, NY: Addison-Wesley Publishers Inc.

Novak, Mark & Campbell, Lori (2006). *Aging and society, A Canadian perspective.* Fifth Edition. Toronto, ON: Thomson/Nelson.

Olson, Laura Katz, Ed. (2001). *Age through ethnic lenses: Caring for the elderly in a multicultural society.* Oxford, UK: Rowman & Littlefield Publishers, Inc.

Rimok, Patricia & Rouzier, Ralph. (2008). Integration policies in Quebec: A need to expand the structures? In John Biles, Meyer Burstein and James Frideres, (Eds.). (2008). *Immigration and integration in Canada in the twenty-first century*. pp. 187-210. Montreal, PQ: McGill-Queen's University Press.

Schaie, K. Warner & Willis, Sherry L. (1996). *Adult development and aging.* 4th Edition. New York, NY: HarperCollins Publishers Inc.

Stone, Leroy O. & Fletcher, Susan. (1980). *A profile of Canada's older population.* Montreal, PQ: The Institute for Research on Public Policy.

Sung, K-T. (2001). Elder respect: exploration of ideals and forms in East Asia. *Journal of Aging Studies, 15*(1). 13-26.

Suzman, R. & Riley, M.W. (1985). Introducing the 'oldest old'. Milbank *Memorial Fund Quarterly: Health and Society. 63.* 177-185.

Ujimoto, K. Victor (1987). The ethnic dimension of aging in Canada. In Victor W. Marshall (Ed.). *Aging in Canada: Social perspectives.* 2nd Edition. pp. 111- 137. Richmond Hill, ON: Fitzhenry & Whiteside.

Verbeeten, D. (2007). The past and future of immigration to Canada. *Journal of International Migration and Integration. 8*(1). 1-10.

Notes

[1]It is acknowledged that close to 1000 years ago, the Vikings attempted a permanent settlement at L'Anse au Meadows, on the northern tip of Newfoundland.

[2]The author is grateful to Mr. Godknows Kumassah for his research work on racism in immigration.

[3]The edited volumes by Cameron (2004) and Biles, Bustein and Frideres (2008) offer an in-depth discussion on multiculturalism and integration in Canada.

[4]The reader is directed to Chapter 3 by Lynn Mcdonald for a more comprehensive discussion on theoretical frameworks.

[5]In this Census data, the foreign-born population does not include non-permanent residents and excludes persons born outside Canada who are Canadian citizens by birth.

[6]The term, "visible minorities," is defined by the federal The Employment Equity Act as "persons, other than Aboriginal peoples, who are non-Caucasian in race or non-white in color." The Act specifies the following groups as visible minorities: Chinese, South Asians (e.g., Indian, Pakistani), Blacks, Arabs, West Asians (e.g., Iranian, Afghan), Filipinos, Southeast Asians (e.g., Vietnamese, Cambodian), Latin Americans, Japanese, Koreans and other visible minority groups, such as Pacific Islanders.

2

Integration Outcomes for Immigrant Seniors in Canada: A Review of Literature 2000-2007 [1]

Herbert C. Northcott & Jennifer L. Northcott, (University of Alberta)

The 2006 Census indicated that 28% of Canadians aged 65 and older were immigrants to Canada. Almost two-thirds (66%) of these immigrant seniors had lived in Canada for more than thirty-five years, while 6% had come to Canada within the last ten years. Almost two-thirds (64%) of all immigrant seniors living in Canada in 2006 had come to Canada from Europe (Statistics Canada, 2010). As immigration from Asia has increased in recent decades, and as these immigrants get older, the percentage of immigrant seniors who are from Asia will increase.

In 2006, most immigrant seniors in Canada (75%) lived in Ontario and British Columbia. Indeed, 41% of seniors living in Ontario in 2006 were immigrants as were 39% of seniors in British Columbia (Statistics Canada, 2010). In 2001, 62% of seniors living in the Toronto CMA were immigrants as were 51% of seniors living in the Vancouver CMA. In any given year from 1995 to 2004, 2%-4% of immigrants arriving in Canada were seniors aged 65 or older, most sponsored by a family member (Turcotte & Schellenberg, 2007, p. 23, p. 274).

It is generally assumed that immigrant seniors who have come to Canada recently are less likely to be integrated into Canadian society relative to immigrant seniors who have lived in Canada for longer periods of time. This review of literature is guided by eight questions posed in 2007 by the Integration Branch of Citizenship and Immigration Canada. These questions focus on "integration outcomes" for immigrant seniors including economic outcomes, social outcomes, and outcomes related to language, education, health, psychological well-being, and so on. These outcomes may be assessed objectively by comparing, for example, the mean incomes of immigrant and non-immigrant seniors. Objective assessments of integration outcomes typically assume that comparisons with Canadian norms are relevant and that integration is

[1] This chapter is based on a report that was originally commissioned by the Integration Branch, Citizenship and Immigration Canada (CIC) in early 2007. The views expressed are those of the authors.

accomplished when differences between immigrant and non-immigrant seniors are minimal. Nevertheless, it may not always be the case that immigrant seniors are better off if they become like other seniors in Canada. Furthermore, Canada is a multi-cultural society that recognizes, values, and encourages social and cultural diversity.

One can ask: what does "integration" mean in a multi-cultural society? Can immigrant seniors maintain cultural beliefs and practices, have a cultural identity, be integrated into their cultural community, and still be integrated into the larger Canadian society? In other words we have to be careful how we conceptualize and operationalize "integration." For example, if immigrant seniors are more likely to live with their extended families and are more likely to report a higher dwelling density, is this necessarily an indicator of low integration, and even if one concludes that this is an indicator of differential integration, is this necessarily an indicator of a social problem in need of fixing? Conversely, if Canadian-born seniors are more likely to live alone, is this necessarily an ideal for immigrant seniors to aspire toward? Nevertheless, despite these limitations, it is important to assess integration outcomes in objective terms.

It is also important to assess integration outcomes subjectively from the point of view of immigrant seniors, themselves. It is important to know if immigrant seniors feel accepted and welcome in Canadian society, and feel free to maintain their cultural identity, beliefs, and practices. Integration, subjectively assessed, may be not so much about minimizing differences between immigrant and non-immigrant seniors, but rather ascertaining that all seniors feel that they are valued members of Canadian society despite all those factors that make one senior different than another. The subjective assessment of integration outcomes then involves focusing on the social acceptance of valued individual and group differences rather than the expectation that differences should become minimized.

Of course, where differences are found that relate to problems such as poverty, abuse, or poor health, the goal should be to eliminate these problems for immigrant and non-immigrant seniors alike. That is, while an integration outcomes approach might identify higher rates of social problems among immigrant seniors, the goal should be the elimination of the problem rather than the reduction of the problem to rates typical of the non-immigrant population.

The purpose of this chapter is to review recent Canadian publications from January 2000 to March 2007 focusing on integration outcomes for immigrant seniors. Initially, academic data bases such as Ageline, EconLit, PsychInfo, and SocIndex were researched. Keyword search terms such as Canada, immigrant, and senior and variations on these terms (for example, senior(s), aged, elder(s), elderly) were used. This produced a listing of possible relevant journal articles. Those articles which were pertinent were selected. Next, all references listed in each of the published articles were selected. This led to additional journal articles and to reports available on various web sites. Also searched were other websites, including a listing provided by Citizen and Immigration Canada (CIC). Finally, books dealing with aging in Canada and immigrant seniors in particular were searched. This review was guided by eight questions posed in 2007 by the Integration Branch of Citizenship and Immigration Canada.

What integration outcomes for immigrant seniors are identified in the literature?

Turcotte and Schellenberg (2007, pp. 271-295) examined a variety of integration outcomes including language (being able to speak English or French), health and well-being, security from crime, financial security, education, labor market participation and retirement, living arrangements, family and social networks, social support, and social participation. Boyd and Vickers (2000) examined income security, noting that elderly immigrants who have come to Canada more recently typically come from developing countries and have a greater degree of income polarization than elderly immigrants from developed countries who tend to have lived in Canada longer. Malenfant (2004) examined suicide in Canada's immigrant population and reported that suicide rates for immigrants in Canada are highest in old age, for both males and females, although lower than for the Canadian-born. Older immigrants who have come to Canada recently are less likely than younger immigrants and long-term immigrants to have become Canadian citizens (Tran, Kustec & Chui, 2005), although immigrants from developing countries are more likely to become citizens.

Spitzer, Neufeld, Harrison, Hughes, and Stewart (2003) explored the experiences of 11 South Asian and 18 Chinese Canadian immigrant women ages 29-75 (mean 50) who provided care to a family member with long-term health problems. Spitzer, et al. (2003) noted that these immigrant women were obligated by cultural values to provide care for family members with long-term health needs. However, as immigrants, they often had less access in Canada than they would in their countries of origin to resources that would help them carry out their obligations. In Canada, they had fewer kin close by, were less likely to hire laborers from outside the family to share domestic obligations, and were more likely to work outside of the home in the paid labor force (often in lower paying jobs), reducing the available time and energy required for family care giving. Ironically, there may be more pressure on these women to follow culturally-prescribed roles in Canada than in their countries of origin. That is, cultural values and norms of ethnic families and communities may be held more rigidly in Canada with little opportunity to negotiate these roles that, in their countries of origin, would have been implemented with greater assistance and more flexibility. Furthermore, there is a reluctance to use available formal services (such as home care) because these are culturally and linguistically unacceptable to elders who expect care to be provided by kin who are obligated to do so rather than by strangers who are paid to provide care. This sense of obligation did not seem to vary substantially with length of residency in Canada. The authors concluded that efforts need to be directed to supporting female family caregivers from diverse cultural backgrounds.

Choudhry (2001) interviewed 10 elderly women who had immigrated to Canada from India. Choudhry suggests that when immigrants in Canada sponsor their elderly parents under the family reunification policy, the elderly parents who then come to Canada and live with their children and grandchildren are at risk for "loss of independence and erosion of their traditional power and authority within the family structure" (p. 377). As a result, these elderly immigrants may experience a sense of loss, disconnection, dislocation, a feeling of being uprooted, isolation, loneliness, hopelessness, desperation, sadness, depression, lack of emotional support, economic dependence, loss of status, intergenerational conflict, and disappointment over erosion of traditional values, beliefs, and practices evident in their children and grandchildren. A lack of proficiency in English, household responsibilities in their child's home, and difficulty with public transportation, and getting around in the winter further exacerbate their isolation and distress.

Choudhry (2001) identified four themes in her interviews with elderly South Asian women immigrants. First, these elderly immigrant women tend to feel isolated and lonely in Canada having left their established network of extended kin, friends, and neighbors in India and because of language barriers, the fast pace of their children's lives, and the lack of time the children have to spend with their parents. Second, family conflict results from the erosion of traditional values, i.e., the Westernization of children and grandchildren. The elder generation tends to feel a sense of regret regarding the loss of traditional culture and the erosion of children's sense of obligation to their parents and the "liberation" of the daughters-in-law who traditionally carried out many of the obligations of the children to the parents. Third, economic dependence results from not having a personal source of income of their own, non-participation in the paid labor force in Canada, ineligibility for old-age income support programs in Canada (for the first 10 years of residence in Canada), widowhood, and dependence on the child who sponsored their immigration and in whose home they live. Finally, attendance at places of worship and seniors clubs, religious practices such as prayer, beliefs, and development of a social network, often within their ethnic community, facilitate adjustment to life in Canada.

Vohra and Adair (2000) studied the life satisfaction of Indian immigrants 18-71 years of age living in Winnipeg. They argued that it is important to assess integration outcomes in terms of immigrants' quality of life and subjective well-being, including measures of positive affect (such as happiness), negative affect, and life satisfaction. Vohra and Adair argued that life satisfaction is self-assessed by evaluating the extent to which one's expectations at the time of immigration have been met and by comparing oneself with Euro-Canadians, Indian and other immigrants in Canada, as well as Indians in India. Life satisfaction tends to be higher for those persons whose expectations have been met and those persons who perceive that they compare favorably with various social referent groups.

Summary

A wide range of integration outcomes for immigrant seniors are discussed in the literature. These can be grouped into several broad categories as follows:

- Economic outcomes (income levels, sources of income, financial dependence/independence, labor market participation/retirement, work history, education and recognition of foreign educational credentials, and eligibility for income security programs such as CPP, private pensions, OAS/GIS/Allowance);

- Language (being proficient in English or French);

- Health outcomes (physical health, mental health, and psycho-social well-being including happiness and satisfaction); and

- Social outcomes (family relationships including inter-generational relationships, social networks and social participation, social supports, living arrangements, transportation, and citizenship).

Note that these various outcomes can be measured both objectively and subjectively. For example, income is an objective measure, and perception of the adequacy of income and resulting sense of security and independence are subjective measures. The recently arrived immigrant senior in Canada is at greatest risk for the following reasons:

- Many are not proficient in English or French and so cannot easily access information, transportation, and needed services;

- Many do not have adequate personal income and so are dependent on their children for support; and

- The resulting social isolation and dependence can undermine psychological well-being and strain family relationships. There is a need not only to support the immigrant senior but also to support the family members who care for their immigrant elders.

What, if any, change over the past two decades in integration outcomes is identified in the literature on immigrant seniors?

Moore and Rosenberg (2001) discussed the increasing diversity of Canada's elderly population and implications for provision of needed services. Moore and Rosenberg noted that the shift from European-dominated immigration "prior to 1967 to an increasingly Asian-dominated immigration since 1978" (p. 146) will have significant consequences in the future as immigrants age. In the short term, because immigrants for the most part are younger rather than older when they come to Canada, changes in immigration patterns will have relatively little impact on the composition of Canada's elderly population, but in the future will have substantial implications for the ethnic, social and geographic characteristics of Canada's elderly population. This will be particularly true for the largest cities in Canada (Toronto, Montreal, and Vancouver) where immigrants concentrate. It follows that there is a growing need for tailoring services to this increasing diversity. The concentration of immigrant seniors in cities such as Toronto and Vancouver in some ways makes this easier. Elsewhere, small numbers increase the difficulty of tailoring services to diverse populations.

Turcotte and Schellenberg (2007, p. 282-283)) observed that both long-term and recent immigrant seniors were more likely to have a post-secondary certificate or university degree in 2001 compared to 1991 and 1981. The percentage of seniors in low income declined from 1980 to 2000 for all categories of seniors (non-immigrants, long-term immigrants, recent immigrants, attached and unattached, male and female). Unattached immigrant seniors who have come to Canada recently are most likely to be in the low-income category in 2000 (57% of male and 70% of female unattached recent immigrant seniors) despite improvements over the past twenty years (Turcotte & Schellenberg, 2007, p. 293).

Harrison (2000) reported that changes in countries of origin for immigrants in the later twentieth century has resulted in a higher percentage of people (of all ages) in Canada who cannot speak either English or French than at any previous time in the twentieth century. Tran, Kustec and Chui (2005) reported that the likelihood of becoming a citizen has increased over the 1981-2001 period. During this time, there has been an increase in immigration from Asia to Canada and immigrants from Asia are more likely to become citizens than immigrants from Europe or the United States.

Summary

Over the past two decades, major changes with respect to immigrant seniors include:

- Increasing diversity with respect to countries of origin (notable shift from Europe to Asia);.

- Increasing percentage of immigrant seniors who are not proficient in English or French;.

- Increasing levels of education (although recent family class immigrant seniors who came to Canada recently may have lower rates of education); and

- Decreasing rates of poverty, although unattached immigrant seniors who have come to Canada recently continue to have very high poverty rates.

The increasing diversity of immigrant seniors and the rising proportion who are not proficient in English or French points to a growing need to tailor services to an increasingly diverse group of seniors including the need for service staff to be able to communicate in various languages.

What, if any, relationship exists between economic outcomes and other outcomes (e.g., social, health, language, education and psychological)?

Turcotte and Schellenberg (2007, p. 277) suggested that immigrant seniors who have come to Canada recently (since 1981) are more likely to have low incomes and more likely to report poor health. Conversely, longer-term residence in Canada is associated with higher incomes and better health.

Summary

Given that economic outcomes are thought to be the primary driver of other outcomes such as health and a sense of well-being, it is perhaps surprising that the literature since 2000 does not focus heavily on the causal effects of economic outcomes. Nevertheless, economic variables are widely incorporated into comparative research (see the next two questions).

What does the literature reveal about the impact of other variables on the integration outcomes for immigrant seniors?

Recent arrival in Canada is associated with low income (Turcotte & Schellenberg, 2007, p. 281) although poverty rates vary depending on ethnic origin and city of residence in Canada (Kazemipur & Halli, 2000). Furthermore, living alone is associated with an increased risk of low income for male and especially female immigrant seniors (Turcotte & Schellenberg, 2007, p. 281).

Basavarajappa (1999; 2000) found that older immigrants from developing regions had more polarized income distributions than older immigrants from developed regions or older non-immigrants, "Thus, the very groups that have the lower average incomes also have a more inequitable distribution of income" (p 15). Basavarajappa noted that this pattern may be explained in part by the fact that immigrants from developing countries tend to have more polarization of educational attainments.

According to Basavarajappa (1998), older immigrants who have come to Canada from developing regions are increasing at a faster rate in Canada, although from a smaller numerical base, than older immigrants from developed regions and that older immigrants from developing regions are less likely to live alone, more likely to live in multi-generational households, and are more likely to experience crowded living conditions (defined as more than one person per room). While these living arrangements may reflect cultural preferences, they may also reflect financial necessity. Immigrants from developing countries are more likely to have come to Canada recently, be sponsored by family members, and depend on family members for financial support.

Gee (2000) examined the relationship between living arrangements and quality of life for elderly Chinese living in Vancouver and Victoria in 1995-1996. While Chinese elders in Canada were much more likely to live in intergenerational households than other Canadian elders, nevertheless, over one-third of married Chinese elders lived with their spouse only and 41% of elderly Chinese widows lived alone. Gee found few differences in the quality of life for married Chinese elders who lived with their spouse only or lived in an intergenerational household. In contrast, elderly Chinese widows who lived alone tended to report a lower quality of life than widows who lived in inter-generational households, although 90% of these widows indicated they did not want to live with a child. Gee concluded that for elderly Chinese in Canada, age, health, and having friends/confidantes were better predictors of quality of life than living arrange-ments. Chappell (2005) reported a study of Chinese seniors living in seven Canadian cities (where 89% of all ethnic Chinese in Canada live). This study focused on subjec-tive well being and in particular perceived change in quality of life as measured by the Chinese seniors' perceptions of the extent to which they felt that life in old age was improved or worse than when they were younger. Chappell concluded that health, socio-economic status, and involvement in traditional culture were related to a more positive experience in one's old age.

Wu and Hart (2002) found that while social support was associated with better health outcomes, it did not vary significantly with length of residence in Canada, abil-ity to speak English or French, or Asian origin; and that "many similarities exist between the determinants of support among Canada's foreign-born elderly and the native-born" (p. 407).

Summary

The recent literature shows that a number of variables are associated with key integration outcomes such as income, health, and subjective well-being for immigrant seniors. For example, recent arrival in Canada, older age at entry, living alone, and being female are associated with higher rates of poverty. Older immigrants from devel-oping regions exhibit more polarization of educational attainments and income distri-butions, are more likely to have come to Canada recently, be sponsored by family members, be financially dependent on family members, are less likely to live alone, more likely to live in multi-generational households, and are more likely to experience "crowded" living conditions. While immigrant seniors are more likely to live in multi-generational households, not all immigrant seniors want to live with their children. Indeed, health and subjective well-being for immigrant seniors may depend more on age, health, income, and social supports (including having a close friend(s) and involvement in one's ethnic community). While social support has positive consequences, social support itself may not depend on length of residence in Canada, English/French language proficiency, or country of origin.

Does the literature suggest variations in the integration outcomes for immigrant seniors when compared to the non-immigrant population?

Turcotte and Schellenberg (2007, p. 276-280) reported that immigrant seniors who came to Canada after 1981 were more likely to report poor health in comparison to longer-term immigrant and Canadian-born seniors, were more likely to need help with daily activities such as getting to an appointment or looking after their personal finances, reported slightly lower well-being although they also reported slightly lower psychological distress, were less likely to be smokers and less likely to be heavy drinkers, made more visits to the doctor and were more likely to report that their health needs were not satisfied. Gee, Kobayashi, and Prus (2004) showed that recent elderly immigrants have poorer overall physical health than Canadian-born seniors. In contrast, recent immigrants 45-64 years of age show a "healthy immigrant" effect having better health than the Canadian-born who are 45-64 years of age.

Pérez (2002) showed that for chronic health conditions, immigrants (of all ages) to Canada report better health than the Canadian-born and converge with the Canadian-born as length of residence in Canada increases. Ali (2002) shows a similar pattern for rates of depression and alcohol dependence. Nevertheless, Pérez and Ali do not disaggregate by age at the time of immigration and therefore do not compare the health status of older versus younger recent immigrants.

Newbold and Filice (2006) compared older immigrants with older non-immigrants and found that "despite some variations between the two groups, the foreign-born do not systematically report *worse/better* health than the native-born" (p. 316, italics in original), although this study does not compare older recent immigrants with older long-term immigrants. Streiner, Cairney, and Veldhuizen (2006) analyzed the prevalence of psychological problems (major depression, bipolar disorder, social phobia, agoraphobia, and panic disorder) and found that prevalence decreased with age and that immigrants were less likely than non-immigrants to report psychological problems, although this study does not compare older recent immigrants with older long-term immigrants.

In contrast, Lai (2004a) examined depressive symptoms of elderly Chinese immigrants living in seven major Canadian cities. Lai found that elderly Chinese immigrants reported a higher prevalence of depressive symptoms than levels thought to be characteristic of older Canadians generally. Lai concluded that: "cultural values maintained by elderly immigrants in combination with the cultural barriers that they face accessing health services are major impediments to mental health . . . thus it is important for the health system to pay attention to cultural uniqueness and cultural appropriateness in service provision to eliminate access barriers and challenges" (p. 825). Lai (2004b) also found that elderly Chinese immigrants in Canada were less likely to use home care services than elderly Canadians. Lai recommended that home care use be promoted among elderly Chinese immigrants and their families. Turcotte and Schellenberg (2007) observed that immigrant and non-immigrant seniors suffering from a long-term health condition were equally likely to have received formal and/or informal care, although recent immigrant seniors, who are less likely to live alone, were more likely to have received care informally from family members.

Tam and Neysmith (2006) convened focus groups with Chinese home care workers serving Chinese seniors in Toronto. These home care workers were asked about elder abuse perpetrated by family members and witnessed in the course of their visits to Chinese elders' homes. This study concluded that elder abuse in the Chinese community typically takes the form of "disrespect" that violates traditional values and norms defining the obligations that children have in regards to their parents.

Malenfant (2004) showed that immigrants of all ages in Canada, regardless of their continent of origin, are less likely than the Canadian-born to commit suicide. Immigrant suicide rates in Canada are closer to suicide rates in their countries of origin than to suicide rates in Canada.

Seniors who have immigrated to Canada are more likely than Canadian-born seniors to experience low income, and this is especially true for recent immigrants (Palameta, 2004; Turcotte and Schellenberg, 2007:281-282, 293; Palameta, 2004. Dempsey (2006, p. 2) showed that "Non-immigrant seniors rely more on contributory retirement income (C/QPP, RRSP and private pensions) while immigrant seniors rely more on non-contributory retirement income (OAS and GIS/Allowance)." That is, immigrant seniors, especially recent immigrants and seniors sponsored under the family reunification category (Dempsey, 2004; 2005), are less likely to have contributed to pension plans and consequently receive a greater proportion of their (lower) income from government transfers such as Old Age Security and the supplement programs for low-income seniors.

Immigrant seniors who came to Canada some time ago are more likely to have a post-secondary certificate or university degree than recent immigrant seniors and non-immigrant seniors. Recent immigrant seniors are more likely to have been admitted to Canada in the family class category that does not have education requirements for qualification (Turcotte & Schellenberg, 2007, p. 282-283).

In 2001, recent immigrant, long-term immigrant, and non-immigrant seniors had virtually identical labor force participation rates; however, recent immigrant seniors were much more likely to be looking for employment. With respect to retirement, immigrants tend to retire later than the Canadian-born. Furthermore, immigrant seniors who have come to Canada since 1980 are more likely to feel that they are not adequately prepared financially for retirement, and immigrants are more likely to retire involuntarily and are more likely to say that they enjoy life less in retirement compared to non-immigrant retirees (Turcotte & Schellenberg, 2007, p. 283-285).

Canadian-born seniors are more likely than immigrant seniors to live alone and immigrant seniors who have lived in Canada for a substantial amount of time are more likely to live alone than immigrant seniors who have come to Canada recently. Recent immigrant seniors who have come to Canada recently tend to have been sponsored by family members and live with these family members when they come to Canada (Turcotte & Schellenberg, 2007, p. 285). Pacey (2002) noted that while having sufficient income may allow some Chinese-Canadian seniors to choose to live alone, not all who are able to live alone choose to do so. Pacey suggested that culture is an important determinant of living arrangements, even after taking income into account.

Contact with family and friends was found to be similar for immigrant and non-immigrant seniors (Turcotte & Schellenberg, 2007, p. 286-287). There was no difference between immigrant and non-immigrant seniors with respect to being a victim of a crime in 2004 (Turcotte &and Schellenberg, 2007, p. 282).

Immigrant seniors who have come to Canada more recently are less likely to have a strong sense of belonging to their local community, are less likely to be members of a voluntary organization, but are more likely to say that their religion is important to them, in comparison to longer-term immigrant and non-immigrant seniors (Turcotte & Schellenberg, 2007, p. 287-288).

Summary

Perhaps the most striking conclusion emerging from studies that compare immigrant seniors in Canada with non-immigrant seniors concerns the "healthy immigrant effect." Immigrants tend to be "positively selected," that is, when they first come to Canada, they tend to be young, better educated, etc. and healthier than the Canadian-born population. This healthy immigrant effect decays over time as immigrant's age in Canada and become more and more like the Canadian-born. However, it appears that seniors who have immigrated to Canada recently at an older age do not exhibit a healthy immigrant effect but instead tend to have worse health than long-term immigrant seniors and non-immigrant seniors. Further, immigrant seniors who have come to Canada recently are more likely to need help with activities such as getting to needed services and managing personal finances. Nevertheless, recent immigrant seniors are less likely to live alone and are more likely to have received informal care from family members.

With respect to economic outcomes, immigrant seniors who have come to Canada recently, especially those coming in the family reunification category, are less likely to have post-secondary education than longer-term immigrant seniors and non-immigrant seniors; more likely to be unemployed and looking for work; more likely to feel unprepared financially for retirement; less likely to have contributed to pension plans; more likely to rely on non-contributory income security programs such as OAS/GIS/Allowance; and are more likely to be poor.

Finally, immigrant seniors who have come to Canada recently are less likely to feel attached to their local community but are more likely to say their religion is important.

Does the literature point to any geographic variation with respect to integration outcomes?

Kazemipur and Halli (2000) show that low-income rates for various immigrant groups (all ages combined) vary not only between immigrant groups but also vary from one city to another in Canada. For example, German immigrants are less likely to be poor than Chinese immigrants and immigrants living in Toronto are less likely to be poor than immigrants living in Winnipeg.

Summary

While there are considerable regional and rural-urban disparities in Canada, it appears that geographic variation in the integration outcomes of immigrant seniors has been understudied in recent years.

What barriers, challenges or needs affect the integration outcomes for immigrant seniors?

Turcotte and Schellenberg (2007, p. 275, Table 7.2) reported that 15% of immigrant seniors in 2001 spoke neither English nor French. This figure varies with length of residence in Canada ranging from 3.6% for seniors who came to Canada forty or more years ago to 50.2% for seniors who came to Canada within the past ten years. Spitzer, et al. (2003) noted that failure to recognize foreign credentials and the tendency to undervalue foreign work experience put immigrant women at a disadvantage in the paid labor force.

Newbold and Filice (2006, p. 306) speculated that barriers to accessing health care for older immigrants include: language, culture, familial roles, access to transportation and ease of personal mobility. Kobayashi (2003) identified barriers to health care for immigrants including health beliefs; ethno-cultural values and beliefs; lack of knowledge, awareness, and understanding; spirituality and religious practices; family relationships; education and income; language; fear of medical facilities; and stereo-types, attitudes, beliefs and behaviors of physicians regarding immigrant groups. Spitzer, et al., (2003) noted that immigrant elders in Canada from East Asia and South Asia expect to be cared for at home by family members, in particular, by daughters and daughters-in-law, and resist formal health care alternatives.

Neufeld,, Harrison, Stewart, Hughes, and Spitzer (2002) noted that some East Asian and South Asian immigrants are able to make connections with formal services while others are less successful in doing so. Access to services is often facilitated by the immigrant's informal network of family and friends. Nevertheless, one's informal network may also function as a barrier to accessing community services when cultural values and norms discourage seeking formal services from outside the kinship and ethno-community network. Additional barriers include: language limitations of either caregiver or elderly care receiver and policy that restricts English-language or French-language training; limited financial resources; transportation barriers including not hav-ing a car, not having a driver's license, and having limited access to persons willing to provide transportation; lack of time or not being able to get off work when services are available; waiting lists for services; cultural values and beliefs and traditional practices; lack of knowledge regarding western medicine and services available in Canada; and limited social ties including absence of a diverse range of "weak ties" outside of one's immediate family and ethnic community.

Leung and McDonald (2001) interviewed Chinese immigrant women who were providing care to aging parents and who were living in three-generational households in Toronto. When parents were in reasonably good health, the relationship between parents and daughters tended to be reciprocal and mutually beneficial. However, when parents were frail and ill, caregiving could become burdensome for the caregivers. Leung and McDonald noted that both caregivers and care receivers experienced barri-ers to care:

> . . . these elderly Chinese immigrants were affected by language barriers, trans-
> portation barriers, isolation, lack of culturally and linguistically sensitive health
> and social services, making care-giving especially challenging. The immigrant
> women who cared for frail elderly parents themselves faced additional challenges
> due to factors resulting from immigration, such as weak informal social networks.
> (p. 1)

Similarly, Grewal, Bottorff, and Hilton (2005) concluded that there is a need for culturally appropriate and women-centred health care for South Asian immigrant women in Canada. Finally, van Dijk (2004) examined elderly Dutch immigrants in southern Ontario and concluded that personal and cultural continuity is important to persons especially in old age and, therefore, staff in senior-care facilities must be aware of personal and cultural preferences and offer appropriate care.

Mulvihill, Mailloux, and Atkin (2001, p. 21) reported that "the most significant challenges for older immigrants are language and communication barriers" and the resulting difficulty these create for accessing health care. They also noted the relative poverty of older immigrant women and their frequent role obligations as informal caregivers. Finally, they suggested that seniors' care requires both family-focused and institutional strategies that are culturally appropriate and effective.

McDonald, George, Daciuk, Yan, and Rowan (2001) examined the needs of recent immigrant seniors. Most of these recently arrived senior immigrants were sponsored by their children, lived with their children, and had no or poor language skills in English or French. The problems identified included: immigrant seniors' lack of proficiency in English and French; and lack of knowledge of available services; "shortage of language specific staff [at service agencies] and language specific informational materials" (p. iii); "a need for more structured programs targeted specifically at older newcomers, more community outreach and a need to connect newcomer seniors with other seniors from their own communities" (p. iii); and immigrant seniors' "over-dependence on their families, financial distress, lack of reliable transportation, the inclement weather and social isolation" (p. iv).

Durst (2005) argued that immigrant seniors should be involved in decision-making regarding issues that affect them; should be encouraged to volunteer in agencies that serve immigrant/ethnic seniors; require interpreters, translated materials, and multilingual staff to facilitate access to services; require services that are culturally sensitive; and finally, "ethno-cultural seniors need to be recognized and valued for their diversity" (p. 268).

Brotman (2003) argued that efforts to offer appropriate services for ethnic elders has tended to focus on language barriers and solutions such as the use of translators but that these efforts do not address racism and indeed tend to make racism invisible. Brotman argues that explicit antiracist agendas should be discussed and addressed. Similarly, Shemirani and O'Connor (2006) argue that endemic racism and ageism influence the experience of older immigrant women in Canada and must be made visible in order to adequately address the needs of older immigrant women. Further, Galabuzi (2004) argues that social exclusion of groups such as immigrants and refugees, visible minorities, women, and the elderly and their unpaid caregivers, lowers health status and should be addressed by healthcare policy-makers.

Chappell, McDonald, and Stones (2008, p. 163-164) noted that there is an ongoing debate as to whether segregated (parallel) services for elderly ethnic minority immigrants are preferable or integrated services which recognize and respond to diversity are best. In either case, these authors pointed to a number of barriers faced by elderly immigrants including a lack of personal income and resulting financial dependence on their children, language problems, lack of knowledge of services, reluctance to use formal Western services, lack of transportation, and a shortage of ethnically sensitive practitioners.

Summary

Barriers, challenges, and needs affecting the integration outcomes for immigrant seniors, especially for those who have come to Canada recently, include:
- language and communication barriers;
- cultural barriers (including culturally and linguistically insensitive service agencies and practitioners on the one hand, and on the other hand, the cultural beliefs and practices of immigrant seniors themselves; lack of knowledge, awareness, and understanding regarding available services and reluctance to use Western formal services);
- economic barriers (poverty/low income, lack of personal income/financial dependence on children, lack of education, undervaluing of foreign credentials and foreign work experience, lack of involvement in labor force or low paying employment, immigration policy that disqualifies sponsored family class immigrant seniors from certain social benefits);
- transportation barriers (e.g., no access to a vehicle, not having a driver's license, lack of persons willing to drive for the senior);
- social barriers (social isolation, lack of "weak ties," familial roles and relationships which can function as either a facilitator or a barrier to integration, lack of support for family caregivers, and systemic racism, sexism, and agism); and
- weather (winter weather in Canada tends to isolate immigrant seniors).

What is needed?
- language training programs for immigrant seniors and the family members who care for them;
- culturally and linguistically sensitive service agencies and practitioners; hiring of practitioners from various ethno-cultural communities and with diverse language skills; outreach and knowledge/awareness efforts in the language of the immigrant senior; where appropriate and possible, services targeted to specific ethno-cultural groups as well as services designed to accommodate a diversity of clientele;
- integration of the older immigrant into the labor force; and
- supportive services targeting senior immigrant households and the multi-generational family members who support senior immigrants, women-centred services given that the bulk of care-giving responsibilities tends to fall to women.

Does the literature suggest ways in which barriers, challenges and needs have changed over time?

McPherson (2004) and Ujimoto, (2002) noted that changing patterns of immigration have increased and will continue to increase the diversity of immigrant seniors in Canada. This means that there is a growing challenge to provide culturally sensitive and appropriate services to this increasingly diverse population of seniors.

Summary

In recent decades, the increasing diversity of immigrant seniors in terms of language, culture, and religion makes it increasingly important to create culturally appropriate and sensitive services for immigrant seniors and their supportive families.

Key Priorities and Recommendations

Focus on immigrant seniors who have come to Canada recently

Immigrant seniors who have been in Canada long-term have needs similar to non-immigrant seniors and therefore services do not have to be differentiated substantially for the long-term immigrant senior. Services need to focus on the recent immigrant senior to determine how their integration needs differ from long-term immigrant and non-immigrant seniors.

Focus on recent immigrant seniors in Toronto, Vancouver, and Montreal

Because recent immigrant seniors tend to be concentrated in Toronto, Vancouver, and Montreal, there is a "critical mass" which presents both a rationale and an opportunity to develop ethno-specific services. Innovative programs piloted in these cities might then spread to other places in Canada where recent immigrant seniors settle in smaller numbers. Alternatively, programs may have to be developed separately to meet the needs of small concentrations of diverse recent immigrant seniors.

Focus on language integration for recent immigrant seniors

Perhaps the leading problem for recent immigrant seniors is lack of proficiency in English or French resulting in difficulty in communication and in accessing services such as health, finances, and transportation as well as difficulty integrating into the labor force (for those who wish to work rather than be "retired"). The language/communication problem can be addressed from two directions. On the one hand, seniors and those family members who care for them need access to language training programs tailored to the older immigrant. Second, service agencies should be staffed whenever possible with multi-lingual speakers and the use of translators (familial or professional) should be facilitated.

Focus on economic integration for recent immigrant seniors

Many recent immigrant seniors, especially those who are sponsored by their family members, have little if any personal income and are often financially dependent on their children. For some recent immigrant seniors this is not problematic; however, for those who wish to be financially independent from their children and who are not ready to be retired, service providers need to integrate these recent immigrant seniors into the labor market. To do this, language skills must be developed, foreign education and foreign work experience must be recognized, training programs must be targeted to the older recent immigrant, and meaningful job opportunities that offer reasonable rates of pay must exist. Where ageism, sexism, and racism constitute barriers to meaningful employment, these problems need to be addressed.

Social support for recent immigrant seniors and their families

It is important to recognize that while recent immigrant seniors who live alone or with a spouse may need support services (such as home care or DATS), recent immigrant seniors who live in multi-generational families, as well as the family members who care for them, may also need support services.

Culturally sensitive and appropriate services for recent immigrant seniors

While all practitioners and programs that serve recent immigrant seniors should be culturally sensitive and appropriate, this may be especially important for health care services and long-term care facilities. Linguistic, cultural, religious, informational, and other barriers must be recognized and managed in order to facilitate service delivery and client satisfaction.

Recognize diversity within diversity

We must recognize that recent immigrant seniors are diverse themselves and they must resist thinking stereotypically. And of course, immigrant seniors' needs tend to be different at 65, 75, 85, and 95 years of age.

Recommendations for Further Research

- What are the demographic implications of elder migration into Canada?
- What are the economic implications of elder migration into Canada?

- To what extent do recently-arrived immigrant elders wish to be incorporated into the labor force and, for those who prefer to be employed, how can their involvement in the labor force be facilitated?

- What are the immediate and long-term implications for the health care system and for health care costs of immigrants coming to Canada who are elderly at the time of arrival?

- There is a need to research elder abuse in its various forms in immigrant and non-immigrant families.

- To what extent do recently-arrived immigrant seniors in Canada wish to gain proficiency in English or French and how effective are language-training programs for immigrant seniors?

- There is a need to examine the process of integration of immigrant seniors who have come to Canada recently, focusing in particular on the first few years in Canada.

- There is a need to examine the discourse of multiculturalism, pluralism, and diversity, on the one hand, and the discourse regarding what it means to be Canadian, on the other hand, with respect to implications for national unity and Canadian identity. In particular, we need to examine the development of Canadian identity and commitment in recently-arrived immigrant seniors.

- There is a need to examine the integration of recently-arrived immigrant seniors within ethnic enclaves in relation to their integration into the Canadian "mainstream."

- There needs to be an examination of what elderly immigrants can reasonably expect of the State and what the State can reasonably expect of elderly immigrants.

- The issues associated with of dual (and triple, etc.) citizenship in the context of an aging population needs to be researched.

Conclusion

Immigrant seniors in Canada include seniors who came years ago as well as seniors who have arrived recently. Furthermore, while earlier immigrants tended to come from Europe, recent immigrants are more likely to come from Asian and other non-European countries. As a result, there is a perception that Canada's aging population is becoming increasingly "diverse" and that this diversity presents challenges for the integration of the aging immigrant, especially the recently arrived immigrant senior. While a research literature is emerging that focuses on the integration of the aging immigrant into Canadian society, there is still much to learn.

References

Ali, J. (2002). Mental health of Canada's immigrants. Supplement to *Health Reports,* Catalogue 82-003-SIE, (1-11). Ottawa: Statistics Canada.

Basavarajappa, K.G. (2000). Distribution, inequality and concentration of income among older immigrants in Canada. *International Migration, 38*(1), 47-65.

Basavarajappa, K.G. (1999). Distribution, inequality and concentration of income among older immigrants in Canada, 1990. Catalogue no. 11F0019MPE No. 129. Ottawa: Statistics Canada.

Basavarajappa, K.G. (1998). *Living arrangements and residential overcrowding: The situation of older immigrants in Canada, 1991.* Catalogue no. 11F0019MPE No. 115. Ottawa: Statistics Canada.

Boyd, M., & Vickers, M. (2000). 100 years of immigration in Canada. *Canadian Social Trends, (Autumn),* 2-12.

Brotman, S. (2003). Limits of multiculturalism in elder care services. *Journal of Aging Studies, 17*(2), 209-229.

Chappell, N. (2005). Perceived change in quality of life among Chinese Canadian seniors: The role of involvement in Chinese culture. *Journal of Happiness Studies, 6*(1), 69-91.

Chappell, N., McDonald, L. & Stones, M. (2008). *Aging in Contemporary Canada* (2nd ed.). Toronto: Pearson.

Choudhry, U.K. (2001). Uprooting and resettlement experiences of South Asian immigrant women. *Western Journal of Nursing Research, 23*(4), 376 - 393.

Dempsey, C. (2006?). *Immigrant Income and the Family.* Ottawa: Citizenship and Immigration Canada.

Dempsey, C. (2005). *Elderly immigrants in Canada: Income sources and self-sufficiency.* Summary. Ottawa: Citizenship and Immigration Canada.

Dempsey, C. (2004). *Elderly immigrants in Canada: Income sources and composition.* Horizons, Policy Research Initiative, 2(7). Accessed 28, March, 2007, from http://policyresearch.gc.ca/-page.asp?pagenm=v7n2_art_10.

Durst, D. (2005). Aging amongst immigrants in Canada: Population drift. *Canadian Studies in Population, 32*(2), 257-270.

Galabuzi, G.E. (2004). Social Exclusion. In Dennis Raphael (Ed.), *Social Determinants of Health: Canadian Perspectives,* (pp. 235-251). Toronto: Canadian Scholars' Press.

Gee, E.M. (2000). Living arrangements and quality of life among Chinese Canadian elders. *Social Indicators Research, 51*, 309-329.

Gee, E.M., Kobayashi, K.M. & Prus, S.G. (2004). Examining the healthy immigrant effect in mid- to later life: Findings from the Canadian Community Health Survey. *Canadian Journal on Aging, 23*, (Supplement), S55-S63.

Grewal, S., Bottorff, J.L. & Hilton, B.A. (2005). The influence of family on immigrant South Asian women's health. *Journal of Family Nursing, 8*(11), 242-263.

Harrison, B. (2000). Passing on the language: Heritage language diversity in Canada. *Canadian Social Trends, (Autumn),* 14-19.

Kazemipur, A. & Halli, S.S. (2000). The colour of poverty: A study of the poverty of ethnic and immigrant groups in Canada. *International Migration, 38*(1), 69-88.

Kobayashi, K.M. (2003). Do intersections of diversity matter? An exploration of the relationship between identity markers and health for mid- to later-life Canadians. *Canadian Ethnic Studies, 35*(3), 85-98.

Lai, D.W.L. (2004a). Impact of culture on depressive symptoms of elderly Chinese immigrants. *Canadian Journal of Psychiatry, 49*(12), 820-827.

Lai, D.W.L. (2004b). Use of home care services by elderly Chinese immigrants. *Home Health Care Services Quarterly, 23*(3), 41-56.

Leung, H.H. & McDonald, L. (2001). *Chinese immigrant women who care for aging parents.* Toronto: Centre for Excellence for Research on Immigration and Settlement.

Malenfant, E.C. (2004). Suicide in Canada's immigrant population. *Health Reports, 15*(2), 9-17.

McDonald, L., George, U., Daciuk, J., Yan, M.C., & Rowan, H. (2001). *A study on the settlement related needs of newly arrived immigrant seniors in Ontario.* Toronto: Centre for Applied Social Research, University of Toronto.

McPherson, B.D. (2004). *Aging as a social process: Canadian perspectives (4th ed.).* Don Mills, Ontario: Oxford University Press.

Moore, E.G. & Rosenberg, M.W. (2001). Canada's elderly population: the challenges of diversity. *Canadian Geographer, 45*(1), 145-150.

Mulvihill, M.A., Mailloux, L. & Atkin, W. (2001). *Advancing policy and research responses to immigrant and refugee women's health in Canada.* Winnipeg: Canadian Women's Health Network.

Neufeld, A., Harrison, M.J., Stewart, M.J., Hughes, K.D. & Spitzer, D. (2002). Immigrant women: Making connections to community resources for support in family caregiving. *Qualitative Health Research, 12*(6), 751-768.

Newbold, K.B. & Filice, J.K. (2006). Health status of older immigrants to Canada. *Canadian Journal on Aging, 25*(3), 305-319.

Pacey, M.A. (2002). Living alone and living with children: The living arrangements of Canadian and Chinese-Canadians seniors. Hamilton: McMaster University, Social and Economic Dimensions of an Aging Population Research Papers. [See M.A. Thesis, Queen's University, Kingston, Ontario. 2001.]

Palameta, B. (2004). Low income among immigrants and visible minorities. Perspectives on *Labour and Income, 5*(4), 12-17.

Pérez, C.E. (2002). Health status and health behaviour among immigrants. In Statistics Canada, Supplement to Health Reports (Catalogue 82-003-SIE) (pages 1-12). Ottawa: Statistics Canada.

Shemirani, F.S. & O'Connor, D.L. (2006). Aging in a foreign country: voices of Iranian women aging in Canada. *Journal of Women and Aging, 18*(2), 73-90.

Spitzer, D., Neufeld, A., Harrison, M., Hughes, K. & Stewart, M. (2003). Caregiving in transnational context: my wings have been cut; where can I fly? *Gender and Society, 17*(2), 267-286.

Statistics Canada (2005). Proportion of foreign-born population, by province and territory (1991 to 2001 Censuses). Accessed 11 March 2007 from http://www40.statcan.ca/101/cst01/demo46a.htm.

Streiner, D.L., Cairney, J. & Veldhuizen, S. (2006). The epidemiology of psychological problems in the elderly. *Canadian Journal of Psychiatry, 52*, 185-191.

Tam, S., & Neysmith, S. (2006). Disrespect and isolation: elder abuse in Chinese communities. *Canadian Journal on Aging, 25*(2), 141-151.

Tran, K., Kustec, S. & Chui, T. (2005). Becoming Canadian: Intent, process and outcome. *Canadian Social Trends, 76*, 8-13.

Turcotte, M. & Schellenberg, G. (2007). *A portrait of seniors in Canada 2006.* Catalog no. 89-519-XIE. Ottawa: Statistics Canada.

Ujimoto, K.V. (2002). Multiculturalism, ethnicity, aging, and health care. In Bolaria, B.S., & Dickinson, H.D. (Eds.), *Health, Illness, and Health Care in Canada* (3rd ed.). (pp. 475-504). Scarborough, Ontario: Nelson Thomson.

van Dijk, J. (2004). The role of ethnicity and religion in the social support system of older Dutch Canadians. *Canadian Journal on Aging, 23*(1), 21-34.

Vohra, N. & Adair, J. (2000). Life satisfaction of Indian Immigrants in Canada. *Psychology & Developing Societies, 12*, 109-138.

Wu, Z. & Hart, R. (2002). Social and health factors associated with support among elderly immigrants in Canada. *Research on Aging, 24*(4), 391-412.

Chapter 3

Theorizing About Aging and Immigration

Lynn McDonald, (University of Toronto)

Social gerontologists have conducted little research on older immigrants and have engaged in theory development to an even lesser extent. Part of the problem reflects the slow development of theory in gerontology generally (Bengston, Putney & Johnson, 2005). The famous statement, "Gerontology is rich in data but poor in theory" (Birren & Bengtson, 1988, p. ix) is especially applicable to aging and immigration. There is a growing body of research but the majority of studies are not guided by theory or attempt to develop theory (e.g., Angel & Angel, 2006; Lai & Surood, 2008; Newbold & Filice, 2006; Wong, Yoo & Stewart, 2007). While social gerontology is not without theory, much of that theory has languished over the years and "newer" developments have rarely been used to explain the lives of aging immigrants. The other half of the problem rests with the complexity involved in studying immigration and aging which does not lend easily to theorizing (Durst, 2005). The objectives of this chapter are to examine the major activities in the development of theory as it applies to aging and immigration starting with the importance of theory, early theoretical developments in the field, specific theory creation in aging and immigration and concluding observations on where gerontological theory is likely headed in the future.

Why Theory?

Most of us have "theories" about all manner of issues which are basically our own hunches. For example, you might hear your colleagues say, "Older adults migrate to Canada because they want to." Overlooking the fact that this statement is not true (about 20 percent of older immigrants do not want to come to Canada), (McDonald, George, Daciuk, Yan & Rowan, 2001), it is not a theory in the way that social scientists would describe it. Bengtson, Rice, and Johnson (1999, p. 5) define theory as "the construction of explicit explanations in accounting for empirical findings." Explanation is the main function of theory which usually takes the form of a causal relationship between two concepts and is expressed as a hypothesis or chains of hypotheses. For example, "If older adults have children living in Canada, then they are more likely to want to immigrate to Canada than are those older adults who do not have children living in Canada." Theories explain phenomena that have been, or can be, observed in interviews, in secondary data, administrative data, textual materials, laboratory trials or observed directly. In the above example about older immigrants, there is no explanation nor is there evidence confirming that all older people want to come to Canada. Even if data confirm a relationship between older people and wanting to come to Canada, there is still no explanation. In the final analysis, all we could do is predict who comes to Canada without knowing why.

Theoretical perspectives or frameworks are terms sometimes seen in the gerontological literature and refer to theoretical thinking that is not as well developed as a full blown theory. Most times, theoretical frameworks are more descriptive and less explanatory than well articulated theories. In practice, however, the distinction between theory and a theoretical framework or perspective is somewhat hazy and the terms are often used interchangeably.

Theory, notwithstanding the lack of attractiveness, is extremely important for many reasons. Here, the most important reason we cite is the obvious – if we know why something happens (we can explain it), then we can do something about it in terms of prevention (Bengston, Putney & Johnson, 2005; Chappell, McDonald & Stones, 2008). A poor theory will generate an inadequate explanation and, in turn, will lead to inappropriate social policy and interventions. For example, the 2002 Ethnic Diversity Study by Statistics Canada indicated that 20% of visible minorities had experienced discrimination in the five years prior to the survey. The black respondents reported the highest levels of discrimination (32%) followed by the South Asians (21% percent) and then the Chinese (18%) (Statistics Canada, 2003c). If we knew what caused this discrimination, different possibilities for prevention would be apparent so that we could eliminate the problem.

The Complexity in Studying Older Immigrants

The complexity inherent in studying aging and immigration can be daunting as some of the following issues would suggest. First, a relatively large proportion of older people in Canada are immigrants; 28.6 percent of the population aged 65 years and over in 2001 were immigrants, compared with only 17.7 percent of the population 64 or under in the same year (Chappell et al., 2008). Canadian history clearly shows that the majority of older immigrants currently living in Canada have been here for a very long time. In fact, 61 percent arrived before 1961; 24 percent came in the 1960s and 1970s, while about 15 percent arrived between 1981 and 1996 (Health Canada, 1998). The current older population "aged in place" or grew older while in Canada. Today, older people immigrate to Canada in smaller numbers. In 2004, about three percent of people (less than 6,000) who immigrated to Canada were 65 years of age or older (Citizenship and Immigration Canada, 2005). Without doubt, the length of time in Canada and age at time of immigration will contribute to very different experiences for older adults (Leu et al., 2008). Those immigrants who came to Canada thirty years ago are more likely to be familiar with one of the two official languages and would be more comfortable with many aspects of Canadian culture.

Second, the limited but growing research in ethno gerontology (the influence of race, ethnicity, national origin, and culture on individual and population aging) has shown that ethnicity and race have a profound influence on the aging experience, whether it be as a consequence of expectations for aging and preferred lifestyles, inter-generational differences, living arrangements, family supports, the use of ethno specific health and social services, or the problems of racism and discrimination, (e.g., Blakemore & Boneham, 1994; Chappell & Kusch, 2006; Collings, 2001; Hooyman & Kiyak, 2005; Keefe, Rosenthal & Beland, 2000; Koybashi, 2000; Lai, 2004; Lai & Surwood, 2008; McDonald et al., 2001). In light of the extensive effect of ethnicity on aging, it is worth noting that the diversity in Canada is huge and is ranked with the United States, Great Britain and Singapore. Over 200 ethnic origins were reported by the total population in Canada in the 2006 Census which included Canada's Aboriginal peoples as well as the groups that came to Canada (Statistics Canada, 2008). It comes as no surprise that as a starting point for understanding, this wide array of ethnic origins has tended to spawn studies that focus on only one ethnic group at one point in time and, in so doing, tend to be a-theoretical (e.g., Chappell & Kusch, 2006; Diwan, Jonnaladda & Balaswamy, 2004; Kalavar & Van Willigen, 2005; Lai, 2004). On the other hand, creating a theoretical perspective that encompasses all ethnic minority groups who have immigrated would be a complicated undertaking. Studies that compare different immigration groups are also a-theoretical and tend to focus on finding differences when commonalities are also important (e.g., Angel & Angel, 2006; Settersten, 2005; Treas & Mazumbar, 2002; Wong, Yoo & Stewart, 2007).

The process of immigration itself can be no less challenging at any time in one's life with settlement and adjustment issues, multiple losses such as friends and family, language barriers and limited resources (Jackson & Antonucci, 2005; Lee, 2007; McDonald et al., 2001; McDonald et al., 2008; Noh & Avison, 1996). In addition, the category of immigration under which the immigrants come is likely to make a difference in experience, especially if the older adult is a refugee compared to someone immigrating under the family reunification category. The life course of immigrants, by definition, stretches from a previous life in the country of origin to a life after in the settlement country but is rarely examined. Scholars usually only make comparisons after immigration has occurred with the most common method being to compare immigrants with the Canadian born which negates a sizable portion of the life of an immigrant, but is an example of the unique requirements for studying older immigrants (Newbold & Felice, 2006).

Third, a number of scholars have warned about stereotyping different immigrant groups. As is the case with the aged in general, the variations within immigrant groups are often overlooked to the detriment of the aging individual (Dietz, John & Roy, 1998; Whitfield & Baker-Thomas, 1999). As an illustration, there are 11 Aboriginal language groups in Canada, made up of more than 65 distinct languages and dialects represented among Aboriginal seniors (Health Canada, 1998a). A study of the involvement of Chinese Canadian seniors in Chinese culture found that different aspects of the culture contributed to a positive experience of aging (Chappell, 2005). A theory, then, has to be mindful of commonalities across groups while at the same time respecting within-group differences (Moriarty & Butt, 2004).

Finally, one of the traps that theory has fallen prey to is related to the issue of generations. Earlier studies often compared immigrant groups with little attention to what generations were being compared (Burr & Mutchler, 1993; Kamo & Zhou, 1994), but today, researchers are more cautious (Hsu, Lew-Ting & Wu, 2001; Kobayashi, 2000; Lowenstein & Katz, 2005). A theoretical perspective that examines older immigrant groups will likely need to consider a generational approach that takes into account socioeconomic and political factors encountered by each generation and, therefore, the different experiences of each generation and the nuances of the inter-generational relationships (Chappell et al., 2008). A study of two generations of Russian émigrés to Israel found that different factors affected life satisfaction in diverse ways according to generation location. For the older generation, subjective health was the most important variable while for the younger generations, standard of living and employment were the most important factors contributing to satisfaction with life (Lowenstein & Katz, 2005)

Current Theories in Gerontology

A cursory review of existing theories in gerontology illustrate how a number of the challenges outlined above, are usually not addressed by most theories. The theories in gerontology can be categorized in a number of ways according to whether they deal with micro or macro issues, interpretative or normative issues or according to the date of their appearance in gerontological scholarship (Chappell et al., 2008). Micro-level theories deal with the aged and the aging process; macro-level theories deal with age as a dimension of social structure. Normative theories assume that individual behavior is determined by social norms or rules where people learn through socialization the norms of their society and generally follow them. Interpretative views assume that people are creative in their use and construction of rules and do not automatically follow them. Here we summarize existing theories in gerontology according to when they appeared in the gerontological literature.

The first generation theories, activity theory, and disengagement theory, both micro theories, focus on the adjustment of individuals to aging. Activity theory hypothesizes that those individuals who are able to meet their social and psychological needs through maintaining the activity level of middle life will be the most adjusted and satisfied with life at older ages (Kart & Kinney, 2001). In an up-to-date take on an "activity society," Katz (2001) addresses the problems of older adults as being treated as "busy bodies" as a part of how professionals manage everyday life in old age, especially in institutions which he labels "management by activity" (Katz, 2001, p. 128). Related to activity theory is the concept of successful aging which some gerontologists view as a reincarnation of activity theory (Litwin, 2005; Rowe & Kahn, 1997). Successful aging generally means that older adults have significant abilities to prevent illness, to minimize losses in physical and mental function and to enhance their engagement in life that are prescriptions proffered by activity theory when proposed over 40 years ago. Torres (2001; 2006) has recently used successful aging theory to explain the situation of Iranian immigrants to Sweden. She found that those who had pre-migration understandings of successful aging that were different than those found in the host society, tended to change to the latter when they immigrated. The problem with successful aging, of course, is that if an older person is sick, chronically disabled, poor and not busy – then they are considered to have failed at aging.

Disengagement theory is concerned with the wider society; it posits that aging is accompanied by a mutual withdrawal of individuals and society (Cumming & Henry, 1961). The controversy emanating from this theory suggests that it provides a negative view of aging. Also, it does not clearly define disengagement because the progenitors of the theory made a number of exceptions, making definition almost impossible. Blakemore (1999) has developed a typology for the comparative study of migration and aging in minority ethnic communities which categorizes the reasons for migration including a reversal of migration. He argues that theories such as disengagement and activity theories and the study of older adults' expectations and aspirations for migration should be combined for a better understanding of the immigration process. He provides several examples from Britain but few theoreticians have followed through on his work or used his typology. In addition, a few scholars have suggested that the idea behind activity theory could apply to immigrants in terms of what activities they did in their country of origin and what they subsequently do in their host country. This long term view of activities may help explain why some older immigrants are lonely and socially isolated since there may be a discontinuity in their activities once they have moved to Canada (McDonald et al., 2001).

The second generation theories move along a continuum from the micro to the macro levels and include continuity theory, social exchange theory, age stratification theory, aging and modernization theory, political economy theory and the life course perspective. Continuity theory holds that as people age, they make choices in an effort to preserve ties with the past as they move into older ages (Kart & Kinney, 2001; Nuttman-Schwartz, 2008), a factor we know that applies to older immigrants who hold on to parts of their past (McDonald et al., 2001). Taking a very different perspective, social exchange theory focuses on the calculations and negotiations that transpire between individuals as they seek to maximize rewards and minimize costs in their interactions. A proponent of this perspective, James Dowd (1975; 1980) argued that older persons find themselves with fewer resources in exchange relationships. Unlike other theories, exchange theory has been used more often in ethnicity and aging. Most recently, Fiori, Consedine and Magai (2008) in a large study of two heterogeneous racial groups in the United States, found that patterns of social exchange represented differences in ethnic group membership and the relational context in which the exchange took place.

Age stratification theory posits that society is structured by age and that people play different roles at different ages, have different capabilities, resources and status as they move through age strata over a life course (Riley, Johnston & Foner, 1972). In a study of Filipino veterans who had been given the option of American citizenship, the veterans chose to immigrate to the United States because of the financial benefits of citizenship and for the status gained in their families (Becker, Beyene & Canalita, 2000). Modernization theory, which was one of the first theories ever applied to older immigrants, links the lower status of older people to the increasing industrialization of a society as when simple societies are transformed into complex urban societies (Cowgill & Holmes, 1972). Older Chinese and key informants were interviewed in a modern new town in Tuen Mun where the researchers found some evidence that traditional Confucian filial piety was on the wane because of changes in traditional values (Ng, Phillips & Lee, 2002).

Moving to a purely structural perspective, the basic premise of political economy theory is that the experience of old age can only be understood within the context of the economy, the state, the labor market, and the intersections of class, gender, age and racial/ethnic divisions in society (Estes, Gerard, Zones & Swan, 1984). The theory seeks to uncover the structural conditions that create age inequalities and the way that older adults are defined and treated (Quadagno & Reid, 1999). Angel and Angel (2006) show how ethnicity-based differentials in health are related to social structures in the United States. This perspective has enormous promise for the study of aging immigrants but has yet to be used systematically. It has been used, however, at the global level to describe population aging in developing countries where the creation of trans-national communities and global families arise as a result of the international migration of workers. People grow old as migrants and go back and forth from one home to another so that there is a new kind of aging where the dynamics of family and social life may be stretched across different continents and across different types of societies (Gardner, 2002; Walker, 2002; Yeates, 2001).

Finally, the life course perspective, often considered the vanguard in gerontological theory, can be defined as sets of trajectories that extend across a person's life such as family, school or work trajectories, and by multiple transitions in the trajectories such as entering or leaving school, acquiring a full-time job, and the first marriage. "Each life course transition is embedded in a trajectory that gives it specific form and meaning." (Elder, 2000, p.1615). A few scholars have begun to apply this perspective to the life course of immigrants although the perspective has been limited to physical and mental health, income security and non-local moves of older adults and does not usually bridge country of origin and host country (e.g., Cornman et al., 2004; Longino et al., 2008; Wilmoth & Chen, 2003). Fry (2003) has argued that time is actually problematic when a life course perspective is applied to another culture because of how time is measured and the cultural knowledge that informs chronological time. According to this scholar, the life course is a cultural construct, based on cultural definitions of time and the uses of age. For example, Fry shows how time is different in East Africa compared to time in industrialized capitalistic societies. In East Africa, time is expressed in terms of generational differences between fathers and sons, not in terms of chronological age (Fry, 2003). At the same time, Settersten (2005) calls for social gerontology to take up the mission of explaining multiple types of aging as in childhood studies that describe and explain multiple childhoods.

The third generation theories include the newer developments in feminist theory, critical theory and postmodernism (Chappell et al., 2008). Calasanti (2004, p. S306) has recently observed, ". . . feminist gerontologists theorize gender relations as forces that shape both social organizations and identities as men and women interact with one another." Calasanti and Slevin continue, "Examining the influence of race and ethnicity implies that we must include majority as well as minority racial status in our analyses. The privileged position of one group relies on the disadvantaged position of another" (Calasanti & Slevin, 2001, p. 3). Gender relations are essentially constructed power relations that are embedded in social processes and institutionalized in ways that have consequences for life chances across the life course. Critical theory zeros in on a critique of the existing social order and its treatment of older adults by exposing assumptions and myths that maintain the status quo. In keeping with the centrality of reflexivity (self examination), critical gerontology seeks to provide an understanding of the meaning of aging and old age (Biggs, Lowenstein & Hendricks, 2003).

Sometimes linked to critical theory, postmodernism is fundamentally anti-theoretical, however, the approach has been recently used in gerontology to "theorize aging" (Katz, 2005; Powell, 2006). Postmodern constructions of aging consider the cultural interaction between the aging body and the social context in shaping the way people experience their lifetimes (Biggs et al., 2003; Katz, 1995). To have omitted the physical signs of an aging body in social and psychological theory is astounding in retrospect, so this postmodern contribution is quite timely. The creation of concepts, like the use of the masquerade where older adults hide behind masks because they cannot express their aging selves in a prejudicial society, are one of the more significant contributions of postmodernism to theory (Biggs, 2005). The development of this idea as it pertains to older immigrants who, not only have to negotiate aging but also biculturalism (their own culture and that of the host society), would probably be productive. While no theory is mentioned, Cantonese and Korean-speaking older immigrants reported how factors such as a changed economic environment, living alone and extending their social network beyond family helped them become more bicultural (Wong, Yoo & Stewart, 2006). Again, applications are beginning to appear that use postmodern approaches, although the material is still fairly new (Katz, 2001).

Torres (2000) contends that ethno gerontologists' research concerns are not entirely consistent with postmodernism. Specifically, it is claimed that the interest of postmodernism in eliminating traditional conceptions of majority and minority populations and power structures with it, threatens the study of ethnicity-based conditions that affect aging processes. In addition, it is maintained that ethno gerontology supports a solution-oriented approach rather than the reflexive perspective favored by postmodernism that may not be useful to older adults. Nevertheless, it is concluded that taking a postmodern approach to critically assessing the ethno gerontological knowledge that has already been accumulated could produce several benefits for future research and theorization (Torres, 2000).

Theories Specific to Aging and Immigration

Modernization and Assimilation Theories

Standard sociological theories underpin both gerontological theory and general theories of ethnicity. One of the first perspectives applied to the study of older immigrants was modernization theory as described before. While the theory has been used in a number of capacities, one of the main uses has been to apply it at the macro societal level to explain disparities among societies at different points along a continuum from developing nations to highly industrialized societies (Olson, 2001). Similarly, it has been used to study various ethnic groups on a continuum of modernization and their specific rank at different points on the continuum. Today, modernization theory has been critiqued as being inconsistent with the research about older immigrants and their families. As an illustration, some researchers have discovered, contrary to what the theory would envisage, that less modernized families do not necessarily support their ethnic elders any more than do modern families (Rosenthal, 1983). Chan (2005) found that the immense economic development in Asia and the rapid aging of the population did not conform to classical modernization theory. Economic development did not result in a decline of older adults' well-being because family support of older persons did not appear to deteriorate as suggested by modernization theory. Longitudinal data for select Southeast and East Asian countries indicated minimal changes in living arrangements over time while cross-sectional data on intergenerational transfers still showed high levels of support for older persons by family (Chan, 2005).

The essentialist approach to ethnicity, with its roots in philosophy, is one of the oldest in sociology and anthropology. Essentialists argue that "ethnicity is something given, ascribed at birth, deriving from the kin-and-clan structure of human society and something more or less fixed and permanent" (Isajiw, 1999, p.30). It involves a set of "ready-made" attributes and an identity that an individual shares with others from birth. Spin-offs from this approach treat ethnicity as a matter of identity, including what forces help maintain it or impel it to change (Chappell et al., 2008). When scholars investigate assimilation and pluralism of ethnic groups, the core issue is about ethnic identity (Li, 1999). For example, Ward (2000) examines the effect of leisure activities on the social identity of marginalized immigrants. In a study of older Iranian women who immigrated to Canada in later life, cultural identity overshadowed the aging process that was rarely acknowledged as a force in these women's lives (Shemirani & O'Connor, 2006).

Stepping back in history, assimilation theories can be traced to the Chicago School of Sociology (e.g., Robert Park, W.I. Thomas & F. Znaniecki) and propose that minority groups will assimilate and lose their separate ethnic identities to a melting pot or through conformity or amalgamation with the dominant group (Driedger & Halli, 2000). As the theories developed over time, they were modified substantially to tap the many possible levels of assimilation or acculturation experienced by immigrant minorities (Glazer & Moynihan, 1963; Driedger & Halli, 2000). In Canada, the first studies of ethnic identity addressed how older persons managed their ethnic identity in the face of aging and how identity changed from first generation to second and third generations, particularly among Japanese Canadians (Sugiman & Nishio, 1983; Ujimoto, 1995). Another Canadian study of first-and second-generation Indo-Guyanese immigrants living in Ottawa found that first-generation immigrants had a greater identification with their Indo-Guyanese identity than the second generation. In public settings, though, first-generation men identified more with Canadians than did first-generation women (Clément, Singh & Gaudet, 2006). A study by Gee (1999) of foreign-born Chinese persons who had immigrated to Vancouver and Victoria later in life, indicated that 49% felt more Canadian than Chinese; 37% felt more Chinese, and 14% felt equally Canadian and Chinese. Aging and identity issues continue to garner the interest of researchers and, in fact, there is a whole journal devoted to aging and identity but with limited material on theory about immigration and identity (Delucchi, 1998).

Assimilation theories lost their sway over time when confronted with extensive variations between and within ethnic groups and in response to multiculturalism policies in Canada that promoted pluralism (Fleras & Elliot, 1992). Driven by the complexity of ethnicity, researchers created a multitude of continuums that ran between assimilation and pluralism on a variety of levels, to include both external and internal processes (Dreidger & Halli, 2000; Li, 1990). Pluralism holds that ethnic groups keep a separate identity and do not always assimilate but still manage to live harmoniously within the Canadian community (Fleras & Elliot, 1992).

The assimilation process may not be as well received as it once was but it is still scrutinized in great detail in Canada. One of the main markers of ethnic assimilation is language and the degree to which people use their language in domestic settings (De Vries, 1995). The assimilation of older ethnic Canadians has been uneven over time. Using 1981 census data, researchers found enormous variation among ethnic groups in the use of mother tongue and home language (Driedger & Chappell, 1987). Because most immigrant older people have spent most of their lives in Canada, they are able to speak English, French or both official languages. In the 2001 Census, only 4 percent of the immigrant elderly who arrived in Canada before 1961 reported that they could not speak either English or French. In contrast, being able to speak one of the official languages is significantly less common among those who have arrived in Canada more recently. Thirty years later, 50.2% of immigrant seniors who arrived in Canada between 1991 and 2001 were unable to speak either English or French (Turcotte & Schellenberg, 2007).

Age and Ethnic Stratification

Additional approaches that cross-cut gerontology and immigrant studies are the structural frameworks used to explain aging and ethnicity. The theories in aging, namely age stratification, political economy and critical theory, and ethnic stratification in ethnic studies, operate on the assumption of inequality in the social structure – because of age in the case of aging and because of immigrant status in the case of immigrant groups. Chappell et al. (2008) state:

> Various ethnic groups are differentially incorporated into the larger society (aided and abetted by prejudice and discrimination) and membership in different groups confers different levels of resources, prestige, and power. The indicators of education, occupation, and income typically have been used to measure these positions. (p. 154)

Age and ethnic stratification converge in the double jeopardy hypothesis, a mainstay in the analysis of older immigrant adults (Gelfand, 1994; Markides, 2001). If a person was old and belonged to an ethnic minority group, especially a visible minority group, that person was doubly disadvantaged. Studies of double jeopardy transformed into studies of multiple jeopardy with the addition of gender and social class to minority status and age (Markides, 2001). The viability of the multiple jeopardy hypothesis is yet to be established (Chan, 1983; Havens & Chappell, 1983; Lubben & Becerra, 1987; Markides, 2001), although it has been tested in many contexts that include income, health, social relationships and psychological well-being. The researchers who first proposed the hypothesis found negative effects for income and self-rated health but no effects for psychological well-being in their study of African, Mexican and Caucasians in the United States (Markides, Liang & Jackson, 1990). Other researchers, however, found considerable evidence that minority older adults expressed high levels of psychological well-being, suggesting that social psychological processes of group identification and interaction were just as relevant as external factors like income or occupation (Koybayashi, 2000; Miner & Montoro-Rodriguez, 1999). The alternative hypothesis, the age-as-leveller hypothesis, maintains that the differences between majorities and minorities may decline over time in so far as age-effects cut across all racial and ethnic lines (Cool, 1981), levelling out inequalities found earlier in life. The underlying premise is that minorities are confronted with prejudice and discrimination over their life course for which they acquire coping skills that may be used to combat age discrimination in later life (Williams & Wilson, 2001).

The buffer hypothesis with its roots in social psychology has been applied to the study of the older immigrants in a limited fashion (Miner & Montoro-Rodriguez, 1999; Olstad, Sexton & Søgaard, 2001). The underlying assumption of this hypothesis is that psychosocial factors buffer stressful events generated by resettlement and life as an older immigrant in a new country. A Canadian study of foreign-born Chinese older adults found that ethnic identity was not a resource that made up for low income (Gee, 1999). The investigation unearthed evidence suggesting Chinese immigrants with lower incomes were less likely to identify themselves as Chinese. The reason offered for the findings was that a Canadian identity, instead of a Chinese identity, may be more accommodating to the descendents of poor older Chinese (Chappell et al., 2008). Using the National Survey of American Life that compared Black Americans and Caribbean Black immigrants concluded that there was little difference between the two groups in so far as intra-familial relations seemed to overcome barriers of geographical distance (Jackson, Forsythe-Brown & Govia, 2007). In contrast, a study of first-generation Somali migrants to London, England, found that family support was the main buffer against depression for this group (Silveira & Alleback, 2001). In the United States, a study of Hispanics compared the role of family psychological factors, to structural factors (acculturation, socioeconomic status) and concluded that collectivistic family values held by older Hispanics were more likely to be related to high levels of well being (Miner & Montoro-Rodriguez, 1999).

Constructing Ethnicity

A recent trend in theorizing about ethnicity and aging is a constructivist perspective. Older adults interpret and construct their social world and, as a result, there are multiple realities that are equally valid (Fivush & Haden, 2003; Gubrium, 2005; Holstein & Gubrium, 2003). The scholarship conducted under the constructionist rubric varies widely and is more a mosaic of theoretical sensibilities. Although meaning-making is central to all of the constructive approaches, different versions of constructionism emphasize different aspects and dimensions of social processes. In the case of immigration and ethnicity ". . . culture is not a shopping cart that comes to us already loaded with a set of historical cultural goods. Rather, we construct culture by picking and choosing items from the shelves of the past and the present" (Nagel, 1994, p.162). Exploration of the various ways in which immigrant minorities construct various aspects of their lives makes up almost all of the literature in this area and is mainly descriptive (e.g., Acharya & Northcott, 2007; Dossa, 1999; Kavala and Van Willigen, 2006; Koybashi, 2000; McConatha, Stoller & Oboudiat, 2001; Wong et al., 2006). For example, a study of 21 elderly immigrant women from India residing in Edmonton, were interviewed to ascertain what they were doing or not doing to reduce the risk of mental distress. The researchers took a subjectivist perspective and came to a number of conclusions, several of which are notable in light of activity theory and the buffer hypothesis, although neither is applied to the study. The women reported that to lower mental distress they exercised strict control over their "inner self" and did this by staying busy while they met their family, social and cultural obligations (Acharya & Northcott, 2007). Their culture provided a number of culturally prescribed ways to stay busy and was thus identified as "moral medicine" that protected them from mental distress (Acharya & Northcott, 2007, p.630).

The Future of Theory

The field of gerontology in the area of aging and immigration has accumulated a number of research findings and has begun to establish certain traditions of theory. It would seem, however, from the glimpse shown that gerontological scholars in this area have lost sight of the vital contributions of theory to the study of older immigrants. At best, the theories addressed before provide several different lenses through which to examine immigration and its effects on the physical, social and psychological aspects of aging, although they usually emerge as tacit assumptions in most research. Unfortunately, the net result is fragmentary resulting in limited theory building and the development of a body of cumulative knowledge to guide policy and practice. Many of the theories assume processes deemed to be the "correct" approach to immigration such as assimilation or pluralism. Most of the theories do not have the capacity to capture the effects of immigration at the structural level and its link to the social, psychological and family levels, let alone the physical aging of individuals or societies. A life course perspective is rarely used which is surprising since immigrants to Canada come with a lengthy history in education, work, family, friends, leisure activities and community involvement. The theories are especially weak in reflecting the effects of multi-generations within immigrant groups.

The overriding complexity of aging in general, and aging and immigration in particular, requires some type of integrating framework which really cannot be accomplished without theories and concepts that are broader and more general in scope (Bengston, Putney & Johnson, 2005). The best possibility to date is the life course perspective which is, at its core, a shell-like framework that can be rounded out with theories and concepts about immigration. The main architect of the approach, Glen Elder, developed five paradigmatic principles that provide a concise, conceptual map of the life course: development and aging as life-long processes, lives in historical time and place, social timing, linked lives and human agency (Elder, 2006). At minimum, this approach can be adjusted to reflect the measurement of time, timing, age and values significant to the life course found in the country of origin and subsequently found in the host country and the continuity or discontinuity created with immigration and resettlement. Studies can be focused on those trajectories of interest like work, education, leisure, family and so forth. In addition, other theories can easily be fit into the framework like the accumulative advantage/disadvantage hypothesis (Dannefer, 2003), a fresh formulation of heterogeneity and inequality over the life course. The disadvantages or advantages created earlier in life are not only perpetrated in later life but are amplified according to this perspective.

The whole edifice of the social construction of a life course as currently proffered by Holstein and Gubrium (2007) is more than amenable to this framework. They take a life course approach and call it *interpretive practice* which is a constellation of practices through which reality is apprehended and conveyed in everyday life and is conditioned by the circumstances within which it unfolds. In their approach, they investigate how social realities like the life course are constructed, what the realities are like, what they are composed from and what social factors condition their production. The application of this approach to immigration would move forward the descriptive studies now available in the research to explanations of aging for various immigrant groups.

The very latest advances in theory development in social gerontology have raised the bar to another level by actually theorizing about how social and psychological forces influence biology based on work linking stress and the shortening of teleomeres (proteins at the end of each chromosome argued by some to be related to aging) and poverty and DNA damage over a life course (Epel, 2007; Ferraro & Shippee, 2007). Ferraro and Shippee (2007) won the Gerontological Society of America's first prize for a new theoretical development in social gerontology. Their theory, called the

"Cumulative Inequality Theory," is a life course process starting in childhood that links DNA damage at older ages to poor health, chronic stress, chronic inflammation and a chronically comprised immune system resulting from accumulated disadvantage over a life course. In the newer theories on aging, the biological and social sciences are connected in a life course perspective.

Although this chapter started on a rather bleak note about theorizing in aging and immigration, the opportunities available to scholars in the field at this juncture are extraordinary. Immigration and aging depends on a range of theories and theoretical perspectives drawn from many disciplines for the reason that a diversity of theoretical perspectives can offer complementary analyses. The life course is simply scaffolding for other theories where seemingly incommensurate, epistemological positions can be easily accommodated. Almost everyone "has a life" in that they pass through time, they are located in specific historical and geographical sites, they are linked to others and they make their own decisions within whatever constrains exist. All theories can be applied to immigration and aging within this framework whether they be at the micro or macro levels or bridging levels. This means leaving the theoretical door open to everyone – the positivists, the constructionists, critical and postmodern scholars – all of whom would do well to refocus some of their interest on theory development or at least declare their theoretical perspectives. At the heart of the matter, however, is the need for interdisciplinary theory building that brings together all manner of gerontologists if the field is to advance in a significant way.

References

Angel, J. & Angel, R. (2006). Minority group status and healthful aging: Social structure still matters. *American Journal of Public Health, 96*(7), 1152-1160.

Archarya, M. & Northcott, H. (2007). Mental distress and the coping strategies of elderly Indian immigrant women. *Transcultural Psychiatry, 44940*, 614-636.

Becker, G., Beyene, Y. & Canalita, L. (2000). *Journal of Aging Studies, 14*(3) 273-291.

Bengston, V.L., Rice, C J. & Johnson, M.L. (1999). Are theories of aging important? Models and explanations in gerontology at the turn of the century. In V.L. Bengston; and K. Warner Schaie (Eds.) *Handbook of Theories of Aging.* (pp 3-20) New York: Springer.

Bengston, V., Putney, N. & Johnson, M. (2005). The problem of theory in gerontology today. In Malcolm M. Johnson (Ed.) *The Cambridge handbook of age and ageing (3-20).* Cambridge, United.Kingdom: Cambridge University Press.

Biggs, S. (2005). Beyond appearances: perspectives on identity in later life and some implications for methods. *The Journal of Gerontology, 60B*, S118-S128.

Biggs, S., Lowenstein, A. & Hendricks, J. (2003). *Need for theory: Critical approaches to social gerontology.* Amityville, New York: Baywood.

Birren, J. & Bengtson, V. (Eds.). (1988). *Emergent theories of aging.* New York, New York: Springer.

Blakemore, K. & Boneham, M. (1994). *Age, race and ethnicity: A comparative approach.* Buckingham: Open University Press.

Burr, J. & Mutchler, J. (1993). Nativity, acculturation, and economic status: Explanations of Asian American living arrangements in later life. *Journal of Gerontology: Social Sciences, 48*, S55-S63.

Calasanti, T.M. & Slevin, K.F. (2001). *Gender, social inequalities, and aging.* New York: AltaMira Press.

Calasanti, T.M. (1996) Incorporating diversity: Meaning, levels of research, and implications for theory. *The Gerontologist, 36*(2), 147-156.

Calasanti, T. (2004). Feminist gerontology and old men. *Journal of Gerontology, 59B*(6), S305-S314.

Chan, A. (2005). Aging on Southeast and East Asia: Issues and policy directions. *Journal of Cross-Cultural Gerontology, 20,* 269-284.

Chan, K. (1983). Coping with aging and managing self-identity: The social world of the elderly Chinese women. *Canadian Ethnic Studies, 15*, 36-50.

Chappell, N. (2005). Perceived change in quality of life among Chinese Canadian seniors: The role of involvement in Chinese Culture. *Journal of Cross-Cultural Gerontology, 6,* 69-91.

Chappell, N. & Kusch, K. (2006). The gendered nature of filial piety - A study among Chinese Canadians. *Journal of Cross-Cultural Gerontology, 22,* 29-45.

Chappell, N., McDonald, L. & Stones, M. (2008). *Aging in contemporary Canada.* Toronto: Pearson, Prentice Hall.

Citizenship and Immigration Canada. (2005). *Facts and figures: Immigration overview, permanent and temporary residents* (No. CI1-8/2004E). Ottawa, Ontario: Research and Evaluation Branch.

Clément, R., Singh, S. & Gaudet, S. (2006). Identity and adaptation among minority Indo-Guyanese: Influence of generational status, gender, reference group and situation. *Group Processes & Intergroup Relations, 9*(2), 289-304.

Collings, P. (2001). If you got everything, it's good enough: Perspectives on successful aging in a Canadian Inuit community. *Journal of cross-cultural Gerontology, 16*, 127-155.

Cool, L. (1981). Ethnic identity: A source of community esteem for the elderly. *Anthropological Quarterly, 54,* 179-181.

Cornman, J.C., Lynch, S.M., Goldman, N., Weinstein, M. & Lin, Hui-Sheng (2004). Stability and Change in the perceived social support of older Taiwanese Adults. *Journal of Gerontology 59B* (6) S350-S357.

Cowgill, D. & Holmes, L. (1972). *Aging and modernization.* New York, New York: Appleton Century-Crofts.

Cumming, E. & Henry, W. (1961). *Growing old: The process of disengagement.* New York: Basic Books.

Dannefer, D. (2003). Cumulative advantage/disadvantage and the life course: Cross-fertilizing age and social science theory. *Journal of Gerontology: Social Sciences, 58B*, S327-S337.

Delucchi, M. (1998). Self & identity among aging immigrants in the joy luck club. *Journal of Aging and Identity, 3*(2), 59-66.

De Vries J. (1995). Ethnic language maintenance and shift. In S.S. Halli, F. Tovato & L. Dreidger (Eds.). *Ethnic demography* (163-177). Ottawa: Carleton University Press.

Dietz, T., John, R. & Roy, C. (1998). Exploring intra-ethnic diversity among four groups of Hispanic elderly: Patterns and levels of service utilization. *International Journal of Aging and Human Development 46*(3), 247-266.

Diwan, S., Jonnalagadda, S. & Balaswamy, S. (2004). Resources predicting positive and negative affect during the experience of stress: A study of older Asians Indian immigrants in the United States. *The Gerontologist, 44*(5), 605-614.

Dosa, P. (1999). (Re) imaging aging lives: Ethnographic narratives of Muslim women in Diaspora. *Journal of Cross-Sectional Gerontology, 14,* 245-272.

Dowd, J. (1975). Aging as exchange: A preface to theory. *Journal of Gerontology, 30*, 584-594.

Dowd, J. (1980). Exchange rates and old people. *Journal of Gerontology, 35*, 596-602.

Driedger, L. & Chappell, N. (1987) *Aging and ethnicity: Toward an interface.* Toronto: Butterworths.

Driedger , L. & Halli, S. (2000). Racial integration: Theoretical options. In L. Driedger & S. Halli (Eds.) *Race and racism* (55-76). Montreal and Kingston: McGill-Queens University Press.

Durst, D. (2005). More Snow on the Roof: Canada's Immigrant Seniors. *Canadian Issues/Themes Canadien: Immigration and the intersections of diversity.* Association for Canadian Studies, Spring 2005, 34-37.

Elder, G. (2000). The life course. In E.F. Borgatta & R.J. V. Montgomery, (Eds.). *The encyclopedia of sociology, Vol. 3* (2nd ed., pp. 939-991). New York, New York: Wiley.

Elder, G., Johnson, M. & Crosnoe, R. (2003). The emergence and development of life course theory. In J. T. Mortimer & M.J. Shanahan (Eds.), *Handbook of the Life Course.* New York: Plenum. pp. 3-22.

Epel, E. (2007). Mind-body connection – Stress and telomeres. Paper presented at The Gerontological Society of America 60th Annual Scientific Meeting, The Era of Global Aging: challenges and Opportunities. San Francisco Nov. 16-20th.

Estes, C., & Associates, (2001). *Social policy and aging: A critical perspective.* Thousand Oaks: Sage Publications.

Estes, C., Gerard, L., Zones, J. & Swan, J. (1984). *Political economy, health and aging.* Boston, Massachussetts: Little, Brown and Company.

Ferraro, K. (1997). (Ed.) *Gerontology: Perspectives and issues. Second edition.* New York: Springer Publishing Company.

Ferraro, K. & Shippee, T. (2007). Aging and cumulative inequality: How does inequality get under the skin? Paper presented at The Gerontological Society of America 60th Annual Scientific Meeting, The Era of Global Aging: challenges and Opportunities. San Francisco Nov. 16-20th.

Fiori, K., Consedine, N. & Magai, C. (2008). Ethnic differences in patterns of social exchange among older adults: The role of resource context. *Ageing and Society, 28,* 495-524.

Fivish, R. & Haden, C. (2003). *Autobiographical memory and the construction of a narrative self: Developmental and cultural perspectives.* Mahwah, New Jersey: Lawrence Erlbaum Associates.

Fleras, A. & Elliot, J. (1992). *Multiculturalism in Canada: The challenge of diversity.* Scarborough, Ontario: Nelson Canada.

Fry, C. (2003). The life course as a cultural construct. In R.A. Settersten (Ed.), *Invitation to the life course: Toward new understandings of later life* (pp. 269-295). Amityville, New York: Baywood.

Gardner, K. (2002). *Age, narrative and migration.* Oxford: Berg.

Gee, E. (1999). Ethnic identity among foreign-born Chinese Canadian elders. *Canadian Journal on Aging, 18*(4), 415-429.

Gelfand, D. (1994). *Aging and ethnicity: Knowledge and services.* New York: Springer Publishing Company.

Glazer, N. & Moynihan, D. (1963). *Beyond the melting pot.* Cambridge, Massachusetts: M.I.T. Press.

Gubrium, J. 92005). Narrative environments and social problems. *Social Problems, 52*(4), 525-528.

Gubrium, J, & Holstein, J. (Eds.). (2003). *Ways of aging.* Boston: Blackwell.

Havens, B. & Chappell, N. (1983). Triple jeopardy: Age, sex and ethnicity. *Canadian Ethnic Studies, 15* (3), 119-132.

Health Canada. (1998a). *Reaching out: A guide to communicating with Aboriginal seniors.* Ottawa: Minister of Public Works and Government Services, Canada. Catalogue No. H88-3/20-1998E.

Health Canada. (1998b). Canada's seniors at a glance. Ottawa: Canadian Council on social Development for the Division of Aging and Seniors, Health Canada. http://www.hc-sc.gc.ca/seniors-aines/pubs/poster/seniors/page5e.htm.

Holstein, J. & Gubrium, J. (2007). Constructionist perspectives on the life course. *Sociology Compass, 1,* 1-18.

Hooyman, N. & Kiyak, H. (2005). *Social gerontology: A multidisciplinary perspective.* (7th Ed.). Boston: Bacon & Allyn

Hsu, h., Lew-Ting, C. & Wu, S. (2001). Age, period and cohort effects on the attitude toward supporting parents in Taiwan. *The Gerontologist, 41*(6), 742-750.

Isajiw, W. (1999). *Understanding diversity: Ethnicity and race in the Canadian context.* Toronto: Thompson Educational Publishing Inc.

Jackson, J. & Antonucci, T. (2005). Physical and mental consequences of aging in place and aging out of place among Black Caribbean immigrants. *Research in Human Development, 2*(4), 229-244.

Jackson, J., Forsythe-Brown, I. & Govia, I. (2007). Age cohort, ancestry, and immigration generation influences in family relations and psychological well-being among Black Caribbean family members. *Journal of Social Issues, 63*(4), 729-743.

Kamo, Y. & Zhou, M. (1994). Living arrangements of elderly Chinese and Japanese in the United States. *Journal of Marriage and the Family, 56,* 544-558.

Kart, C. & Kinney, J. (2001). *The realities of aging. (6th Ed.)* Boston, Massachusetts: Allyn and Bacon.

Katz, S. (2005). *Cultural aging: Life course, lifestyle and senior worlds.* Peterborough, Ontario: Broadview Press.

Kavalar, J. & Van Willigen, J. (2006). Older Asian Indians resettled in America: Narratives about households, culture and generation. *Journal of Cross-Cultural Gerontology, 20,* 213-230.

Keefe, J., Rosenthal, C. & Béland, F. (2000). Impact of ethnicity on helping older relatives. *Canadian Journal of Aging, 19,* 317-342

Kim, H., Hisata, M., Kai, I. & Lee, S. (2000). Social support exchange and quality of life among Korean elderly. *Journal of Cross-Cultural Gerontology, 15*(4), 331-347.

Kobayashi, K. (2000). The nature of support from adult Sansei (third generation) children to older Nisei (second generation) parents in Japanese Canadian families. *Journal of Cross-Cultural Gerontology, 15,* 185-2000.

Lai, D. (2004). Health status of older Chinese in Canada: Findings from the SF-36 health survey. *Canadian Journal of Public Health, 95*(3), 193-197.

Lai, D. & Surood, S. (2008). Predictors of depression in aging South Asian. *Canadians. Journal of Cross-Cultural Gerontology, 23*(1) 57-75.

Lee, Y. (2007). The immigration experience among elderly Korean immigrants. *Journal of Psychiatric and Mental Health Nursing, 14,* 403-410.

Leu, J., Yen, I., Gansky, S., Walton, E., Adler, N. & Takeuchi, D. (2008). The association between subjective social status and mental health among Asian immigrants: Investigating the influence of age at immigration. *Social Science and Medicine, 66,* 1152-1164.

Li, P.S. (1990). Race and ethnicity. In P. S. Li (Ed.). *Race and ethnic relations in Canada* (3-17). Don Mills, Ontario: Oxford University Press.

Li, P.S. (1999). Race and ethnicity. In P.S. Li (Ed.), *Race and ethnic relations in Canada* (2nd ed., 3-20). Don Mills, ON: Oxford University Press.

Litwin. H. (2005). Correlates of successful aging: Are they universal? *The International Journal of Aging and Human Development, 61*(4), 313-333.

Longino, Jr. C.F., Bradley, D.E., Stoller, E. & Haas, W. H. III (2008). Predictors of non-local moves among older adults: A prospective Study. *Journals of Gerontology: Series B Psychological and Social Sciences 63B* (1), S7-S14.

Lowenstein, A. & Katz, R. (2005). Living arrangements, family solidarity and life satisfaction of two generations of immigrants in Israel. *Ageing and Society, 25,* 749-767.

Lubben, J. & Becerra, R. (1987). Social support among Black, Mexican, and Chinese elderly. In D. E. Gelfand & C. M. Berresi (Eds.) *Ethnic dimensions of aging* (130-144). New York: Springer Publishing Company.

Markides, K., Liang, J. & Jackson, J. (1990). Race, ethnicity and aging: Conceptual and method-ological issues. In R.H. Binstock & L. K. George (Eds.). *Handbook of Aging and the Social Sciences* (3rd edition, 112-129). New York: Academic Press.

Markides, K.S. (2001). Minorities and aging. In G. L. Maddox, Editor-in-Chief. *The Encyclopedia of Aging* 691-693). (3rd Edition) New York: Springer Publishing Company.

McConatha, J., Stoller, P. & Oboudiat, F. (2001). Reflections of older Iranian women adapting to life in the United States. *Journal of Aging Studies, 15,* 369-381.

McDonald, L., George, U., Daciuk, J., Yan, M. & Rowan, H. (2001). *A Study on the settlement related needs of newly arrived immigrant seniors in Ontario.* Toronto: Centre for Applied Social Research, University of Toronto.

McDonald, L., George, U., Cleghorn, L. & Karenova, K. (2008). *An Analysis of Second Language Training Programs for Older Adults Across Canada.* Toronto: Citizen and Immigration Canada, Ontario Region.

McMullin, J.A. (2000). Diversity and the state of sociological aging theory. *The Gerontologist, 40*(5), S517-530.

Miner, S. & Montoro-Rodriguez, J. (1999). Intersections of society, family, and self among Hispanics in middle and later life. 423-552. In C.D. Ryff & V.W. Marshall (Eds.) *The self and society in aging processes* (423-552). New York: Springer Publishing Company.

Moriarty, J. & Butt, J. (2004). Inequalities in quality of life among older people from different ethnic groups. *Ageing and Society, 24,* 729-753.

Nagel, J. (1994). Constructing ethnicity: Creating and recreating ethnic identity and culture. *Social Problems, 41,* 152-176.

Newbold, K. & Felice, J. (2006). Health status of older immigrants to Canada. *Canadian Journal on Aging, 25*(3), 305-319.

Ng, A., Phillips, D. & Lee, W. (2002) Persistence and challenges to filial piety and informal support of older persons in a modern Chinese society: A case study in Tuen Mun, Hong Kong. *Journal of Aging Studies, 16*, 135-153.

Noh, S. & Avison W. (1996). Asian immigrants and the stress process: A study of Koreans in Canada. *Journal of Health and Social Behaviour, 37*(2), 192-208.

Nuttman-Schwartz, O. (2008). Bridging the gap: The creation of continuity by men on the verge of retirement. *Ageing and Society, 28*, 185-202.

Olson, L. (Ed.) (2001). *Age through ethnic lenses: caring for the elderly in a multicultural society.* Lanham, Maryland: Rowan & Littlefield.

Olstad, R., Sexton, H. & Søgaard, A. (2001). The Finnmark study. A prospective population study of the social support buffer hypothesis, specific stressors and mental distress. *Social Psychiatry Psychiatr Epidemiol, 36,* 582-589.

Penning, M. (1983). Multiple jeopardy: Age sex and ethnic variations. *Canadian Ethnic Studies, 15* (3), 81-105.

Powell, J. (2006). *Social theory and aging.* Lanham, MD: Rowan & Littlefield.

Quadagno, J. & Reid, J. (1999). The political economy perspective in aging. In V.L. Bengston, & K.W. Schaie, (Eds.). *Handbook of theories of aging* (344-358). New York, New York: Springer Publishing Company Inc.

Riley, M., Johnston, M. & Foner, A. (1972). *Aging and society, Vol.3: Sociology of age stratification.* New York, NY: Russell Sage Foundation.

Rosenthal, C.J. (1983). Aging, ethnicity and the family: Beyond the modernization Thesis. *Canadian Ethnic Studies, 15* (3), 1-16.

Rosenthal, C.J. (1987). Aging and intergenerational relations in Canada. In V.W. Marshall (Ed.). *Aging in Canada: Social perspectives,* (2nd edition, 311-342). Markham, ON: Fitzhenry and Whiteside.

Rowe, J. & Kahn, R. (1997). Successful aging. *The Gerontologist, 37*(4), 433-440.

Shemirani, F. & O'Connor, D. (2006). Aging in a foreign country: Voices of Iranian women aging in Canada. *Journal of Woman and Aging, 18*(2), 73-90.

Settersten, R. (2005). Linking the two ends of life: What gerontology can learn from childhood studies. *The Journals of Gerontology, 60B,* S173-S180.

Silveira, E. & Allebeck, P. (2001) Migration, ageing and mental health: An ethnographic study on perceptions of life satisfaction, anxiety and depression in older Somali men in East London. *International Journal of Social Welfare, 10,* 309-320.

Statistics Canada (2003). *Ethnic diversity survey: Portrait of a multicultural society.* (catalogue number 98-593-XIE). Ottawa: Ministry of Industry.

Sugiman, P. & Nishio, H. (1983). Socialization and cultural duality among Japanese Canadians. *Canadian Ethnic Studies, 15* (3), 17-35.

Torres, S. (2000) A postmodern ethnogerontology why not? what for? *Contemporary Gerontology, 6*(4), 115-118.

Torres, S. (2001). Understandings of successful aging in the context of migration: the case of Iranian immigrants to Sweden. *Ageing and Society, 21*(3), 333-355.

Torres, S. (2006). Different ways of understanding the construct of successful aging: Iranian immigrants speak about what aging means to them. *Journal of Cross-Cultural Gerontology, 21,* 1-23.

Treas, J. & Mazumdar, S. (2002). Older people in America's immigrant families: Dilemmas of dependence, integration and isolation. *Journal of Aging Studies, 16,* 243-258.

Turcotte, M. & Schellenberg, G. (2006). *A portrait of seniors in Canada.* Ottawa: Statistics Canada, Social and Aboriginal Statistics Division.

Ujimoto, K. (1995). Ethnic dimension of aging in Canada. In R. Neugebauer-Visano (Ed.), *Aging and Inequality: Cultural Constructions of Difference.* pp. 3-29. Toronto: Canadian Scholars' Press.

Walker, A. (2002). *Globalisation and policies on aging. Paper to 55th Annual Scientific Meeting,* Gerontological Society of America, Boston.

Whitfield, K. & Baker-Thomas, T. (1999). Individual differences in aging minorities. *International Journal Aging and Human Development, 48*(1), 73-79.

Williams, D., & Wilson, C. (2001). Race, ethnicity and aging. In R.H. Binstock & L.K. George (Eds.) *Handbook of Aging and the Social Sciences.* (5th ed., 160-178). New York: Academic Press.

Wilmoth, J.M, & Chen, Pei-Chun, (2003). Immigration status, living arrangements and depressive symptoms among middle-aged and older adults. *Journals of Gerontology: Series B* Pyschological and Social Sciences 58B (5) S305-S313

Wong, S., Yoo, G. & Stewart, A. (2006).The changing meaning of family support among older Chinese and Korean immigrants. *The Journals of Gerontology, 61BB* 1. S4-S9.

Wong, S., Yoo, G. & Stewart, A. (2007). An empirical evaluation of social support and psychological well-being in older Chinese and Korean immigrants. *Ethnicity and Health, 12*(1), 43-67.

Wong, P. & Reker, G. (1985). Stress, coping and well-being in Anglo and Chinese elderly. Canadian *Journal on Aging, 4,* 29-37.

Yeates, N. (2001). *Globalisation and social policy.* London: Sage.

Chapter 4

Promises, Promises: Cultural and Legal Dimensions of Sponsorship for Immigrant Seniors

Sharon Koehn, Charmaine Spencer and Eunju Hwang,
(Providence Health, B.C.)

Introduction

In every society, the family forms the nucleus for social, physical, psychological and spiritual well-being. A healthy family is both a barometer of and a mechanism to promote the well-being of society. The right to apply to unite family members in this country has long been a cornerstone of Canada's immigration policy. Both immigrants and Canada are well served by this laudable principle and the resulting policy goals (MOSAIC, 2005). Immigration is a joint federal/provincial/territorial responsibility, with the federal government controlling the numbers and types of immigrants, and provincial-territorial laws and policies significantly affecting their day-to-day lives. The primary focus in Canadian immigration has shifted significantly in the past decade and a half to economic immigrants. However many older immigrants arrive under the family reunification program. For example, during the years 2002-2006, 88% of senior immigrants arrived under the Family Class (Multiculturalism and Immigration Branch, Government of British Columbia, 2007). Nationally, seniors comprised almost half of the all Family Class immigrants to Canada in 2006 (CIC, 2007)[1] As a condition of their arrival, sponsors (usually children) of senior Family Class immigrants are required to make an unconditional promise to the federal government to support them financially for a period of ten years, a significantly longer period than for any other Family Class group.

The process by which sponsored parents and grandparents come to and live in Canada, the circumstances of their lives, and the mechanisms by which federal and provincial laws and policies shape their experiences and identities during and post-sponsorship has received little research attention. Sponsored older immigrants are not only legal dependants during sponsorship when they come to Canada, they may be left financially and socially vulnerable by a constellation of cultural, situational and structural factors. As a result, sponsored older immigrants often suffer role reversals and a significant drop in status within families. During this period, they are excluded from the social resources that generally provide some security to Canadians in later life.

This chapter introduces some of the tensions of immigration status and explores how these issues are connected to family sponsorship laws and related policies. It describes the lived experiences of older Family Class (or sponsored) immigrants and their sponsors as well as the law's role in shaping identities and changing relationships. It considers these in the context of isolation, access to health care and housing, sponsorship breakdown and the potential for abuse or neglect within the sponsorship. The chapter concludes with several policy recommendations, including domains of inquiry to include in future studies of older adult immigrant populations.

Overcoming Invisibility

"It's important to stress that they haven't chosen this country themselves; they would have preferred to stay where they were" explained a Punjabi community leader referring to many older adults from the Punjab[2] who came to British Columbia as Family Class immigrants (Koehn, 1993). He continued:

> They only get benefits, such as pensions and so on, after they have been here for ten years. They are not angry about this, they have accepted it, but it makes them sad. In India, they have worked their entire lives, now they have to start over again working on farms. If they were more economically independent, it would help them build better relationships with their children. It would save a lot of misery, since they would be able to contribute more. Now, life is just survival. They have contributed to Canada in the sense that they have raised productive sons and daughters who work here – there should be some consideration for this. (*Punjab Leader*)

Immigration status has significant implications for sponsored parents and grandparents and has emerged as a central theme in qualitative research conducted by Koehn (1993; 1999; 2006) over a sixteen-year period with Punjabis in British Columbia. Especially relevant to this chapter is Koehn's (1993) study of late-in-life immigration which entailed the collection of in-depth interviews with sixty-two participants that included elderly Punjabi Sikh women (n=12), elderly Punjabi Sikh men (n=14), younger Punjabi Sikh women (n=12), South Asian community leaders (n=8), and South Asian service providers (n=16).

Hwang's (2008) research with Chinese seniors who have moved out of their sponsors' homes illustrates the ongoing struggle that many seniors face even after they have been in Canada for more than the initial ten-year dependency period. Aimed at identifying unique demographic, housing, and neighborhood characteristics of

Chinese seniors who reside in Chinatown, Hwang's data was derived from a survey of 50 seniors, 24 of whom resided in Vancouver's Chinatown and 26 who lived elsewhere in the Greater Vancouver Regional District. This material was supplemented by a focus group with Chinese community leaders, health and social service providers, housing advocates, and senior volunteers (n=8).

The challenges associated with sponsorship of older family members have also been identified by other immigrant communities, such as the Vietnamese in British Columbia (Nguyen, 2008). Despite an apparent consensus among seniors, family members, settlement workers and health care providers that more attention to concerns around sponsorship in later life is required (Koehn, 2006; 1993), this topic has not caught the imagination of many researchers, particularly in Canada.

Côté, Kérisit and Côté (2001) have made the best effort to date to discern the hegemonic "reality" constructed by different levels of government and understand how it influences and frames family sponsorship policy in Canada vis-à-vis women. But interpretations of their lived experiences by older sponsored immigrants of the sort that this chapter provides, have been glaringly absent, with the notable exception of McLaren (2006a; 2006b).

The inclusion of the voices of Koehn's and Hwang's respondents speaks to McLaren and Black's (2005) call for alternatives to prevailing discourses that frame family class immigration as beset by "deadbeat sponsors" and immigrant parents, as undesirable burdens on society (Collacott, 2006). In this regard, the interstices between the hegemonic text that the policies and laws represent and the culturally mediated negotiations of identity by the sponsored parents and grandparents draw our attention to "borderlands," wherein the potential for supportive intervention as well as conflict and misunderstanding may be realized (Anzaldúa, 1987; Hinton et al., 2006).

Literature Review

Despite the aging and increasing diversification of Canada's population, "aging-related programs and policies continue to treat the seniors population as a homogeneous group and the variety of needs, concerns and histories of ethno cultural minority seniors often go unrecognized" (National Advisory Council on Aging, 2005). The blindness to "race" or ethno cultural identity and immigrant status in studies of aging is one part of the problem, argues Patel (1999); the failure of studies on immigrants to differentiate by age is another.

Other writers have also noted that studies of immigrants too often focus on the individual rather than relationships within families or social networks that may facilitate integration and appropriate access to essential services, such as health care (Bailie &

Denis, 2006; VanderPlaat, 2006). Yet familial networks can be important sources of the social capital necessary to facilitate successful migration.

Drawing on the Longitudinal Survey of Immigrants to Canada (Statistics Canada, 2005), Bergeron and Potter (2006) report that "seniors' social networks tend to be dominated by kin" and that "immigrants landed in the family class appear to be the best connected," which may lead people to assume immigrant seniors will have access to sufficient social capital to secure the services that they need and avoid social isolation. This argument appears to be supported, at least for the younger Family Class immigrants in Lewis-Watts' (2006) study, who relied heavily on family networks for pragmatic advice as well as economic support, particularly in terms of securing employment. In-depth qualitative studies nonetheless reveal additional nuances. For example, Grewal et al. (2005) found that family members were pivotal to the health of immigrant South Asian women, but in two directions. Families may provide direct and indirect assistance that benefits the women's health, but families also expect that women will fulfill certain prescribed roles and responsibilities that can have negative health consequences. For sponsored older adults, knowing only that relatives may limit the available strategies used to solve problems and hence may increase their vulnerability to harm within relationships or from broader systems.

The connections between policy and health outcomes specific to immigrants are increasingly becoming recognized. Health and social policy changes in some provinces have been found to negatively influence immigrant and refugee health – most especially in the domains of mental health and spousal abuse (Steele, Lemieux-Charles, Clark, & Glazier, 2002). Côté et al. (2001) also suggest that family power imbalances are constructed in part by sponsorship policies and practices. Up to 1997, sponsored persons were not involved in the sponsorship agreement process, and their consent was not required. As a result, they were often ill informed about their rights; with many believing that their sponsor had the power to withdraw the sponsorship. McLaren (2006a) has also noted the role of Canada's immigration policy in creating conditions of vulnerability, not only for sponsored parents and grandparents, but also for their families upon whom the responsibility for providing a social safety net falls.

At issue here is not the value of sponsored immigrants to the families with whom they are reunited and Canada as a whole; as Thompson (2005) reminds us, "We seem to have forgotten somewhere along the way that immigration is a social program that helps define our society, not just an economic program that brings in workers." Rather we argue that the configuration and cumulative effect of laws and policies themselves create vulnerabilities.

A shifting immigration policy that focuses heavily on immigrants' potential economic value as workers risks framing sponsored parents as an economic deficit (McLaren, 2006a). Thinly veiled bigotry poses as academic discourse in commentaries on elderly Family Class immigrants, characterizing them as undesirable burdens on society incapable of integration and ill prepared for the Canadian labor market (Grubel, 2005). Sponsored elderly immigrants have been represented as an "indirect" burden on taxpayers, and portrayed as "diverting" resources from the sponsor's children and "hindering" the economic assimilation of their adult children (Baker & Benjamin, 2002).

A Thumbnail History of Family Sponsorship in Canada

Canada has a long-standing tradition of giving priority to family reunification in immigration policies (CIC, 2006). Family reunification is an important factor in "promoting newcomer integration and it is part of our international legal obligations" (MOSA-IC, 2005, p. 4). The extent to which sponsored older immigrants have been welcomed at a federal and provincial policy level has nonetheless fluctuated over time, as evinced by a drop in admissions in this category from 18% of all immigrants in 1994, to only 5% a decade later (McLaren, 2006a).

Throughout the early nineteenth century, Canada took a number of measures to restrict the right of entry of newcomers likely to become public charges due to race, sickness, age or destitution (Côté et al., 2001).[3] Modern sponsorship law emerged post-war when a 1949 statutory order set out the conditions of entry for the relatively extended family members of a principal applicant: the guarantor had to agree to "care for" the sponsored relatives. For the two decades prior to 1966, just over a third of newcomers to Canada arrived as sponsored relatives.

Debate around the inclusion criteria of different family members emerged in the late 1950s and early 1960s when some began to voice fears of an "invasion" by large numbers of unskilled workers from non-European countries (Côté et al., 2001). At the turn of the twenty-first century, economic immigration has swelled in response to current economic conditions, and resistance to admission of older Family Class immigrants is now framed in terms of a concern, accurate or not, about a potential strain caused by demographic aging and Canada's ability to "take care of our own, especially our own elderly." Missing from this discourse is any recognition of the significant social and financial investment already made by working immigrants' parents in raising families to adulthood, from which Canadian society benefits, as noted by the Punjabi community leader cited above.

In recent years, tight control over family sponsorship has been exacerbated by significant procedural delays, leading to a class action lawsuit initiated in 2005, representing 100 000 affected parental applicants (as documented by the lobby group, Sponsor Your Parents, 2006)[5] and comments in the Legislature by concerned politicians (Government of Canada, 2006a).[6] These delays have significant psychosocial and financial impacts on the family and older immigrants in particular. People are left in administrative and legal limbo for years at a time after paying the processing fees, even though the files may not be opened for two years, and may not be processed for many more. Immigration lawyer, Pansula (2007), argues that that by delaying the entry of parents, CIC creates undue hardships on new immigrant families who rely on parents as an essential aspect of running a household.

The Undertaking

As Family Class immigrants, sponsored parents and grandparents are not subject to the education, language, and employability criteria of economic immigrant categories. They must, however, meet the general health and security criteria. As a condition of their arrival, sponsors (usually adult offspring) of Family Class immigrants must make an unconditional promise of support in the form of an Undertaking with the Minister of Citizenship and Immigration (2005). This is essentially a promise made by the sponsor to the federal government to financially support the older immigrant for a period of ten years. During the initial dependency period, seniors may not be eligible for public pensions such as the Allowance, Old Age Security or the Guaranteed Income Supplement, social services, subsidized housing or housing subsidies or other local benefits such as reduced fare bus passes. In addition many older immigrants remain economically disadvantaged even after sponsorship ends, because of the way the residency criterion for Old Age Security is calculated.

As part of the undertaking, sponsors must agree to cover the sponsored individual's "food, clothing, shelter, and other goods or services, including dental care, eye care, and other health needs not provided by public health care" to all Canadian citizens and permanent residents of Canada (Shelton, 2003). This list of responsibilities is not exhaustive and the government may refuse to cover other basic needs, such as language programs if the person is not considered destined for the labor market (Côté et al., 2001). The ten-year clock starts ticking at the point where the person is granted entry into Canada as a permanent resident.

While the ten-year criterion for financial support is the same as sponsored dependent children, it is markedly different than the 12 to 36 months stipulated for privately sponsored refugees or the three years of support required for a sponsored spouse. In the face of evidence that the policy created power imbalances and dependency, and increased the risk of abuse or exploitation, the conjugal sponsorship period for women was reduced in 1994 in Quebec from ten years to three, and the federal government has since followed suit (CIC, 2005; Côté et al., 2001).

Financial Ability to Sponsor

In addition to the other eligibility criteria, a prospective sponsor must meet minimum income requirements for the twelve months prior to application. This amount is based on the number of people already in the sponsor's family plus those they intend to sponsor and reflects the Low Income Cutoffs (CIC, 2005). A couple with two children wanting to sponsor the husband's mother, for example, would need to earn a minimum of $41 642 annually. Providing the sponsor's spouse is willing to co-sponsor, the income can be jointly earned. Prospective sponsors must also prove that they have not been on any form of government assistance in the last twelve months, except for reasons of disability. In this regard, the policy requires a significant feat of prognostication; sponsors must consider their current position plus project their financial ability for ten years from the point the sponsored immigrant lands in Canada. The job security and financial stability of many Canadians is often unpredictable for any period, let alone a decade, due to numerous factors beyond their control.

Dependency and Self-Esteem

Intergenerational relationships are key to the success of sponsorship but pre-existing relationships between the sponsors and sponsored seniors, family structure, the seniors' resources (economic, language, etc.), the gender of the senior, motivations for sponsorship, the immigration experience (degrees of volunteering and familiarity, and so on) and sponsorship regulations all contribute to familial harmony or discord.

In Koehn's (1993) Punjabi sample, elderly women who sought to maintain the upper hand over acculturated daughters-in-law were said to cause considerable tension in the sponsoring household and/or could be extremely vulnerable, depending on the direction of the son's/husband's support in favor of either his mother or his wife. Arriving into a household in which the children were already of school age and more acculturated toward Western values, styles of dress and manner of speaking was also associated with higher levels of friction. Intergenerational tension was often exacerbated when grandchildren and grandparents did not share a language. Seniors who did not speak English, more often women, were disadvantaged both in relation to navigating their new environment, and within their own families. In another study by Koehn (1999), elderly vegetarian Punjabi Hindu women reported considerable tension when their sons married non-vegetarian, non-Hindu wives.

While differences in cultural orientation, language and religion are more commonly encountered in the immigrant context, urban Hindu Punjabi seniors living in India also reported intergenerational tension for the same reasons (Koehn, 1999). Yet in India, unlike Canada, elderly parents typically have greater social capital. There they are more likely to control resources, are relatively at ease and able to navigate their physical environments and institutional structures, and draw on a network of friends and relations for support. Subject to a ten-year period of dependency on their sponsors, immigrant seniors are rendered both economically and socially dependent on their families, which can place a tremendous strain on even the most positive of intergenerational relationships. Nor is this phenomenon limited to immigrants from India, as a Chinese service provider interviewed in Hwang's (2008) study attests:

> When living with the younger generation, conflicts are inevitable. Shortly after [older Chinese] moved to Canada, they started to have depression and started to want to go back to where they came from – a lot of problems. The problems also extend to the next generation and affect their work. How to solve this problem? The seniors just need a place to settle. It doesn't matter even if the place is small. They just need a place. Probably they can take care of the grandchildren when they have time. Many conflicts with the younger generation will be prevented. It creates harmony. (Chinese service provider, as cited in Hwang, 2008, p. 6)

Most significantly, sponsored seniors surrender their status as heads of the family. An experienced multicultural social worker succinctly echoed the comments of numerous participants in Koehn's (1993) study, particularly the service providers among them, when she commented that with their married children running the home, [sponsored elderly parents] lose their traditional position of domestic control. This reversal of traditional patterns of dependence and authority can cause conflicts and a loss of self-esteem and depression in the elderly (Assanand, Dias, Richardson & Waxler-Morrison, 1990).

The diminished respect shown to sponsored elderly parents by family members, especially evident in their attenuated decision-making powers, has been found in studies of South Asians in British Columbia and Ontario (Joy, 1989; Koehn, 2006; 1993; 1999; McLaren, 2006a; Rahim & Mukherjee, 1984; Stephenson, 1991), and among Chinese Canadians (Costa & Renaud, 1995) and older immigrant women in general (Boyd, 1991). Efforts by sponsored seniors to control or manipulate family members can thus be interpreted as a strategy to counter the dependency that the sponsorship role imposes upon them.

Isolation

Although they live with family members, these seniors can be incredibly lonely and isolated from the supports and services that they need (Koehn, 2006; 1993; Rahim & Mukherjee, 1984; Sadavoy, Meier & Ong, 2004). Often, parents are sponsored so that they can provide childcare for young grandchildren (Koehn, 1993; 1999).

Most, but not all, of the elderly women interviewed by Koehn (1993, p. 112) did not complain about tending their grandchildren; rather, they said that they enjoy it because they love them, because it keeps them busy, or simply because they see this as their role – the reason they are in Canada. Indeed, some young children succeed in validating their grandparents, particularly "if they seek their advice, treat them as a source of wisdom, acknowledge and respect them" (service provider, as cited in Koehn, 1993). Yet some of the elderly women and the majority of the participants in the other subsets painted a less rosy picture of the older woman's childcare responsibilities, commenting that elderly women view the childcare and domestic labor that they contribute as a means of compensation for their sponsorship:

> Elderly women assume the responsibilities of raising their grandchildren . . . They feel obligated, duty bound. If they don't, they may have a problem with the daughter-in-law. This duty almost constitutes payment for her own care – she's earning her keep. (Service provider, as cited by Koehn, 1993, p. 112)

Unremitting dedication to the care of grandchildren often serves to deprive elderly women of contact with their peers, preventing the establishment of support networks essential to their mental well-being; 78% of the elderly women interviewed by Koehn (1993) said that their responsibilities at home prevented them from getting out. These women were therefore less likely to participate in ethno-specific support groups that are important as a forum for social interaction and information exchange about essential services and rights (Koehn, 2006). Chappell and Lai (1998) have commented on similar patterns of isolation and the resulting limitations to health care access for Chinese seniors who were late-in-life immigrants to British Columbia. Sponsored elders are thus likely to position themselves as vulnerable both in the family and in the new country.

Almost half of the elderly Punjabi women in Koehn's sample (1993) also admitted to feeling lonely. Participants in the other subsets saw the problem of loneliness and isolation among senior Punjabi women as being even more significant: one service provider estimated that as many as "ninety per cent of them are probably depressed. They're not involved in enough activities to sustain their creativity" (Koehn, 1993, p. 78).

Isolation can be further reinforced by a combination of cultural mores, language limitations and sponsorship regulations that limit transportation options. Extended family members in the Punjabi community generally view the transportation of elderly women as a duty, but the women are forever waiting for someone to take them somewhere; men are more independent and often ride bicycles (Koehn, 1993). Already conscious of their extreme dependency, sponsored seniors hesitate to ask busy children for rides unless they are absolutely essential (Koehn, 2006). Women especially lack the language skills and information to successfully navigate public transit (Koehn, 1993).

This reflects both gender discrepancies in education opportunities in the home country, but also the limited availability of English as a Second Language classes for seniors and the inability of women to attend them unless childcare is provided. The sponsored seniors' use of public transit is also limited by a lack of income and their ineligibility for senior's bus passes during their first ten years in Canada (Koehn, 2006).

Housing Challenges

The stipulation that sponsors ensure that their sponsored parents or grandparents are adequately housed for the first ten years following immigration to Canada encourages co-residence, but it is not required (Baker & Benjamin, 2002). And while it accomplishes, in part, the task of providing for the sponsored parents' material needs, it does not guarantee that the seniors' emotional needs are met. Punjabi and Chinese seniors alike have commented on the distance they feel from grandchildren who do not speak their language adequately and children who work long hours (Hwang, 2008; Koehn, 2006; 1993).

Some seniors thus seek out an independent living arrangement separate from their adult children, but moving out of a sponsor's home isn't easy: limited by their financial dependency on their children or minimal incomes, and because housing at market rates is out of reach. Add to this the difficulty of accessing affordable housing and negotiating their environment with limited English and it is hardly surprising that many of the seniors in Hwang's study looked for government-assisted or government-owned housing in Chinatown:

> Sponsored Chinese [elders] may move out and live in the senior houses, like those provided by the government. Because of the language problem, most of them prefer living near Chinatown. If they can speak English, or have been working and have good social skills, they don't mind living somewhere else because it takes longer to get a place in Chinatown. Another reason they want to live in Chinatown is because of the resources they can get here. It's easy to buy food and go to the Chinese restaurants. Of course it's getting better now because now Chinese food and Chinese restaurants can be found everywhere. But like a decade ago, many people really like living in/around Chinatown, even now. In Chinatown, government provides low-rental housing or subsidized housing. Like Mr. [C] used to living in the housing provided by the city government and he may want to share more about it later. In Chinatown, there are also many societies, restaurants, SUCCESS and Chinese Cultural Centre. There are many resources here and it is very convenient. They don't need to worry about the language barriers when accessing the services. SUCCESS really did a lot to help the seniors and it is like a big family. I also know there's the Lion's Club and other

organizations. They also provide senior housing at a low cost. (Chinese service provider, Hwang, 2008, p. 3)

Hwang's findings indicate that government resources such as subsidized housing, as well as community organizations, and local amenities, enable Chinese seniors to live separately from their adult children. Wong, Yoo, and Stewart (2006) have similarly found that the elderly Chinese immigrants in their study gained independence more quickly when they had access to a large network of Chinese-speaking community resources.

Among the most recently sponsored seniors, the availability of subsidized housing adjacent to a concentration of ethnic business districts was more likely to be associated with increased residential autonomy. For these new immigrants, the ethnic business district played an integral role in providing social and recreational activities, case management, congregate meals, and home care services. With increasing time living in Canada, Hwang found that seniors became more aware of their service options and focused increasingly on more negative features of their environment, such as safety concerns. While it is difficult to discern the causality in this small sample, seniors living in Chinatown appeared to be less healthy than their counterparts living elsewhere in the city. Hwang did not find any correlation with other variables such as age, income or education to explain this local level phenomenon.

Potential for Abuse or Neglect

There is a gradually developing literature on abuse of older persons in ethnic minority and immigrant families which has identified factors such as isolation, dependency, and ethno-structural change as factors that increase the risk of harm from within the immediate extended family (Anetzberger, Korbin & Tomita, 1996; CANE [Clearinghouse on Abuse and Neglect of the Elderly], 2007; Carefirst Seniors and Community Services Association, 2002; Moon, 1999; Park, 2006; Tam & Neysmith, 2006; Yan, So-Kum & Yeung, 2002). We argue there are two components of the legal obligation to provide for all of the sponsor's needs that significantly increase the seniors' susceptibility to abuse or neglect.

The first component is the length of time of the sponsorship obligation during which the financial status of the sponsor and the health status of either the sponsored parents or the sponsor may decline through no fault of their own. The result may be extreme financial hardship and sometimes, emotional or physical abuse, or passive or active neglect. If a family finds itself in financial dire straits, the elderly parents may be treated badly; they may be subject to emotional abuse. They are more likely to be negatively affected if they are dependent such as if they do not have a pension and they are not self-sufficient. This may happen within the ten-year dependency period, especially if they are not [in paid employment] (Service provider, Koehn, 1993, p. 125).

A younger woman interviewed by Koehn (1993, p. 105) related how parents may be "questioned about the type of food they eat constantly so they are afraid to even go to the fridge." She also commented on financial abuse whereby the "son's family may take the money the elderly parents get from farm work, or from their pensions," a phenomenon also observed by Sethi in Prince George (Koehn, Assanand & Sethi, 2007). The issue here is not whether or not sponsored parents should contribute to a family's living expenses, but the manner by which that contribution is extracted.

The second component of sponsorship related policies that may increase the potential of abuse is through the intensification of the dependency and resultant power imbalance between family members that the policies invoke. Among Punjabis, this imbalance is especially evident in the familial role reversals occurring between the mother-in-law and daughter-in-law who is the sponsor or co-sponsor living in Canada, with daughters-in-law seen as now having "the upper hand" (Koehn, 1993). Dependent on their sponsors in every respect, including access to information, South Asian sponsored seniors often do not have accurate information about their rights. They are often fearful that the sponsorship can be withdrawn, and they do not know where to turn for help if problems do occur. Moreover, any public admission of abuse or neglect occurring in the family brings shame on all of the family members – something the elders would prefer to avoid at almost any cost. In Koehn's (2006) Barriers to Access study, a health care provider further commented on how language barriers complicate the detection of abuse:

> From an elder abuse and neglect perspective certainly that makes things a lot harder when you can't communicate. I mean, you always deal with people being reluctant to admit that their daughter- or son-in-law or whatever is abusing them. But with the language difficulty it is really hard to pick up on the situation. And very often it's a mother-in-law and daughter-in-law friction. Mother-in-law ends up in the basement with a bowl of rice once in a while. We've seen a lot of that sort of situation as well. (Health care provider, Koehn, 2006, p. 2; see also Koihn, 2009)

Work and Exploitation

During the ten-year dependency period, between 25 – 40% of elders who arrive in Canada after the age of 60 have no source of income (Dempsey & CIC, 2004). This reflects the fact that almost 80% of this group came as Family Class immigrants. The bulk of their income (approximately 60%) during this period is derived from income earned through participation in the labor market.

Participants in Koehn's (1993) study agreed that at least 50% of all elderly Punjabi Sikh women participate in farm labor during the summer months. This is extremely arduous work, typified by long hours, low wages, and pitiful working conditions. To some extent, the social milieu is reminiscent of the Punjabi village, but most elderly participants, both male and female, reported the desire for freedom from financial dependence on their sponsors as the primary incentive for working:

> Even though elderly women are not seen as a financial burden, the fact that they have no income is really a hindrance to their psychological well-being. In India, they have economic control in the household . . . If they are able to manage some income, even a small amount, elderly women regain some degree of self-esteem. (Service provider, Koehn, 1993, p. 145)

While some are forced to use this income as their primary means of support, the majority spend this money on family members, on culturally mandated gift-giving essential to the preservation of social networks, and so on. Work performed by sponsored seniors is as much an effort to preserve their self-esteem and dignity and to secure a more respected position in the family as it is a means to access material benefits: "If they can't work, they won't ask the family for money. They are already sponsored, so they feel obligated as it is" (Younger woman, Koehn, 1993, p. 105).

The service provider cited here went on to describe the value of pensions to sponsored seniors: "They are much happier when they get a pension. It gives them some sense of independence if they are able to give something to their sons – say, towards the mortgage – some contribution to the household" (Koehn, 1993, p. 145). It should be noted, however, that even after ten years in Canada, sponsored seniors are only eligible for partial pensions. At the ten-year mark, this translates into one quarter of the base Old Age Security (OAS) amount (or $125.50 per month, as of March 2008) (Service Canada, 2006; 2007). Exclusive of cost-of-living inflation increases,[7] the OAS amount received by the sponsored immigrant will remain the same no matter how long they live in Canada or contribute to Canadian society.

Once in receipt of the OAS, sponsored seniors are also eligible to apply for the Guaranteed Income Supplement (GIS), "a monthly benefit paid to residents of Canada who receive a basic, full or partial Old Age Security pension and who have little or no other income" (Service Canada, 2006). At $634 a month for single individuals in March 2008, the maximum amount of GIS still leaves many sponsored immigrants below the poverty line (Service Canada, 2007).

Other Canadians and immigrants who arrived in Canada prior to the age of 60 are more likely to receive some contributory pension income (CPP/QPP) after the age of 65. CPP/QPP eligibility is contingent on making one valid contribution to the plan; the amount received is directly related to the length of time worked in Canada. After twenty years in Canada, the income of Family Class immigrants is comprised primarily of non-contributory retirement sources (OAS and GIS) (Dempsey & CIC, 2004), from which we can infer that, even after the ten-year sponsorship period, many older Family Class immigrants have very limited financial resources.

Agism and racism can intersect for older sponsored immigrants. Member of Parliament, Penny Priddy, has pointed out that older Family Class immigrants can face discrimination in government policy based on their country of origin (Government of Canada, 2006b). For example, immigrants from countries such as Australia, New Zealand, and the United Kingdom do not face the same burden as do immigrants from countries such as India, Pakistan, and Sri Lanka, because the former group has recip- rocal agreements on social security with Canada. The agreement can have a benefi- cial effect on residency credits which determine the eventual amount of Old Age Security the person will receive. On its face this appears to violate equality protections of human rights law in many provinces as well as section 15 of the Canadian Charter of Rights and Freedoms (Government of Canada, 1982).

Access to Health Care

An obvious impediment to health care access for sponsored seniors is their lack of eligibility for any more than basic health services during their first ten years in Canada. Although in a broad sense, the *Canada Health Act*[8] delineates federal and provincial or territorial responsibilities, what is covered within the "basic health serv- ices" will vary considerably with province and territory. A health care provider partici- pating in a focus group in Koehn's (2006, p. 2) study of barriers to access to health care for ethnic minority seniors provided the following example of inequities in health care experienced by a sponsored South Asian senior in her care:

> We find it real difficult to work with sponsored immigrants . . . We had a lady who had a CVA [cerebrovascular accident] and she'd been in the country for less than two or three years. She had a stroke and basically became wheelchair- bound so she needed access to good equipment to improve her functioning and she had the drive and the motivation to return to a level of functioning but unfor- tunately, the finances from the family [were insufficient] . . . there was no sup- port from the government meant that she didn't have access to this equipment, which is a huge problem for anyone under that 10-year program. Where do you go and why can't we get this equipment? (Healthcare provider)

More subtly, the responses of sponsored seniors to sponsorship laws and policies that render them dependent can reduce the likelihood that they will seek medical assistance when ill. The extreme dependency and the associated status demotion that seniors experience in relation to their sponsors makes them hesitate to ask their adult children for anything unless absolutely necessary. As a result, some seniors do not ask sponsors to take time off work to provide the transportation and interpretation they need in order to attend a medical appointment, and health care providers tend to see them in crisis (Koehn, 2006). Sponsors may be unwilling or unable to take an elderly parent or to relieve them of child minding responsibilities to enable them to attend appointments (Sadavoy et al., 2004). Working on farms, seniors also find it difficult to take the time off to attend a medical appointment. Each of these factors, in combination with language barriers and their unfamiliarity with Canada's institutions limits their access to information about health and social services. As a result, they are less likely to benefit from the health promotion and prevention approach that regional health authorities are now advocating (e.g., Busse, 2007).

Sponsorship and Long Term Care

The criteria and process for accessing long term care varies with province and territory. An older immigrant who becomes frail or whose health deteriorates may need home support, an alternative living environment such as assisted living or a special care home, or skilled nursing care of a licensed care facility. In some cases sponsoring families will keep an elderly sponsored parent who has dementia or other significant health problems at home because they have been told they would be required to pay the costs and they cannot afford care. The result is inequitable access to health care, family stress, and the potential for passive neglect or, in some cases, abuse. Ho et al. (2000) have also identified relationships between non-care giving stresses, such as low income, and unmet service needs among ethnic minority families aiding a family member with dementia.

In the case of licensed facilities, all residents are co-payers and the resident's contribution is based on his or her personal income. This is normally considered the personal responsibility of the resident (i.e., the individual needing care). The facility cannot legally require the sponsor to guarantee costs and the health authority in the province may have a process for exempting the health care cost component, but the family is seldom informed about the possibility (Advocacy Centre for the Elderly, 2003).

Broken Promises: When Sponsorship Breaks Down

Declaration of sponsorship breakdown, whether because the sponsor is unable or unwilling to continue to support their senior family during their first ten years in Canada, amounts to an infraction of the sponsor's legal undertaking. Unless they have an income or other relatives willing to support them, sponsored immigrants will need to apply for social assistance, a process which varies considerably across provinces and territories and which is by no means guaranteed.

While some jurisdictions such as the Northwest Territories (2002) preclude any sponsored immigrant from applying for social assistance, other jurisdictions (for example Saskatchewan and Alberta) allow the application, pending notification of Canada Immigration and Citizenship that the immigrant is no longer receiving any support from the sponsor (Alberta Income Supports, 2003; Saskatchewan Ministry of Social Services, 2007). However, some jurisdictions, such as British Columbia (2007), treat the social assistance payments to the sponsored immigrant, and the accruing interest, as a debt that sponsors must repay to the province. The federal and provincial governments collaborate to facilitate repayment under a memorandum of agreement (CIC, 2004).

Government views the social assistance paid to a sponsored immigrant as an "overpayment," which thereby empowers it to place a lien on the "debtor's" (sponsor's) house and endows it with special priority rights to debt repayment, including garnishment. One could argue that this putative "debt" does not respect the fundamentals of providing public social assistance for need, nor does it distinguish between bad faith and natural events that may prevent sponsorship from being observed, such as cases wherein there has been illness, job loss or marital breakdown.

In Ontario, for example, exceptions to the requirement that sponsors repay the debt are made only if the sponsor dies or falls ill, is living below the poverty line, or if the sponsored immigrant is being abused (Jiménez, 2007). At the federal level, however, an appeal of the decision that a sponsored immigrant was not eligible for the Guaranteed Income Supplement because "[t]he illness of an applicant's immigration sponsor does not result in a sponsorship breakdown" was dismissed and the ruling of the Minister of Human Resources Development Canada was confirmed (The Office of the Commissioner of Review Tribunals (OCRT), 2004). In Saskatchewan, even the death of the sponsor is not sufficient to guarantee eligibility for assistance since the sponsor's estate is held responsible to support the sponsored immigrant providing there are sufficient funds (Saskatchewan Ministry of Social Services, 2007).

The assistance that different jurisdictions provide for housing assistance is also inconsistent. Ontario's discriminatory practice of providing less assistance for housing costs to sponsored immigrants was recently reformed due to litigation, but the rules for obtaining assistance nonetheless remain complex (Shields & isthatlegal.ca, 2007). Similarly, the stipulation that seniors in British Columbia who have been resident in the province for less than ten years are not eligible for the Shelter Aid for Elderly Renters – a subsidy for low and middle income renters – has only recently been revoked (Government of B.C., 1977).

Estimates as to the rates and causes of sponsorship breakdown within the Punjabi community of British Columbia also vary. One of the service providers interviewed by Koehn (1993) claimed that it is not unusual to come across seniors who have been asked to move out when the sponsor is under economic duress. Another service provider and a younger woman placed greater emphasis on the family dynamics that precipitate the breakdown of extended household units and ultimately, the sponsorship agreement. As we have demonstrated already, however, it is the enforcement of sponsorship regulations and associated policies that introduces financial strain and intensifies power imbalances that together render the sponsored seniors dependent, demoralized, and vulnerable to abuse. Charan Gill (2007), who is well known in British Columbia for his social justice work with Punjabi farm workers and seniors issues, has commented that in the majority of cases in which sponsorship breakdown has been declared, it is because the senior has become ill and the family cannot pay for the treatment that is not covered by provincial health insurance during the ten-year dependency period. Gill (2007) maintains that pressure on families to repay the social assistance "loans" is contributing to their disintegration.

In addition to the bureaucratic and legal barriers to declaring a breakdown in sponsorship relations, seniors are inhibited from doing so by their own socio-culturally informed ethics and mores. These can include their own pride and desire to avoid shaming the family (the willingness of Punjabi seniors to engage in gruelling menial labor, so as to be able to ease the financial strain and uphold their self-esteem in the family is a case in point), their inability to return to the home country to which they have already "burnt their boats" by immigrating to Canada (Punjabi community leader, Koehn, 1993), the difficulty of negotiating health and social service systems to secure health care and housing without language skills or familiarity with Canada's infrastructure and the cultural inappropriateness of depending on certain categories of relatives. For Punjabis, for example, living with a daughter is usually not an option:

> There are a lot of gaps in the system, which help perpetuate abuse of these seniors. For example, if elderly women are abused by their sponsor's family, and they go to family court, they may be told that they have to go and live with a daughter who lives here, instead of their son, the sponsor. The courts are insensitive to the cultural inappropriateness of this recommendation; they do not understand why this is next to impossible for some of these people. There's also a huge stigma of showing up the son, exposing the family's honor to public shame, in taking him to court. Some do this out of desperation, but it's very rare that they want to go ahead with this sort of action. (Punjabi service provider, Koehn, 1993, p. 110)

Sponsored seniors living in families in which they experience considerable tension have also commented that they would not declare a breakdown in sponsorship because this would prevent their sponsor from sponsoring additional family members with whom the senior has a better relationship and could feasibly co-reside in the future (Koehn, 1999).

Conclusions: A Constellation of Vulnerabilities

Family Class immigration policy, culture, and the migration experience combine to create vulnerabilities for sponsored seniors. Sponsored parents and grandparents have invested and continue to invest their time and resources in their children (their sponsors) and their grandchildren. In the face of declining birth rates, Canada is dependent on immigrants for its demographic stability. Yet the past and present contributions of older family members go unrecognized in Canada's immigration laws and social service policies. The ten years of complete dependency on their sponsors, and limited access to health care services, transportation and housing options to which sponsored older adults are subjected magnifies the intergenerational shift in roles and status within the family. The consequences can be profound. Many seniors are isolated from social supports, particularly when family members are financially stressed and /or communication between family members breaks down. This in turn can affect the seniors' mental health while at the same time reducing the likelihood that they will be able to access appropriate health care. In extreme circumstances, the potential for abuse or neglect and the likelihood of sponsorship breakdown are increased.

Seniors should not be portrayed as entirely lacking in agency, however. They attempt through their contributions to the household as child-minders, housekeepers, and income-earners to raise their self-esteem and position within the family. Yet none of these strategies is without a cost. While domestic responsibilities prevent seniors from interacting with their peers and familiarizing themselves with their new environment, the farm labor that Punjabi immigrants typically engage in has deleterious health consequences.

Cultural stigma combines with legal and policy obstacles to prevent seniors from declaring a breakdown in the sponsorship relationship. In some cases, this is necessary to escape an abusive environment; in others, the sponsor has experienced unforeseen circumstances, such as illness, that preclude their ongoing provision for the senior. Yet the road to obtaining assistance following a sponsorship break down is a difficult one and the outcome is inconsistent across different jurisdictions. The requirement that sponsors repay the "debt" incurred as a result bespeaks a purely economic motivation for the admission of immigrants and incurs extreme hardship on families already stretched beyond their limit.

Affordable housing that is located in ethno linguistically-dense neighborhoods with strong social supports can facilitate the transition of seniors, if desired, to independent living once the ten-year period of dependency is attained. The non-contributory retirement income of sponsored seniors is nonetheless extremely limited and continues to place them at risk for poor health, social isolation and so forth.

The interpretations of the hegemonic reality to which Family Class older immigrants are subjected will vary from one ethno cultural group to another, depending on socio-cultural mores, family structure, language spoken, education, familiarity with Western institutions (such as health care), existing infrastructural supports within both mainstream and ethnic communities and so on. Variation can also be seen across gender. The impact of geography (living in urban versus rural or remote environments) is also critical. Further research in each of these domains is essential.

These findings also suggest directions for policy change. Most importantly, the authors applaud Penny Priddy's call for an end to the discriminatory ten-year waiting period applied to some new Canadians (Government of Canada, 2006b); the period of time that elderly parents are dependent on their sponsors should be reduced to five years or less. Idealized expectations and assistance with adjustment should be facilitated through orientation sessions for both sponsors and their elderly parents prior to reunification. There is also a need for the development and support of programs that reduce the dependency of sponsored older adults on their children. Examples include flexible housing arrangements (e.g., re-zoning to facilitate in-law suites), the provision of free or reduced rate bus passes for newcomers, job orientation and placement of able-bodied seniors in work that is less harmful to their health than farming, or affordable English as a Second Language classes tailored to seniors. Finally, a complimentary approach is to build the rights knowledge of both sponsors and those they sponsor.

References

Advocacy Centre for the Elderly. (2003). *Admission of sponsored immigrants into long-term care facilities.* Retrieved 12/04, 2007, from www.advocacycentreelderly.org/pubs/nursing/spon-imm.pdf.

Health and Training Benefits Regulation, Alberta. Reg. 60/2004, Enabled by *Income and Employment Supports Act,* S.A. (2003).

Anetzberger, G.J., Korbin, J.E. & Tomita, S.K. (1996). Defining elder mistreatment in four ethnic groups across two generations. *Journal of Cross-Cultural Gerontology, 11*(2), 187-212.

Anzaldúa, G. (1987). *Borderlands/La frontera: The new mestiza.* San Francisco: Aunt Lute Books.

Assanand, S., Dias, M., Richardson, E. & Waxler-Morrison, N. (1990). The South Asians. In N. Waxler-Morrison, J. Anderson & E. Richardson (Eds.), *Cross-cultural caring: A handbook for health professionals in Western Canada* (pp. 141-180). Vancouver: University of British Columbia Press.

Bailie, L. & Denis, J. (2006). Statistics Canada's data sources on immigrants and immigrant families. *Canadian Issues, 21*.

Baker, M. & Benjamin, D. (2002). Are elderly immigrants a burden? Unpublished manuscript, Prepared for the conference, Canadian Immigration Policy for the 21st Century, Kingston, Ontario, October 2002.

Bergeron, J. & Potter, S. (2006). Family members and relatives: An important resource for newcomers' settlement? *Canadian Issues, 76*.

Boyd, M. (1991). Immigration and living arrangements: Elderly women in Canada. *International Migration Review, 25*(1), 4-27.

Busse, B.A. (2007). *Access to health care for ethnic minority seniors.* Speaking to the Interface: A Symposium on Access to Care for Ethnic Minority Seniors, Surrey, B.C. Retrieved 02/15, 2008, from http://www.hccrn.com.

CANE (Clearinghouse on Abuse and Neglect of the Elderly). (2007). Annotated bibliography: Cultural issues in elder abuse. Retrieved 13/02, 2008, from http://www.ncea.aoa.gov/N-CEAroot/Main_Site/Library/CANE/CANE_Series/CANE_cultural.aspx

Carefirst Seniors and Community Services Association. (2002). *In disguise: Elder abuse and neglect in the Chinese community.* Toronto: Carefirst Seniors and Community Services Association.

Chappell, N.L. & Lai, D. (1998). Health care service use by Chinese seniors in British Columbia, Canada. *Journal of Cross Cultural Gerontology, 13*(1), 21-37.

CIC. (2004). *Agreement for Canada-British Columbia co-operation on immigration – 2004 annex E: Sponsorship of family classes.* Retrieved 29/2, 2008, from http://www.cic.gc.ca/ENGLISH/about/laws-policy/agreements/bc/bc-2004-annex-e.asp

CIC. (2005). You asked about immigration and citizenship 2005 (Cat. No. Ci63-16/2005). Ottawa: Minister of Public Works and Government Services Canada. Retrieved 30/11, 2007, from http://www.cic.gc.ca/EnGLIsh/pdf/pub/you-asked.pdf

CIC. (2006). *Annual report to parliament on immigration.* Retrieved 30/11, 2007, from http://www.cic.gc.ca/english/resources/publications/annual-report2006/index.asp

CIC. (2007). *Immigrant overview: Permanent residents.* Retrieved 21/12, 2007, from http://www-.cic.gc.ca/english/resources/statistics/facts2006/permanent/11.asp

Collacott, M. (2006). Family class immigration: The need for a policy review. *Canadian Issues, 90*.

Costa, R. & Renaud, V. (1995). The Chinese in Canada. *Canadian Social Trends, 39*, 22-26.

Côté, A., Kérisit, M. & Côté, M. (2001). *Sponsorship…For better or for worse: The impact of sponsorship on the equality rights of immigrant women.* Ottawa: Status of Women Canada. Retrieved 15/10, 2007 from http://www.swc-cfc.gc.ca/pubs/pubspr/0662296427/200103-_0662296427_2_e.html

Dempsey, C. & CIC. (2004). Elderly immigrants: Income sources and compositions. *Horizons, 7*(2), 58-65.

Gill, C. (Executive Director, Progressive Intercultural Community Services (PICS) Society) (2007). Personal communication with Sharon Koehn. Surrey, B.C. July 4, 2007.

Government of British Columbia. (2007). *Family class sponsorship: Defaulting on an undertaking* (brochure). Victoria: Provincial Government of British Columbia. Retrieved 18/2, 2008, from http://www.cserv.gov.bc.ca/women/sponsorship/documents/english.pdf

Government of Canada. (1982).*The Canadian Charter of Rights and Freedoms,* Schedule B *Constitution Act,* (1982).

Government of Canada (2004). *S-75500 v. the Minister of Human Resources Development Canada.*

Government of Canada. (2006a). *Statements by members: Hon. Raymond Chan* (Richmond, Lib.). 39th parliament, 1st session: Edited Hansard (No. 036). Retrieved 16/2, 2008, from http://www2.parl.gc.ca/HousePublications/Publication.aspx?pub=hansard&mee=36&parl=39&ses=1&language=E&x=1#toc1583120

Government of Canada. (2006b). *Statements by members: Penny Priddy* (Surrey North, NDP). 39th parliament, 1st session: Edited Hansard (No. 036). Retrieved 29/2, 2008, from http://www2.parl.gc.ca/HousePublications/Publication.aspx?pub=hansard&mee=36&parl=39&ses=1&language=E&x=1#toc1583120

Government of Northwest Territories. (2002). Department of education, culture and employment: *Income assistance program policy manual.* Retrieved 29/2, 2008, from http://www.ece.gov.nt.ca/PDF_File/IncSuptPolicyMan.pdf

Grewal, S., Bottorff, J.L. & Hilton, B. A. (2005). The influence of family on immigrant South Asian women's health. *Journal of Family Nursing, 11*(3), 242-263.

Grubel, H. (2005). *Immigration and the welfare state in Canada: Growing conflicts, constructive solutions* (No. 84). Vancouver, BC: Fraser Institute.

Hinton, L., Flores, Y., Franz, C., Hernandez, I. & Mitteness, L.S. (2006). The borderlands of primary care. In A. Leibing, & L. Cohen (Eds.), *Thinking about dementia: Culture, loss and the anthropology of senility* (pp. 43-63). New Brunswick/New Jersey/ London: Rutgers University Press.

Ho, C. J., Weitzman, P.F., Cui, X. & Levkoff, S.E. (2000). Stress and service use among minority caregivers to elders with dementia. *Journal of Gerontological Social Work, 33*(1), 67-88.

Hwang, E. (2008). Chinese seniors in Chinatown, Vancouver, BC. Unpublished manuscript.

Jiménez, M. (2007, 1 May). Sponsors balk at paying. [Electronic version]. *Globe and Mail,* pp. 148.

Joy, A. (1989). *Ethnicity in Canada: Social accommodation and cultural persistence among the Sikhs and the Portuguese.* New York: AMS Press.

Koehn, S., Assanand, S. & Sethi, B. (2007). *Immigration status workshop.* Speaking to the Interface: A Symposium on Access to Care for Ethnic Minority Seniors, Surrey, BC. Retrieved 02/15, 2008, from http://www.hccrn.com.

Koehn, S. (2006). Ethnic minority seniors face a double whammy in health care access. *GRC News, 25*(2), 1-2.

Koehn, S. (1993). *Negotiating new lives and new lands: Elderly Punjabi women in British Columbia.* M.A. Thesis. University of Victoria, Victoria, B.C.

Koehn, S. (1999). *A fine balance: Family, food, and faith in the health worlds of elderly Punjabi women.* Ph.D. Dissertation. University of Victoria, Victoria, B.C.

Lewis-Watts, L. (2006). Speaking with families from within the 'family class'. *Canadian Issues, 81.*

McLaren, A. T. (2006a). *Parental sponsorship – whose problematic? A consideration of South Asian Women's immigration experiences in Vancouver* (Research on Immigration and Integration in the Metropolis Working Paper Series No. 06-08). Vancouver, B.C.: Research on Immigration and Integration in the Metropolis.

McLaren, A.T. (2006b). Immigration and parental sponsorship in Canada: Implications for elderly women, *Canadian Issues, 34.*

McLaren, A.T. & Black, T.L. (2005). *Family class and immigration in Canada: Implications for sponsored elderly women* (Research on Immigration and Integration in the Metropolis Working Paper Series No. 05-26). Vancouver, B.C.: Research on Immigration and Integration in the Metropolis.

Moon, T. (1999). Elder abuse and neglect among the Korean elderly in the United States. In T. Tatara (Ed.), *Understanding elder abuse in minority populations* (pp. 109-118). Philadelphia: Brunner/Mazel.

MOSAIC. (2005). *A submission re: Family reunification issues.* Testimony to the House of Commons standing committee on citizenship and immigration (April 7, 2005). Unpublished manuscript.

Multiculturalism and Immigration Branch, Government of British Columbia. (2007). *Immigrant seniors to British Columbia: 2002-2006* (Fact Sheet, May 2007). Retrieved 30/01, 2008 from www.ag.gov.bc.ca/immigration/pdf/FACT-Seniors.pdf

National Advisory Council on Aging (Canada). (2005). *Seniors on the margins: Seniors from ethnocultural minorities.* Ottawa: Minister of Public Works and Government Services Canada. Retrieved 12/07, 2006 from http://www.naca.ca/margins/ethnocultural/pdf/margins-ethnocultural_e.pdf

Nguyen, H.P. (secretary, Vietnamese-Canadian Seniors Society of BC). (2008). Personal communication with Sharon Koehn. Vancouver, B.C. February 11, 2008.

Pansula, G. (2007, February 06). *Sponsoring parents -unacceptable delays.* Message posted to http://www.entercanada.ca/blog/2007/02/sponsoring-parents-unacceptable-delays.html

Park, H.J. (2006). *Scoping the issues of elder abuse among Asian migrants.* The Second International Asian Health and Wellbeing Conference: Prevention, Protection and Promotion – Conference Proceedings, Auckland, New Zealand.

Patel, N. (1999). *Black and minority ethnic elderly: Perspectives on long-term care (a report to the Royal Commission on Long Term Care for the Elderly). With respect to old age: Long term care - rights and responsibilities* (Vol 1 ed., pp. 257-304). London: The Stationary Office.

Rahim, A. & Mukherjee, A.K. (1984). *South Asians in transition: Problems and challenges.* Scarborough, Ontario: Indian Immigrant Aid Services.

Sadavoy, J., Meier, R. & Ong, A.Y. (2004). Barriers to access to mental health services for ethnic seniors: The Toronto study. *Canadian Journal of Psychiatry, 49*(3), 192-199.

Service Canada. (2006). *Overview of the old age security program.* Retrieved 2/15, 2008, from http://www.hrsdc.gc.ca/en/isp/oas/oasoverview.shtml

Service Canada. (2007). *Old age security (OAS) payment rates.* Retrieved 2/29, 2008, from http://www1.servicecanada.gc.ca/en/isp/oas/oasrates.shtml

Shelter Aid for Elderly Renters Act [Includes Amendments Up to B.C. Reg. 144/2006, July 1, 2006], Shelter Aid for Elderly Renters Regulation U.S.C. 4 (d) (1977). Victoria, B.C. Retrieved 13/2, 2008, from http://www.qp.gov.bc.ca/statreg/reg/S/298_77.htm

Shelton, L. (2003). *Sponsorship breakdown (2nd ed.).* Vancouver, B.C.: Legal Services Society.

Shields, S. & isthatlegal.ca. (2007). *Welfare (Ontario works): Chapter 6 - income rules. Legal guides to Ontario and Canadian law* (online). Retrieved 15/01, 2008 from http://www.isthatlegal.ca/index.php?name=income.owa#Immigration%20Sponsorship%20Income

Social Assistance Program: *Policy Manual,* Section 2.4.11 (2007). Retrieved 28/01, 2008, from http://cr.gov.sk.ca/social-assistance-policy.pdf

Sponsor Your Parents. (2006). *Sponsor your parents.* Retrieved 07/27, 2006, from http://www.sponsoryourparents.ca/about.htm

Statistics Canada. (2005). *Longitudinal survey of immigrants to Canada: A portrait of early settlement experiences* (No. 89-614-XIE). Ottawa: Minister of Industry. Retrieved 10/07, 2006 from http://www.statcan.ca/bsolc/english/bsolc?catno=89-614-XIE

Steele, L.S., Lemieux-Charles, L., Clark, J.P. & Glazier, R.H. (2002). The impact of policy changes on the health of recent immigrants and refugees in the inner city: A qualitative study of service providers' perspectives. *Canadian Journal of Public Health, 93*(2), 118-122.

Stephenson, P.H. (1991). *The Victoria multi-cultural health care research project: Final report.* Victoria, BC: Secretary of State, Multiculturalism Canada.

Tam, S., & Neysmith, S. (2006). Disrespect and isolation: Elder abuse in Chinese communities. *Canadian Journal on Aging, 25*(2), 141-151.

Thompson, A. (2005, May 28). *Family class backlash ignores history.* Toronto Star, pp. L.04.

VanderPlaat, M. (2006). Immigration and families: Introduction. *Canadian Issues, 3.*

Wong, S.T., Yoo, G.J., & Stewart, A.L. (2006). The changing meaning of family support among older Chinese and Korean immigrants. *The Journals of Gerontology. Series B, 61*(1), S4-9.

Yan, E., So-Kum, C. & Yeung, T. D. (2002). No safe haven: A review on elder abuse in *Chinese families. Trauma Violence Abuse, 3*(3), 167-180.

Endnotes

[1]Out of approximately 12 000 Family Class immigrants to Canada in 2006, 5 700 were seniors (i.e., 47.5%).

[2]Punjabis trace their origins to the productive agricultural state of Punjab in North West India (and Pakistan) and speak the Punjabi language. Linguistic continuity binds even second (plus) generation Punjabis to a Punjabi identity, even though they may have moved away from the state prior to moving to Canada. Pre-partition Punjab was considerably larger than it is today, hence many people from neighboring states in India such as Haryana, identify themselves as Punjabis. Punjabis can be further subdivided by religion into Sikh, Hindu and Muslim communities. Representative of British Columbia's South Asian population overall, almost all of the participants in Koehn's (1993) study were Punjabi Sikhs.

[3]The Immigration Act of 1910, amended in 1919, prohibited the settlement of immigrants whose race was considered "unsuitable to the Canadian climate." These laws were the first to allude to the families' undertaking to be responsible for newcomers who were "dumb, blind or otherwise physically defective" (An Act Respecting Immigration, 1910, ch. 38, s. 3, as cited in Côté et al., 2001).

[4]Of the 2.5 million newcomers to Canada between 1946 and 1966, 900 000 were sponsored (Côté et al., 2001).

[5]Other lawsuits have been filed in the past for writs of mandamus to get government immigration department to address delays of this nature (e.g., Dragan v. Canada (Minister of Citizenship and Immigration) (T.D.)).

[6]"Canada has an estimated 800 000-person backlog in our immigration system and the wait time for citizenship in urban centres is close to a year. Not only is this important for my riding of Richmond, but it is also very important to the rest of Canada.

The previous Liberal government designed a multitude of efficient and effective immigration policies, allocated $700 million over five years to reduce the application inventory, signed a

$920 million Canada-Ontario immigration agreement, and invested over $2.4 billion in immigration policies in 2005 alone. It was a government working for Canadians.

The Conservative government has pledged that it would improve Canada's immigration policy, but instead it has cut the $700 million in funding to reduce the backlog, has failed to formally ratify the Canada-Ontario agreement and has failed to allocate funds for the other eight provinces' immigration strategies."

[7] Old Age Security increases are tied to the Consumer Price Index.

[8] R.S.C. 1985, c. C-6. Available at http://www.canlii.org/ca/sta/c-6/

5

Service Use by Immigrant Families Caring
for an Older Relative:
A Question of Culture or Structure?

Jean-Pierre Lavoie, Nancy Guberman (l'Universite du Québec a Montréal)
and Shari Brotman, (McGill University)

Introduction

The growth and aging of the immigrant population, combined with the deinstitutionalisation of aged care in Western societies, have resulted in a major interest by researchers regarding the family-oriented practices of immigrant families caring for relatives living with chronic illness and disability. Numerous studies have attempted to explain to what extent these families distinguish themselves from those in the host country with regards to their accessing of formal ser-vices (Synthesis of these studies have been carried out in the last years, e.g., Angel & Angel, 1999; Janevic & Connell, 2001; Pinquart & Sörensen, 2005). What emerges from these studies is that immigrant families tend to provide more care and resort less to formal services than do non-immigrant families, although the differences appear to vary, and may well be exaggerated (Lum, 2005; Tennstedt, Chang & Delgado, 1998).

While some consensus has emerged that both cultural and structural factors influence family strategies of care for disabled members, many questions remain as to their relative importance. It should be pointed out that some methodological constraints certainly contribute to maintaining this confusion. The majority of the (mostly American) studies were based on secondary analyses of data stemming from large-scale national investigations of a quantitative nature, most of which mixed recent immigrants with immigrants of longer standing (i.e., those who might already be well-integrated in their host country) (Calderon-Rosado et al., 2002; Mausbach et al., 2004; Wilmoth, 2001). Length of stay and English proficiency are considered by some researchers as an indication of the degree of acculturation, though the former is also an indication of a change in status (from that of 'immigrant' to "citizen," for example) (e.g., Burr & Mutchler, 1993; Wilmoth, 2001). Also, the very nature of these studies often makes it impossible for the immigrant families themselves to give explanations and justifications of their practices that do not allow researchers to differentiate cultural from structural barriers. Also, it is often difficult to distinguish between what constitutes a "cultural" or "structural" factor: for example, is a lack of knowledge of services (such as homecare) by immigrant families a cultural trait, or is it a reflection of a lack of effort on the part of services to make themselves known to immigrant populations? Do language barriers in accessing and using services point to a cultural obstacle (due to a high proportion of newly-immigrated seniors who do not speak English nor French (Turcotte & Schellenberg, 2007)), or to a structural one (due to the inaccessibility of language courses, as well as a lack of multilingual resources in organizations (Brotman, 2003; Brotman, 2001; Forbat, 2003; Gelfand, 2003; Kalavar & Van Willigen 2005; Liu, 2003))? Lastly, little is known about the experiences of immigrant families utilizing services over a long period of time, especially homecare services; therefore, judging the accessibility and appropriateness of such long-term services in meeting the needs of immigrant populations is rendered problematic.

In spite of the difficulty in distinguishing cultural factors from structural ones, we will attempt, in this chapter, to specify their respective role, first with regard to the disabled individual being able to access services, and then with regard to these individuals and their families' experiences of these same services. To do this, we will use a recent review of the literature and four qualitative studies conducted with disabled older immigrants and their families in Quebec and Ontario. The first study, conducted between 1992 and 1996, with families of Italian and Haitian descent, aimed to understand the experience of caregivers of older adults in these families (Guberman & Maheu, 1997). These two groups differed as to length of stay in Québec, the visibility of their phenotype, linguistic problems and the degree to which their communities were organized. Semi-structured interviews were conducted with 49 caregivers of 22 Italian families and 20 Haitian families. In addition to this, group interviews were conducted with staff from the home care agencies in the neighborhoods where numerous Italian and Haitian families reside. The second study was conducted between 1995 and 1997 with older adults of Chinese origin residing in downtown Montreal. It aimed to understand the way social and health resources were used by these older adults as well as identify the elements taken into account that facilitated their access to health and social services. Thirty-two Chinese older adults, including six couples, were met in individual interviews and nine others in a group interview. The third study (Brotman, 2001, 2002, 2003) was undertaken in 1998 and 1999 and addressed the problem of access for ethnic elderly women through an examination of the working processes of a publicly-funded community care organization in Ontario. Thirty separate interviews and three focus groups were completed during the study with a total of 43 participants. Participants included 10 older ethnic women and 3 family members, 16 staff of the health care organization in which the study was conducted, and 14 people who worked in multicultural or ethno-specific organizations in the community. The older women interviewed represented both white ethnic women (of Greek and Italian origins) and women of color (of South Asian, Black and Chinese origins) and all were immigrants to Canada (five having immigrated between 1950 and 1965 and five having immigrated after 1985). Seven out of ten of the participants spoke neither English nor French. The fourth study (Lavoie et al., 2006) was conducted between 2003 and 2005 with 33 persons belonging to 15 families of recent immigrants in Québec. A third of these families were from Latin America and another third from North Africa and the Middle East. Two families originated from the African continent and two were from South-East Asia. Using semi-directed interviews, the study aimed to research what strategies of care were used by these families to understand how migratory patterns influenced these strategies and finally, to see what impact these strategies had on their integration into Quebec society.

A Question of Culture: Family Solidarity and Reluctance to Use Formal Services

Numerous studies report strong feelings of solidarity and reciprocity among immigrant families (e.g., Angel & Angel, 1997; Aranda & Knight, 1997; Wilmoth, 2001). As an older woman from the Middle East stated: ". . . they're my kids and they're sort of responsible for me . . ." A son from Sri Lanka said that not caring for his older impaired mother would be a "sin." Among East-Asian families (Chinese, Japanese, Korean, etc.) a strong sense of filial obligation to care for the older parents, referred as "filial piety," has been reported (Dai & Diamond, 1998; Wong, Yoo & Stewart, 2005; Yeo & Galagher-Thompson, 1996). Filial piety could be reinforced by the social pressure – sekentei – to behave according to this norm (Asai & Kameoka, 2005). This strong belief in family solidarity and proximity has an impact upon living arrangement choices and, according to Wilmoth (2001), most immigrant families choose to share multigenerational dwellings. According to authors cited above, a process of acculturation occurs with the gradual integration to the society of adoption. Such a process results in an erosion of these norms of family and filial responsibility to care for elders with immigrant family members adopting beliefs and attitudes of the native-born population. As one older immigrant woman stated:

> I notice here in the West actually, it's very different from what we do culturally. Uh, we wouldn't think of putting our elderly in a senior home. No, we look after our own. Which is very different. . . . almost not there . . . I mean this culture (Western) does not call for that kind of thing . . . young people, who are getting, who think that by trying to get away from their culture or religion they can get educated and become modern and westernized. (Iranian woman)

This strong belief in family solidarity and obligation to care for older relatives lead most families to be reluctant to use formal services according to many authors (Balgopal, 1999; Kosloski, Montgomery & Karner, 1999; Ma & Chi, 2005; Radina & Barber, 2004). In our studies, a few respondents from Italian and Haitian families were quite reluctant to resort to services, especially homecare services. Having a stranger in the home was viewed as intrusive and something to be wary of: "We can manage on our own. It's not easy to accept strangers in our midst, especially people with a mentality different from us" (an Italian woman). In that respect, the evalua-tion process, that opens the door to services, reinforces this impression of intrusion with questions pertaining to income, employment or again, family environment. "Those people don't like it when we question them. It's as if we're seeking to intrude, as if we wanted to take a part of their privacy and put it on public display . . ." (staff worker regarding Haitian families). Older Italian parents are especially reluctant about having strangers, that they consider a source of fear and anxiety, intrude. For older Haitian persons, the greater stake is receiving care from a person towards whom they feel no attachment. Lai (2004) reports similar fear and preference in Chinese families in Canada.

Furthermore, resorting to services takes on a symbolic value, embedded in a culture that sometimes confronts family values. Resorting to services is seen as something shameful. For some Japanese families, using services is in contradiction with the obligation to care for older parents (Kitano, Shibusawa & Kitano, 1997) and might be harmful to the reputation of the family (Asai & Kameoka, 2005). For a few Italian and Haitian persons, this recourse is a sign of failure that highlights the family's inability to take care of the older parent's well-being: "At the hospital, we [were offered] a volunteer to help out at home. [. . .] My father refused because he viewed it as a failure, he felt quite capable of taking care of his wife" (Italian woman). This symbolic dimension of using services derives from the context of the country of origin or from the context of immigration. For Italians, health and social services are there for the poor. Ma and Chi (2005) make the same observation in Chinese famllies as well as Strumpf et al. (2001) among Asian and East-European refugees. For Haitians, the experience of living under a dictatorship and of being oppressed leads them to be distrustful, even fearful, of anything that has to do with public services. For recent immigrants, asking for services means begging or bothering, as was the case with an older Chinese woman who stated: "I do not want to trouble [them]. I feel embarrassed." Fears regarding being seen as a bother are more acute when one's immigrant status is not clear, as in the case of this woman originally from the Middle East: "Because their situation, their papers, they're not immigrants. We thought that we were going to be like, like asking or begging to the government or CLSC (home care organization) or

any organization. We don't want to bother people. We don't want to, to make trouble
. . ."

Besides homecare services, nursing homes and psychosocial services are especially viewed with reluctance. Long-term institutional care is seen as abandonment, an
abdication of one's duty, which can be guilt-inducing (Balgopal, 1999). Besides, there
is this negative view of services and the fear of racism. The institution is seen as a solution of last resort. "I think we wait until the very end, when we are really forced to . . ."
one Italian woman tells us. As to psychosocial services, a few Italians told us about
their fear of having to see a stranger. For Haitians, these services raised the fear of
being seen "as crazy." The reluctance might also be linked to the stigmatization associated with the illness of the older parent such as Alzheimer's disease (Dillworth, Ander
& Gibson, 1999; Samaoli, 2000).

The concept of "familism" was adopted by some researchers to capture this cultural orientation toward strong family bonds and solidarity. "Familism" is an expression
describing the importance given to family ties, mutual aid, and an identity derived from
the family rather than from the individual, a certain mistrust of the outside world, and
a will to resolve family problems privately (Clément et Lavoie, 2001; Luna et al., 1996).
Thus, persons belonging to ethnic minorities – especially recent immigrants – are more
likely to be living in extended families, with much value placed on family responsibility
for caring for relatives with a disability (Firbank & Johnson-Lafleur, 2007; Janevic &
Connell 2001), and would therefore be more reluctant to resort to public and private
services, especially as they pertain to institutional care and psychosocial services
(Dillworth-Anderson & Gibson, 1999; Patterson, 2004; Turner, Christie & Haworth,
2005). One of the obvious by-products of this "familism" would therefore be an overall lack of knowledge of available formal aged-care services.

It comes as no surprise then that organizations that dispense front line long term
services are, for the most part, little known by recent immigrants (Salari, 2002;
Samaoli, 2000; Strumpf et al., 2001). As a Haitian woman notes: ". . . I do not know
the other services except the nursing homes for older adults, so I do not know what
else I could ask for." An 83-year-old woman from Jamaica comments on her lack of
awareness regarding how to reach a homecare worker:

> I've been trying to reach her and the number on the card she gave me must be
> wrong, because every time I call they say no one by that name works there. Oh
> I don't know about all that, when they tell me she doesn't work there I just hang
> up. (Jamaican woman)

Also, not knowing the language limits the ability to learn about services available
(Wong, Yoo & Stewart, 2005). Language sometimes complicates things so that it is difficult to understand the information that one gains access to, as in the case of an Asian

family: "Lack of knowledge of the essential services and the language were two main barriers for us. I did not have sufficient knowledge to whom and where I should ask and go about. Also, the information is mostly in French which I do not understand." Furthermore, not knowing the language also impedes fully understanding the actual nature of services and their use. This Asian family cannot get their elderly mother to understand that the rehabilitation centre (nonexistent in their country of origin) is not a nursing home. It becomes not only necessary to be able to understand the sense of the words used, but also to know how to formulate the problem using the right terms. The precarious or marginalized status of immigrant families may lead to a kind of resignation in the face of health care encounters. As one older Chinese woman stated:

> It would be nice if we spoke the same language . . . but that's what happens when you leave your country . . . your homeland . . . we've been dealing with this our whole life now . . . what do you expect when you leave your homeland? (Chinese woman)

A strictly culturalist interpretation of the gaps between immigrant and non-immigrant families has been criticized in recent years, on three major fronts. First, many researchers underline that differences between immigrant populations and the population of the host country have been overemphasized. Families did not provide as much care as was expected (Delgado & Tennstedt, 1997; Wong, Yoo & Stewart, 2005). Immigrant populations also have quite important expectations of the formal services and governmental help (Tennstedt, Chang & Delgado, 1998; Lan, 2002; Wong, Yoo & Stewart, 2005). In our research projects, very little reluctance to accept formal services is found among immigrant seniors and their families from a variety of ethnic back-grounds, and most notably, in recent immigrant families. On the contrary, the latter have great expectations towards services. How does one explain these high expectations? The majority of recent immigrant families that were met had an image of Canada as a country of services. In the study by Lavoie et al. (2006), five families with a family member with a disability came to Canada/Québec with great expectations regarding available services for this person. In other respects, in spite of the sharp reluctance shown by most of the Italian and Haitian families in one study, more than half of these were using homecare services, either because they were unavailable to take care of their relative or the level of care required was too high. As to recent immigrant families, their expectations may possibly be due to the fact that they feel unable to rely on the support of an already reduced family network and even less so from the one in their neighborhood. Had health problems surfaced in their countries of origin, the latter would have been much more involved: "we would have received the physical support from the relations and neighbors" (an Asian man).

According to some of the persons interviewed, it would have mostly been neighbors rather than family that would have helped out. In addition, expectations for care may also emerge as an expression of reciprocity within families. In fact, many older immigrants stated that they ask for formal services in an effort to relieve their children from the burden of care, a reality that may be more intense among immigrant families, as this desire is directly tied to their own experience of hardship as a result of immigration and, more importantly, to their reasons for choosing to immigrate in the first place. It appears that a central component of ethnic minority people's identity as immigrants is bound up with the desire to improve the life chances of their children and to provide opportunities to their children which were unavailable to them. Thus, central to their sense of self and purpose is the notion of sacrifice for the sake of their children. An Iranian woman stated, "I came for my boys, to make a better life for them."

Older immigrants shared their realities of economic hardship and spoke about the difficulties that face immigrants in society. As a result, older immigrants have expressed that children may have less time available to engage in support of elderly family members and may face greater barriers to economic security which would require them to forego family care for paid employment. As these two older women stated:

> But coming here most of the ethnic people are busy working, trying to be able to make . . . maybe double income families so it's very difficult for them even to give too much time to each other. (Iranian woman)

> My children had a few children of their own and they lived very far away. I did not want to complain to them. They worked very hard. They got up at five o'clock in the morning to go to work and they did not return home until after five in the evening. How could they help me? (Chinese woman)

Second, strictly cultural interpretations have tended to convey a homogenizing and static conception of immigrant cultures and important intra-cultural variations are underestimated (Durst, 2005; Fung & Wong, 2007; Lai & Kalyniak, 2005; Liu, 2003; Markides, 1998), including the extent to which individuals conform to their culture's prevailing norms and identities (Chiu & Yu, 2001).They also have failed to recognize that cultural "norms" themselves evolve, including, of course, within the countries of origin themselves (Kalavar & Van Willigen, 2005) and may be interpreted differently when those populations immigrate. Lan (2002) as well as Wong, Yoo, and Stewart (2005), for example, have shown that the concept of "filial piety" is often (re)interpreted by Chinese and Korean-American families to include extra-familial help that is hired and paid for by the children or public funds.

The third major reproach of the culturalist explanation is the correspondingly little attention that is paid to structural barriers when explaining immigrant families' less frequent accessing of formal services (Gelfand, 2003; Guberman & Maheu, 1997; Markides, 1998). To take one example, that of the aforementioned prevalence of intergenerational cohabitation, certain researchers have argued that the decision to cohabit has less to do with culture than it does with the economic hardships resulting from, among other things, the exclusion of immigrants (especially those sponsored) from receiving welfare assistance, and by difficulties related to integration (Gelfand, 2003; Turcotte & Schellenberg, 2007).

A Question of Structure: The Barriers to Accessing Formal Services

The difficulties accessing long-term services, mostly homecare services, are certainly tied to linguistic and cultural barriers and, as was mentioned earlier, to a lack of knowledge of services. But immigrant families having high expectations to formal services still receive little services. In their conversations, most of the families participating in our studies emphasized the difficulties they encountered, the obstacles in their path and the repeated requests without answesr. When faced with rejection from homecare services, families get lost in conjectures, especially when no justification is given by the home care agency. In fact, with some families, their steps can best be summarized by images of struggle and fighting to obtain the desired services: "By continuing to *fight* [our emphasis], to take steps, to get information, I got hold of a rehabilitation centre [. . .], very good!" (Latin-American woman).

More often than not, they are confronted with a host of obstacles that limit access to non-medical help and services. First of all, immigration laws have a direct impact on the accessibility to long term care by restricting eligibility to services for the immigrant population. In the United States, the law has been structured in such a way that, even when formal services are desired by a family (including homecare and nursing home), the costs are often not eligible to be covered by governments, thus leading to their lesser use (Angel, Angel & Markides, 2000; Fung & Wong, 2007; Gelfand, 2003). It appeared in one of our studies on recent immigrant families that the immigration status of various family members played a major role in their difficulty to access long term care and other types of governmental supports. Indeed, according to their status, families and their members with disabilities are given limited access to services by immigration law. Added to these legal and administrative obstacles, is the reality that institutions differentially interpret eligibility criteria for service based upon legal status and staffs often apply agency policies more or less strictly.

Thus, in Canada, immigrant persons with a status of independent immigrant or convention refugee have access to services and an economic support system that sponsored persons or those with a permit of stay for humanitarian reasons (not to mention those without legal status) do not have. Convention refugee and independent immigrant status allows access to health and social services. As well, such status allows adult members of these familes to benefit from government financial programs such as welfare. Problematic in the current context is that older immigrants are most likely to enter the host country under the status of sponsorship. Sponsors must take on the economic responsibility of those family members they sponsor and must commit to their upkeep (by providing shelter, food and clothing) for 10 years (3 if it is a spouse) in Canada. Some older persons might have an even more precarious legal status: the right to stay for humanitarian reasons. This status institutes conditions of admissibility similar to those of the sponsored person, except there is no fixed limited time. Thus, even after 10 years, these persons do not have a chance of benefitting from welfare assistance programs or financial aid to which other immigrants have a right. Such status limits access to certain services, mainly financial aid. As to homecare services and low-cost housing, our most recent study showed that policies vary from one agency to the other; some are rather restrictive regarding access to homecare services and low-cost housing. Thus, one family is refused homecare services because two members with disabilities are sponsored. Yet, another family from a different neighborhood receives services from the local home care agency even though the family is temporarily residing illegally in Canada. Finally, in our study, two older persons with disabilities were living in Québec with an expired tourist visa and one of them had twice been refused sponsorship. None of the services, not even the medical ones, are accessible to these people without costs involved. For one of these families, the fear of being discovered and eventually deported curbs their resolve to resort to formal services.

Regardless of the immigrant senior's legal status, agency policies and professional interventions regarding entitlement to services is often premised on the presence of families to provide support. In the context of assumptions regarding the preference and availability of ethnic families to provide care among health care professionals, immigrant families may be differentially treated with respect to entitlement to services or in the number of hours of service provided. For example, the following case managers had this to say about the role of ethnic families in providing care and subsequent decisions about entitlement to services:

> Because people can have large support systems and that is on the chart and people look through the chart. So we don't need to put in as much [service]. I think it's an unspoken expectation that if a person has family, the family should put in their fair share . . . for some of the care. And again that's fine and good.

> I just recently had an incident here where someone was referred but they were referred by the family. The family had brought up the need for services at home to the resource nurse and he came to me "Oh, by the way the family of so and so wants home care. I don't know what they want homecare for, really. There's a very supportive family. I don't know what they want. (Case manager)

Adding to the interpretations that institutions and their staff give to the rights of older immigrants, immigrant persons themselves have different understandings of the rights they have with their different statuses and these understandings come into play with their actual rights (Strumpf et al., 2001). In our study, three families told us of their surprise at obtaining a service that they thought they were not entitled to receive or their hesitation at requesting the services that they thought they were not eligible for, as their relative was either sponsored or had a permit of stay for humanitarian reasons.

Other obstacles are linked to access to services for immigrant seniors and their families. These obstacles are not specific to immigrants, but might affect them particularly. The first stems from the costs that are incurred regarding certain services. Indeed, some health care is not covered by medicare while some other at-home services, such as housework, or placement in a nursing home require a monetary contribution from the client. Thus, an elderly refugee woman who presently resides in Québec receives home care services without any problem. As to house cleaning, this woman refuses to resort to a social economy business since she considers the costs too high. A Latin American woman, who holds a special minister's permit, is obliged to stop the chiropractic treatments for her son since she can no longer afford them. Such economic barriers to recourse to services have seldom been reported in existing literature (Angel & Angel, 1997; Angel, Angel & Markides, 2000; Min, 2005).

Access to homecare services is also framed by a series of criteria that might vary from one agency to the other. Thus, one daughter's request for homecare services for her older mother is denied because she is available for care, working only part-time. Another woman's request for respite is rejected only because the activity that is planned during the respite, to go out with her teenage daughter, is not deemed eligible:

> You see, with a teenage daughter, she would like that I go to the movies with her, but I can't, I can't leave my mother all alone. I made a request at the (home care agency) but they told me that it is not the (home care agency) but volunteers. They can accompany her to the grocery store or to the bank but it is out of the question that they come here while I go out to enjoy myself. I don't think that this is a question of enjoyment. (Latin-American woman)

While it would seem that some of the obstacles mentioned are not just the lot of immigrant families, it is clear that they are most certainly affected by them, especially when it comes to costs. The literature describing systemic barriers in aged care chronicle a number of factors that affect all seniors, native-born and not including lack of transportation, inconvenient location and/or hours of operation, and physical accessibility considerations (Gelfand, 2003; Kalavar & Van Willigen, 2005; Patterson, 2004). So it is not surprising that immigrant seniors have a special difficulty accessing services, considering the number of additional unique barriers they face, including not being able to access publicity for services in languages other than English or French (assuming that they are even literate in their native tongue), difficulties in communicating with services, the perceived (and intimidating) invasive evaluation process, and reported experiences of racism (Baker, 2006; Brotman, 2003).

Assessing the Experience of Formal Care Utilization

In spite of these problems with access, many immigrant elders and their families do use long term care services. Yet, besides numerous papers on the importance of implementing culturally sensitive services, little research focuses on the experience and assessment of utilization of services by immigrant elders and their families (Liu, 2003; Ma & Ambrose, 2005). Studies conducted by the authors did focus on the experience of such utilization.

As an intitial observation, our respondents' overall assessment is rather mixed; the stories related include both positive and negative experiences. The appreciation is globally more positive with medical, hospital or some rehabilitation services than with long-term care services, homecare, adapted transportation and rehabilitation services.

Concerning medical and hospital services, as well as rehabilitation services, the majority of families give them positive reviews. These touch on professional quality and the competency of staff as well as on the fact that care is free. A few persons are grateful for the services. If this gratitude towards services and hospital staff is found in a great number of persons of all origins in Québec and Ontario, it is more greatly expressed by recent immigrants, since having access to a free hospital stay and the latest technology are often taken for granted by non-immmigrants. The human side of these services, especially regarding physicians, is an important aspect of the overall assessment given by respondents as it is with a majority of users (Dubé, Ferland & Moskowitz, 2003). However, if there are some persons who are quick to emphasize the empathy, listening and encouragement received on the part of certain physicians, nurses and social workers, there are just as many who highlight a lack of listening and coldness from professionals. A lack of humanity in organized care and the little time that is given by physicians during appointments are frequent complaints in the health system (Armstrong et al., 2007) and cannot be attributed to issues of culture. Another complaint shared by our respondents and quite a few users in the healthcare system, deals with the authoritative manner of health professionals and their sometimes guilt-inducing attitude. For other persons who have been in Québec and Ontario for more than 10 years, we also hear a similar refrain to the one found with most of the populations regarding the deterioration of the quality of care in hospitals. These often speak of their dissatisfaction with the inappropriateness and insufficient level of hospital services often caused by budget cuts and cuts in staff. It would therefore seem that once the wonder felt for a modern and free healthcare system passes, the structural gaps found in that very system become more apparent for all users and that the cultural elements underlying its appreciation become less important.

Regarding long-term care services, most notably homecare, the overall assessment given by our respondents looks much like the one given by non-immigrants. Thus, while it is for the most part positive for some families, others are much more critical and any appreciation seems to rest on aspects of a structural order, even if, for some respondents, the issue of quality refers as well to linguistic and cultural dimensions. However, as indicated at the beginning of this chapter, these dimensions also have a structural component (lack of translation services, lack of staff belonging to minority ethnic groups). As one professional stated:

> Well I think what I would say is . . . because of the uncertainty in the last few years, pennies had to be watched very very carefully. And although we had a translation service we were not really all that encouraged to use it. But you would first try and find an individual, a family member. That isn't always the best scenario, but that's what we have to do. (Professional)

Respondents, who like the whole of the population, consider that the services they receive are sufficient and are of good quality, tend to give a positive overall assessment. For some respondents, the ability of services to meet their needs is what gives them satisfaction. Thus, when one benefits from many hours of homecare, as in the case of this family of Asian origin, praise is given to the amount of service given and to the equipment made available:

> Initially the nurse (family aid) came home to take care for my mother 3 days a week. Now they are coming 5 days a week. Everyday they clean my mother and once change the diaper too . . . Immediately, they gave us a hand and we are very happy about this. Also they have given her a sliding bed for her to be comfortable, a table and a chair. It was a big help and we feel very good about this. (Asian family member)

Other families highlighted the skills of the social worker and the referrals to the proper service. Day centres, either those in the public sector or the community sector, seem to rate high providing, on the one hand, a place for for the senior with disabilities to interact socially and on the other, respite for caregivers: "If we hadn't had the help of the day centre, we would have been in trouble for a long time. Since she's been going, she only lives for that! Plus, it really saved us, I can't really say, there are no other words" (Italian woman).

In other respects, some respondents will emphasize the staff's empathy, the warm relationships that exist between people that mostly stem from services that have been put in place again. The social and family aids are especially appreciated and are praised for fostering meaningful relationships. For one Haitian woman, the family aid provides care that is almost as if she were a part of the family: "she (the family aid) is in every respect matchless. I have no problem with her. It is as if she were my own daughter." It is interesting to note that these satisfied accounts do not at all make reference to cultural aspects, to whether or not values were respected or to the specific behaviors of immigrant families.

Negative criticism does focus as well on the difficulties linked to the respect or lack of respect of cultural values and norms. There may be an insistence on the meaningfulness of the relationship with staff in which one may find cultural overtones, yet this same criticism is also echoed by the rest of the population. Haitian sisters tell of the difficulties encountered by their grandmother when they tried to send her to the day centre: "She didn't like it because she found that they greeted her coldly, the atmosphere was also cold."

However, it is not so much in these areas that lay the main elements of dissatisfaction concerning long-term care services. As Mai & Chi (2005) report, structural aspects such as not enough services offered and waiting lists, as well as inadequate services to meet the needs constitute the main sources of dissatisfaction. One man from North Africa qualifies the homecare services as a real "bluff," since for him; these services "have nothing to offer." One woman tells us of the well-known issue of baths: "In the beginning, they would only come twice a week to give a bath. I couldn't get more" (Latin American woman). When they have access to services, a few persons note that these simply do not meet their needs and that it is impossible for them to get the needed help:

> They want to come to give my mother a bath. That's not it, what my mother needs. She's capable of taking her bath. It's a cultural issue, one of modesty, etc. She takes her bath. She's capable of doing so. But the way things work at the (homecare agency). It's written that she should get help to take a bath . . . We need other services that we can't get. We can't get what we want. (Middle-East woman)

Other structural problems are also denounced like staff turnover, the complex nature of a bureaucratic system and the lack of flexibility regarding services such as adapted transportation. Older Chinese Canadians interviewed by Ma & Chi (2005) also complained about complicated procedures when using services.

In the overall assessment of services given by respondents who participated in one of the four studies, most of the praise and the problems described ressembled, on every point, the assessment that was given by French Canadian persons (Guberman et al., 1991; Lavoie, 2000), and all were attributed to the structural problems found within the health and social services system. With regard to the criticism, immigrant persons denounced as much as Canadian-born persons, the insufficient human and material resources, the difficulty in accessing services and the fact that services were not adapted to meet the needs of persons with disabilities and their relatives. That said however, immigrant persons do face specific realities related to their language, their culture and their situation as immigrants.

Linguistic, Cultural and Migratory Dimensions in Assessing Services

Problems owing to linguistic barriers and cultural distance that affect communication and mutual understanding greatly complicate the relationships between older immigrants and their families and staff (Capitman, 2002; Fitzpatrick & Freed, 2002). This problem was indeed reported by some of our respondents. But again, the distinction between culture and structure is not that clear as certain services seem to have found ways to overcome barriers.

With regard to linguistic barriers, many of the persons that we met highlighted the efforts made by some institutions to offer them services in their language. Others were of the opinion that language barriers can be overcome; that with good faith, from everyone it can be done:

> Q.: But how does your brother manage [to participate at the day centre] if he doesn't speak French, if he only speaks Armenian?

> R.: I don't know. [. . .] I called and they said: "Everybody understands him, though I don't know what language he's speaking." (Family originally from the Middle-East)

The study conducted with older Chinese persons reveals similar attitudes. Obviously, having staff speak Chinese with them helps when interacting, but many positively appreciate the services and the homecare family aids, just as long as their gestures can be understood by them.

In spite of this, other respondents deplore the lack of services in their language, notably the way it impacts the quality of services. One family of recent immigrants and a few persons of Italian and especially Haitian descent attribute the lack of attention and inadequate supervision received in hospitals to a lack of their older relative's knowledge of French. These problems in communication between the ill person and staff forces other members of the family to be present at all times, which adds to their responsiblities: "And our elderly parents, we need to defend them against the negligence of staff who sometimes, voluntarily or not, tend to sometimes discriminate against them, not meet their needs under the pretext that when spoken to, they don't understand or I don't know" (Italian woman). A Chinese woman from Ontario stated:

> When the doctor, the physiotherapist and the doctor had a meeting, they asked me to attend. I sat there like a piece of wood and I did not understand their conversation. I did not know what has happened, I just sat there like a block of wood. (Chinese woman)

Is this solely a language problem or is it racism? In fact, in line with Brotman (2003), in the four studies, it is alluded to, although some respondents explicitly make note of the racism of some of the staff. Two women of Haitian origin link poor quality and lack of care to racism:

> From the start, I told the nurse to bring a bed pan for mother. She was using a bed pan then . . . a good thing that I came back. The bed pan was never given to mother. Poor her, there she was praying and in her anguish, she even forgot that she could ring . . . I returned to the station and asked the nurse if she was paid to take care of all the patients or just some of them. I don't know what kind of Negro story she told me. (Haitian woman)

> Also, I have to say that the fact that the nurses are overworked doesn't help much. To constantly cut services and positions doesn't make things better. They then have all the more reason to push us along, to not meet our needs, and to make us believe that we ask too much, especially when we are black or immigrant. (Haitian woman)

And even then, the possibility of racism leads family members to be constantly present with their elderly parents. Experiences with homecare support staff are not exempt of examples of racism either:

> This nurse came here it seems, with already preconceived notions . . . She was acting all high and mighty . . . she even insinuated that we were lying . . . She searched the house, the fridge, and the tone she used to speak to us . . . Believing us to be lying, she increased, I don't know how much, the dose of insulin and my father almost died. And why, without any proof, would she think that we were lying? Because that's what racism is, it's word that we don't like to use, but that's where we should look for in, in the public services. (Haitian woman)

The problems inherent to a lack of services and their inappropriateness to meet the needs are seemingly made worse by language barriers and a lack of cultural sensitivity on the part of staff. These last two elements do not just refer to cultural factors but also, if not more so, to the ability of services to adapt. In other respects, it should be noted that these barriers do not just touch on putting into place new services, but also the latter's ability to meet the needs of immigrant persons, as some accounts would seem to indicate.

What to Come Away With? Some Recommendations for Practice.

With its diversified origins that are less and less European, the marked growth of the immigrant population has been a major source of inquiry for researchers and health and social service agencies alike. Important research, of great value, has shown us what is specific about immigrant populations regarding their aging, health, family practices and ways of using services. Such research has not only been able to direct and transform services offered but also ongoing professional practices as well (Bennett, 1986; Cohen-Emérique, 1984; Devore & Schlesinger, 1987; Kadushin, 1983). Based on this research, services as well as staff have been encouraged to develop approaches and methods of practice that take into account ethnocultural differences. We have thus been able to put into place services that are culturally appropriate, all the while devoting important efforts to training staff. The latter has allowed them to gain the knowledge and needed skills to better understand these differences and adapt their practices to these new clients. This trend, which places emphasis on ethnocultural diversity, has allowed us to confront those views on assimiliation that see immigrants, especially those of the second and third generations, as needing to adapt as quickly as possible to become more like the dominant culture of Western Europe). However, by placing the emphasis on these differences and on the development of culture-based skills in staff, this trend has earned criticism from some (Devore & Schlesinger, 1987; Ivey et al., 1997; Jenkins, 1988).

In this quest for open-mindedness concerning diversity and sensitivity for difference, a danger exists that we view the immigrant person as the "other" rather than as "another," that is, as a person who experiences many commonalities with those born in the host country. And these points in common may be more important than the differences. Based on literature and on the studies we did, it would seem, in fact, that between those older immigrant persons and their families and the ones from Canada that we met in other studies (Guberman et al., 1993; Guberman et al., 2005; Lavoie, 2000), the similarities found in both come across as more important than their differences. Also, it seems that the difficulties experienced by immigrant persons accessing services, stem largely from obstacles of a structural nature rather than from those related to culture. Language barriers, clearly more important for immigrant populations, distinguish the two groups. However, language barriers are structural in nature, reflecting the lack of resources available to provide people with interpretation rather than as a problem with the older people's lack of English or French comprehension. However, we find in immigrant and Canadian-born older people and their families, open-mindedness to services. Where reluctance exists (notably concerning home-care services and institutional care), it is based both upon cultural concerns regarding seeing a lack of care as abandonment and upon structural concerns regarding the inaccessibility of services. Either way, there is a claim to know little about services or not understand how these function. Moreover, when assessing services, immigrant persons denounce as much as Canadian-born persons, the lack of long-term homecare services, their rigidity and inability to meet their needs. In spite of their skills, the turnover, coldness and rudeness of staff and professionals are a recurring critique.

Furthermore, by placing emphasis on ethnocultural differences between immigrant populations and host country-born populations, we risk putting forward a view that these two groups are homogeneous. For us, the studies that were presented highlight important differences among immigrant populations: some were reluctant about the services; others had high expectations towards the latter; for some language was an issue, for others, not. For host-country-born populations, there are also cultural gaps, especially between the more disadvantaged groups and professionals from the health and social services network (Massé, 1995).

From what we have been able to observe, we find it important to draw three conclusions. First, researchers and professionals must develop an approach that emphasizes similarities among, as well as differences between, older immigrant persons and their families and those of the host society. Next, researchers and professionals must move beyond the development of a cultural analysis for ethnic and immigrant born persons only. Rather attention must be paid to culture within all populations and communities. To that effect, as noted by Clément and Lavoie (2001) and Guberman and Maheu (1997), many of the values, beliefs and practices that have to do with the family, illness or services that are linked to immigrant populations can also be found in the disadvantaged populations of host societies. Finally, with the same degree of importance that they give to cultural factors, our studies and the literature invite researchers and professionals to address the structural problems that delay access to services and to look to the ways in which organizations design and deliver services that hinder both access and satisfaction with services and lead to further barriers among clients and their families.

Indeed, one restriction of culturalist interpretations is that they distract researchers and staff from focusing on structural factors such as the social conditions in which immigrant families find themselves, the immigration policies of the host society and the policies and services destined for persons with disabilities. The insufficient income, the restrictions in rights to services that some immigration statuses impose or again, the interpretations that certain organizations or their staff will give to these restrictions, the insufficient long-term services owing to chronic underfunding, the rigidity of criteria for the allocation of services, all of these contribute to limit access for older immigrant persons with disabilities and their families. Most factors related to not being satisfied with the services received, either because they are insufficient or rigid, or do not meet the needs of clients, have more to do with their underfunding and their bureaucratic functioning than with culture. Besides, as we stated in the introduction, it is difficult to distinguish between that which stems from culture from that which stems from structure. Is the lack of knowledge regarding long-term services due to culture or rather to the fact that there is no hurry to make these services known and to the absence of screening of those in need? Can we not partly explain language problems and the lack of cultural adaptation to the underfunding of services that limits access to translation services or to the training of staff? Moreover, as Brotman (2001; 2003) indicates, placing emphasis on the ethnocultural gaps can mean keeping silent about the issue of institutional racism. Does giving culturally-related explanations, where language plays a dominant role, to problems that deal with access to services or that relates to the interactions between staff and immigrant persons not place the burden of adaptation on immigrant persons rather than on the host society that should be adapting its services to the populations that it serves? How does one explain the problems encountered by immigrants who have a strong command of the language of the host country?

It is essential that researchers and staff, while taking into account cultural differences, put them into their social, economic and political context. We need to arrive at a model that gives a conception of the issues as to consider ethnicity without pretending that it explains everything. This model will have to consider structural factors with an emphasis on the dialectic relationships between the latter and ethnicity.

In short, if our studies reinforce the importance of developing a certain cultural competency within our organizations and with our staff, this means going beyond using the tool box (knowledge and skills) when intervening with persons identified as belonging to ethnic minorities. This approach, qualified by Kaufert (1990) as the "boxification" of culture, gives way to the idea that cultural competency is restricted to one enormous matrix of values, beliefs and attitudes that should be consulted in order to know how to intervene with a person belonging to such or such ethnic group. On the contrary, this competency must rest on an analysis that, while taking into account cultural differences, places them in the socio-economic context of the groups in question. As McCall and his colleagues indicate, the more staff know about their clients, the more they consider in their analyses of their clients' problems the complex nature of existing relationships and social conditions, the less they will include culture in that analyses:

> We are less differentiated by our cultures of origin than united by the conditions in which we live: conditions of housing, inequalities of income, health problems, aging, isolation, conjugal violence, single parenthood, despair of being out of work. (McCall et al., 1997)

By taking an approach that ignores structural factors, we run the risk of reducing the problems of immigrant persons with disabilities and their families to problems of a cultural nature. By doing so, we risk blaming immigrant families for their reluctance to use services or by further limiting their access to needed services already available based upon the assumption that they do not want or need formal support. By implicitly excluding immigrant people from mainstream services they will have no other choice but to do without or to begin setting up their own culturally-specific services. This can lead to self-managed exclusion (Massé, 1995) in which immigrants with disabilities and their families are seen as being resistant to support, an assumption that our research suggests is highly problematic. It ignores the potential reality that immigrants with disabilities and their families, like all people with disabilities and their families, have difficulty accessing services or are ambivalent about doing so, given the current climate of scarcity and medicalization of formal care in public sector agencies across Canada.

References

Angel, J.L., Angel, R.J. & Markides, K.S. (2000), Late-Life immigration, changes in living arrangements, and headship status among older Mexican-origin individuals. *Social Science Quaterly, vol 81*, no 1, p. 389-403.

Angel, R.J. & Angel J.L. (1997). Health service use and long-term care among Hispanics. In Markides, K.S. & Miranda, M.R. (Eds). *Minorities, aging and health.* Thousand Oaks (California), Sage Publications, 343-366.

Angel, R.J. & Angel, J.L. (1999). *Who will care for us? Aging and long-term care in multi-cultural America.* New York, University Press.

Aranda, M.P. & Knignt, B.G. (1997). The influence of ethnicity and culture on the caregiver stress and coping process: A sociocultural review and analysis. *The Gerontologist, 37*, 342-354.

Armstrong, Pat, Boscoe, Madeline, Clow, Barbara, Grant, Karen R., Guberman, Nancy, Haworth-Brockman, Margaret, Jackson, Beth E, Pederson, Ann, Seeley, Morgan & Willson, Kay, It's about time: women defined quality care. Under review, *Time and Society* (submitted August 2007).

Asai, M.O. & Kameoka, V.A. (2005). The influence of Sekentei on family caregiving and underutilization of social services among Japanese caregivers.. *Social Work, 50*, 111-118.

Baker, PA. (2006). *The living arrangements of older west Indian migrant women in the United States.* Unpublished PhD thesis, Case Western Reserve University, Cleveland, OH.

Balgopal, P.R. (1999). Getting Old in the U.S.: Dilemnas of Indo-Americans. *Journal of Sociology and Social Welfare, 26*, 51-68.

Bennett, J.M. (1986). Modes of cross-cultural training: conceptualizing cross-cultural training as education.. *International Journal of Intercultural Relations, 10*, 117-134.

Brotman, S. (2003), The limits of multiculturalism in elder care services. *Journal of Aging Studies,* vol 17, p. 209-229.

Brotman, S. (2002). The primacy of family in elder care discourse: Home care services to older ethnic women in Canada..*Journal of Gerontological Social Work 38*(3), 19-52.

Brotman, S. (2001). The dilemma of prolonged engagement: Building opportunities for reciprocity among ethnic women and workers in elder care. In D.N. Weisstub, D.C. Thomasma, S. Gauthier & G.F. Tomossy (eds.) *Aging: Caring for our elders* (pp. 139-163). Volume 11 of the

International library of ethics, law, and the new medicine. Dordrecht: Kluwer Academic Publishers.

Burr, J.A. & Mutchler, J.E. (1993). Nativity, acculturation, and economic status: Explanations of Asian American living arrangements in later life. *Journal of Gerontology: Social Sciences, 48*, S55-S63.

Calderon-Rosado, V. Morrill, V., Chang, B.H. & Tennstedt, S. (2002). Service utilization among disabled Puerto-Rican elders and their caregivers: Does acculturation play a role? *Journal of Aging and Mental Health, 14*, 3-23.

Capitman, J. (2002). Defining diversity: A primer and a review. *Generations, 26,* 8-14.

Chiu, S. & Yu, S. (2001). An excess of culture: the myth of shared care in the Chinese community in Britain. *Ageing and Society, 21*, 681-699.

Clément, S. & Lavoie, J.P. (2001). L'interface formel-informel au confluent de rationalités divergentes (pp. 97-119). In Henrard, J.C., Firbank, O., Clément, S., Frossard, M., Lavoie, J.P. & Vézina, A. (Eds). *Personnes âgées dépendantes en France et au Québec. Qualité de vie, pratiques et politiques.* Paris, INSERM.

Cohen-Emérique, M. (1984). Choc culturel et relations interculturelles dans la pratique des travailleurs sociaux. Formation à la méthode des incidents-critiques. *Cahiers de Sociologie économique et culturelle, 2*, 183-218.

Dai, Y-T & Diamond, M.F. (1998). A cross-cultural comparison and its implications for the well-being of Older Parents. *Journal of Gerontololgical Nursing, 24,* 13-18.

Delgado, M. & Tennstedt, S. (1997). Making the case for culturally appropriate community services: Puerto Rican elders and their caregivers..*Health and Social Work, 22,* 246-255.

Devore, W. & Schlesinger, E. (1987). *Ethnic-sensitive social work practice.* Columbus, Ohio, Merrill.

Dilworth-Anderson, P. & Gibson, B.E. (1999). Ethnic minority perspectives on dementia, family caregiving, and interventions. *Generations, 23,* 40-45

Dubé, L., Ferland, G. & Moskowitz, D.S. (2003). *Emotional & interpersonal dimensions of health services.* Montreal, McGill-Queen's University Press.

Durst, D. (2005). Aging Amongst Immigrants in Canada: Population Drift. *Canadian Studies in Population, 32,* 257-270.

Firbank, O.E. & Johnson-Lafleur, J. (2007). Older persons relocating with a family caregiver: processes, stages, and motives. *Journal of Applied Gerontology, 26,* 182-207.

Fitzpatrick, T.R. & Freed, A.O. (2000). Older Russian immigrants to the USA. Their utilization of health services. *International Social Work, 43,* 305-323.

Forbat, L. (2003). Concepts and understandings of dementia by 'Gatekeepers' and minority ethnic 'service users.' *Journal of Health Psychology, 8,* 645-655.

Fung, K., & Wong, Y-L. (2007). Factors influencing attitudes towards seeking professional help among East and Southeast Asian immigrant and refugee women. *International Journal of Social Psychiatry, 53,* 216-231.

Gelfand, D.E. (2003). *Aging and ethnicity: Knowledge and services. 2nd Edition.* New York, NY: Springer Publishing Company, Inc.

Guberman, N., Lavoie, J.P. & Gagnon, É. (2005). *Valeurs et normes de la solidarité familiale: Statu quo, évolution, mutation?* Côte-St-Luc, CSSS Cavendish – CAU.

Guberman, N., Maheu, P. & Maillé, C. (1993). *Travail et soins aux proches dépendants.* Montréal, Les éditions du remue-ménage.

Guberman, N., Maheu, P. & Maillé, C., (1991). *Et si l'amour ne suffisait pas?: Femmes, familles et adultes dépendants.* Montréal, Les éditions du remue-ménage.

Ivey, A.E., Ivey, M.B. & Simek-Morgan, L. (1997). *Counselling and psychotherapy: A multicultural perspective,* 4th Edition. Boston, Allyn & Bacon.

Janevic, M.R. & Connell. C.M. (2001). Racial, Ethnic, and Cultural Differences in the dementia caregiving experience: Recent findings. *The Gerontologist, 41,* 334-347.

Jenkins, S. (1988). *Ethnic associations and the welfare state.* New York, NY: Columbia University School of Social Work.

Kadushin, A. (1983). *The social work interview.* Washington, Columbia University Press.

Kalavar, J.M., & Van Willigen, J. (2005). Older Asian Indians resettled in America: Narratives about households, culture and generation.. *Journal of Cross-Cultural Gerontology, 20,* 213-230.

Kaufert, P.A. (1990). The boxification of culture: The role of the social scientist. *Santé-Culture-Health, 7,* 139-48.

Kosloski, K., Montgomery, R.J.V. & Karner, T.X. (1999). Differences in the perceived need for assistive services by culturally diverse caregivers of persons with dementia. *The Journal of Applied Gerontology, 18,* 239-256.

Lai, D.W.L. (2004). Use of home care services by elderly Chinese immigrants. *Home Health Care Services Quarterly, 23,* 41-56.

Lai, D.W.L., & Kalyniak, S. (2005). Use of annual physical examinations by aging Chinese Canadians. *Journal of Aging & Health, 17,* 573-591.

Lan, P.C. (2002). Subcontracting filial piety. elder care in ethnic Chinese immigrant families in California. *Journal of Family Issues, 23,* 812-835.

Lavoie, J.P. (2000). *Familles et soutien aux parents âgés dépendants.* Paris, L'Harmattan.

Lavoie, J.P., Guberman, N., Battaglini, A., Belleau, H., Brotman, S., Montejo, M.E. & Hallouche, K. (2006). Entre le soin et l'insertion. L'expérience de familles d'immigration récente qui prennent soin d'un proche. *Côte St-Luc, CREGÉS,* CSSS Cavendish – CAU.

Liu, Y-L. (2003). Aging service need and use among Chinese American seniors: Intragroup variations. *Journal of Cross-Cultural Gerontology, 18,* 273-301.

Luna, I., Torres de Ardon, E., Lin, Y.M., Cromwell, S.L., Phillips, L.R. & Russell, C.K. (1996). The relevance of familism in cross-cultural studies of family caregiving. *Western Journal of Nursing Research, 18,* 267-283.

Lum, T.Y. (2005). Understanding the racial and ethnic differences in caregiving arrangements. *Journal of Gerontological Social Work, 45,* 3-21.

Ma, A. & Chi, I. (2005). Utilization and accessibility of social services for Chinese Canadians. *International Social Work, 48,* 148-160.

Markides, K.S. (1998). Challenges to minority aging research in the next century. *The Jour-nal of Applied Gerontology, 17,* 129-132.

Massé, R. (1995). *Culture et santé publique.* Montréal, Gaétan Morin Editeur.

Mausbach, B.T., Coon, D.W., Depp, C., Rabinowitz, Y.G., Wilson-Arias, E., Kraemer, H.C., Thompson, L.W., Lane, G. & Gallagher-Thompson, D. (2004). Ethnicity and time to institutionalization of dementia patients: A comparison of Latina and Caucasian female family caregivers. *Journal of the American Geriatrics Society, 52* 1077-1084.

McCall, C., Tremblay, L. & Le Goff, F. (1997). *Proximité et distance,* Montréal, Éditions Saint-Martin.

Min, J.W. (2005). Preference for long-term care arrangement and its correlates for older Korean Americans. *Journal of Aging and Health, 17,* 363-395.

Patterson, F.M. (2004). Policy and practice implications from the lives of aging international migrant women. *International Social Work, 47,* 25-37.

Pinquart, M. & Sörensen, S. (2005). Ethnic differences in stressors, ressources, and psychological outcomes of family caregiving : A Meta-analysis. *The Gerontologist, 45,* 90-106.

Radina, E.M. & Barber, C.E. (2004). Utilization of formal support services among Hispanic Americans caring for aging parents. *Journal of Gerontological Social Work, 43,* 5-23.

Salari, S. (2002). Invisible in aging research: Arab Americans, Middle Eastern immigrants, and Muslims in the United States. *The Gerontologist, 42,* 580-588.

Samaoli, O. (2000). *Vieillesse, démence et immigration. Pour une prise en charge adaptée des personnes âgées migrantes en France, au Danemark et au Royaume-Uni.* Paris: L'Harmattan.

Strumpf, N.E., Glicksman, A., Goldberg-Glen, R.S., Fox, R.C. & Logue, E.H. (2001). Caregiver and elder experiences of Cambodian, Vietnamese, Soviet Jewish, and Ukrainian Refugees. *International Journal of aging and human development, 53,* 233-252

Tennstedt, S.L., Chang, B.H. & Delgado M. (1998), Patterns of long-term care: A comparison of Puerto Rican, African-American, and Non-Latino white elders. *Journal of Gerontological Social Work, 30,* 179-199.

Turcotte, M. & Schellenberg, G. (2007). *A portrait of seniors in Canada: 2006.* Ottawa: Statistics Canada. Retrieved January 29, 2008, from Statistics Canada: http://www.statcan.ca/english/freepub/89-519-XIE/89-519-XIE2006001.pdf.

Turner, S., Christie, A. & Haworth, E. (2005). South Asian and white older people and dementia: A qualitative study of knowledge and attitudes. *Diversity in Health & Social Care, 2,* 197-209.

Wilmoth, J.M. (2001). Living Arrangements Among Older Immigrants in the United States. *The Gerontologist, 41,* 228-238.

Wong, S.T., Yoo, G.J. & Stewart, A.L. (2005). Examining the types of social support and the actual sources of support in older Chinese and Korean immigrants. *International Journal of Aging and Human Development, 61,* 105-121.

Yeo, G. & Gallagher-Thompson, D. (Eds.) (1996). *Ethnicity and the dementias.* Washington (D.C.), Taylor and Francis.

6

*The Incidence of Poverty Among Canada's Elderly Immigrants**

Hugh Grant and James Townsend, (The University of Winnipeg)

Introduction

A dramatic decline in the incidence of poverty among the elderly is heralded as "one of Canada's biggest success stories in social policy during the latter part of the 20th Century" (National Council of Welfare, 2002, p. 129). In 1980, 34% of elderly Canadians lived below the poverty line, a rate roughly twice that for all Canadians; by 1998, poverty among the elderly had fallen to 18%, approximating that among the population as a whole.

This accomplishment is largely attributed to the expanded coverage of both public and private pension plans, as well as the impact of Registered Retirement Savings Plans (RRSPs) on personal savings. By international standards, Canada was relatively slow to adopt publicly-funded pension plans; it did so 35 years after the United States and some eighty years later than Germany (Osberg, 2001) but the resulting reduction in the rate of poverty among its elderly population is no less remarkable. Myles, however, offers a cautionary note:

> Earnings-related pensions are not the usual policy instruments one thinks of
> when considering reducing income inequality or low-income rates among seniors.
> They are aimed, after all, at reproducing the income differentials created during
> the working years. Since a large share of benefits in all such plans goes to mid-
> dle and upper income families, it is often argued that the social insurance (i.e.,

*This chapterr is based upon research originally prepared for the Law Commission of Canada. The document expresses the views of the authors and does not necessarily represent the opinion of the Law Commission of Canada. The accuracy of the information contained in the papers is the sole responsiblility of the authors. Also acknowledged is the generous support of the Prairie Centre of Excellence for Research on Immigration and Integration.

earnings-related) model creates welfare states for the middle class that do little
to help the poor or achieve more equality. (Myles, 2000, p.2)

If Myles' intuition is correct, the vulnerability of the elderly without significant previous employment earnings, and, therefore without substantial employment-based pension benefits, is likely to remain high.

One such group is elderly immigrants to Canada. There are several reasons why their incomes, in general, and their receipt of pension benefits in particular, are expected to be relatively modest. First, since many immigrants arrive with little savings by virtue of a disruption in their working lives or because their pension entitlements are not portable between countries, they have a relatively short window in which to accumulate sufficient savings for their retirement. Second, there is a substantial literature that documents the different labor market experience of immigrants. Compared to non-immigrants with similar education and employment experience, they tend to receive lower annual earnings upon first entering the Canadian labor market, and while their annual income may gradually "catch-up" to and exceed what native-born Canadians receive, it is unlikely that it does so at a fast enough rate to generate equivalent career earnings (Baker & Benjamin, 1994; Bloom et al., 1995; Grant, 1999). Third, among the immigrant population 60 years of age and older, Basavarajappa (1999) observes extreme inequality in income. Taken together, it is likely that many immigrants do not accumulate sufficient savings during their employment career to provide an adequate income upon retirement. Existing data confirms that elderly immigrants are at greater risk of living in poverty. In 1995, the incidence of poverty among elderly immigrant men (17.5%) and immigrant women (26.5%) was much higher than that for non-immigrants (among men 11.5% and among women 23.0%). Nor is this a minor exception. In 1995, immigrants composed 27% of Canada's population 65 years of age and older and this percentage is expected to grow over the next two decades (Statistics Canada, 1996).

This chapterr examines the determinants of poverty among Canada's elderly immigrants and the implications for social policy. First, the published data is reviewed on the rate of poverty among the elderly in the context of Canada's social policy and then examine the economic status of elderly immigrants to Canada and the extent to which they are particularly vulnerable to poverty. The 2006 Census microfiles are used in order to apply a binomial logit analysis of the determinants of low-income status among Canada's elderly people.

This analysis finds that gender, family structure and the standard proxies for human capital play a significant role in determining one's likelihood of poverty after reaching age 65, and that immigration status and the age of arrival in Canada tend to intensify this vulnerability. The results suggests that less emphasis must be placed on employment-based benefits if further improvements in the living standards of elderly Canadians are to be achieved.

Poverty Rates Among Canada's Elderly

The most readily available poverty data in Canada, published annually by the National Council of Welfare, is derived from Statistics Canada's analysis based on the Low-Income Cut Off (LICO) line (National Council of Welfare 2006, p. 126). Figure 1 displays the rapid decline in the incidence of poverty among elderly Canadians between 1976 and 2007. While the rate of poverty for the entire Canadian population fluctuated between 14 and 18% over the period, it fell from 43 to 13% among the elderly. Since 1995, poverty rates for the elderly have been similar to those for the general population.

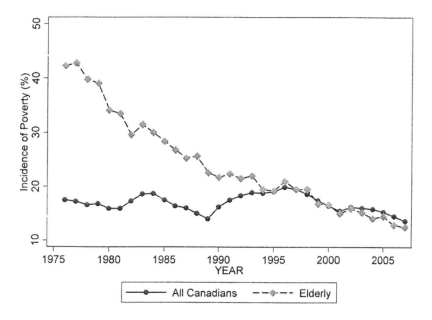

Figure 1: The Incidence of Poverty in Canada – All Canadian and the Elderly.
Source: Statistics Canada, Table 202-0802

There are four well-known caveats with respect to the effort to identify the poor and measure the inadequacy of their income (Hagenaars, 1991) and each merits consideration when applied to the elderly. The first is the extent to which annual income – rather than consumption or wealth – is the relevant focus of analysis. Following Sen (1976), poverty can be defined in terms of "capability deprivation," or one's inability to participate fully in community life. While this deprivation may have several causes, the most prevalent is the lack of an adequate level of income. Since earnings vary over the life cycle, however, individuals tend to smooth out their annual consumption by saving during periods of high income, and dis-saving when their annual income is lower. Since wealth tends to increase with age, the elderly are expected to enjoy more in-kind benefits in the form of housing services.

The second caveat pertains to the appropriate unit of analysis, whether it be by individual, different family types or the household. The two most commonly-adopted units of analysis are "unattached individual" (defined as "a person living either alone or with others to who her or she is unrelated") and "economic family" ("a group of two or more persons who live in the same dwelling and are related to each other by blood, marriage, common-law or adoption") (Statistics Canada, 2005). Figure 2 disaggregates the data for elderly people according to family status and gender. For elderly couples, the incidence of poverty fell from 29.3 to 4.2 per cent, the latter figure well below that for the Canadian population as a whole (13.6%). In contrast, elderly unattached individuals continue to experience alarmingly high rates of poverty despite the significant decline since 1980 (from 72 to 35% for women, and for 61 to 28% for men). Phipps and Burton (1995), however, emphasize the extent to which the sharing of income and other resources within families can have a profound influence on the standard of living of individuals. To the extent that the elderly are more likely than the

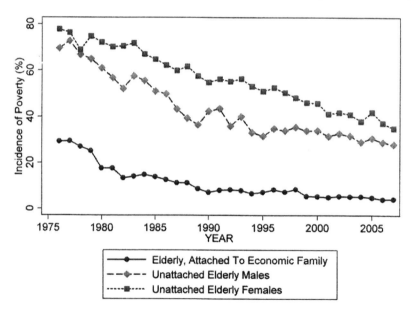

Figure 2. The Incidence of Poverty by Family Status – Elderly Canadians. Source: Statistics Canada, Table 202-0802.

general population to receive income transfers from their immediate relatives, poverty data may not properly reflect the inadequacy of their own income, but overstate the degree to which their consumption is beneath a socially-defined minimum. Using administrative data, Baker and Benjamin (2002) find that immigrants arriving later in life are most likely to be admitted under the "family class," which requires sponsorship by family members within Canada that have achieved either citizenship or permanent residence status. In the case of such sponsorship:

> Sponsors must sign a contract with the Ministry of Citizenship and Immigration called an Undertaking. This contract outlines the sponsor's promise to financially support the sponsored immigrant for a period of up to 10 years. The contract is intended to ensure that the sponsored immigrants do not become dependent on Canadian social assistance. (Baker & Benjamin, 2002, p. 4)

This suggests that income transfers from family members may be of particular importance for elderly immigrants that arrive to Canada late in life.

The third concern is with respect to the often-visited debate around the appropriate standard of the minimum income necessary to be free of poverty. Statistics Canada offers two definitions of the low-income threshold. The LICO is

> an income threshold below which a family will likely devote a larger share of its income to the necessities of food, shelter and clothing than an average family would. When the cutoff was first established on the basis of the 1959 Family Expenditures Survey (FAMEX), an average family spent 50% of its pre-tax income on these necessities. Twenty points were added to this percentage on the assumption that a family spending 70% of its income on those items would be "in strained circumstance." (Paquet, 2001, p. 10).

By focusing on the basic necessities of life, the LICO may be seen as an attempt to provide an absolute measure of the poverty threshold; however, the 70% benchmark has been regularly recalculated downward (in 1969, 1978, 1986 and 1992) according to observed spending behavior of the average family on basic necessities. The LICO, therefore, is a hybrid concept, resting rather uneasily on both a relative and absolute conception of poverty. In contrast, the Low Income Measure (LIM) offers a purely relative measure of poverty. Defined as 50% of the median income according to an individual's family and community size, as the median income rises, so too does the LIM. It tends to generate a higher minimum income threshold and a lower rate of poverty than the LICO.

Osberg (2001, p. 18) observes that estimated rate of poverty among the elderly is particularly sensitive to the choice of low-income threshold. Since incomes of a large proportion of the elderly are solely dependent on government transfers and public pension benefits, many have the same income which yields a "spike" in the income distribution. This clustering of incomes around a fairly low level of income, may result in the small differences in the low-income cutoff yielding large differences in the estimated rate of poverty. Figures 3a and 3b display the distribution of income in 2005 among elderly unattached and attached (living in a family) individuals respectively. The impact of government transfer payments and pension benefits is most apparent among unattached individuals: less than 5% of elderly persons received less than $12 500; 13.9% received between $12 500 and $14 999; and 17.2% received between $15 000 and $17 499. In comparison, the LICO for an unattached individual living in Toronto in 2005 was $21 199. Income distribution among the elderly living in families is less concentrated; however, a much higher proportion received less than $10 000.

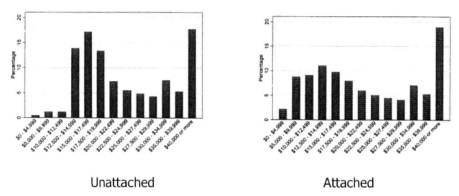

Unattached   Attached

Figure 3. 2000 Income Distribution of Elderly Individuals, by economic family structure

Fourth, while the incidence of poverty provides the important preliminary insight of identifying the number of poor, Sen (1976) argues that it is not sufficient to capture the intensity of poverty. Specifically, the former does not indicate the extent that the incomes of the poor fall below the minimum threshold or, stated from a policy perspective, how much of income would be needed to eradicate poverty by bringing the incomes of the poor up to the threshold. This distinction can be important. Osberg (2000), for instance, finds that although the poverty rate has generally been lower in Canada compared to the United States, the depth of poverty, or the relative hardship experience by those below the low-income threshold, is worse.

These qualifications notwithstanding, there is little doubt that overall poverty among Canada's elderly has been significantly reduced. Since the early 1970s, there has been a steady expansion in the value and coverage of the Canada and Quebec Pension Plans (CPP/QPP) in employer-sponsored pension plans and in investment income derived from RRSPs. When added to universal Old Age Security (OAS) and means-tested Guaranteed Income Supplement (GIS) benefits, the average income of elderly Canadians grew more rapidly than that of the population as a whole between

1971 and 1986 (Oja and Love, 1988). Women benefited less than men from these pension changes. Despite the rising participation rate of women in the paid labor force, the expanded provisions for survivor benefits in pension plans, and legal changes that require pension entitlements to be split upon divorce, the income of many elderly women remained largely untouched by the expansion in employment-based pension benefits (Boyd, 1989). Instead, it was the growth in investment income that caused the gap in average income between elderly men and women to narrow from roughly one half to one third between 1971 and 1985 (Oja and Love, 1988).

Myles suggests that "trends in the next decade are more likely to be dominated by continued maturation of employer pensions and personal retirement accounts" (2000, p. 19). Since employment-based benefits tend to affect disproportionately individuals that enjoyed a relatively high income during their work career; however, increasing inequality among the elderly may be anticipated. One group likely to benefit less from the increasing impact of pension benefits are immigrants to Canada.

Poverty Among Elderly Canadian Immigrants

The "economic integration" of immigrants or the capacity of the host economy to "absorb" new immigrants has been the major focus of research on the economics of immigration. In Canada, this has spawned an extensive literature that compares the labor market behavior and age-earnings profiles of immigrants relative to their native-born counterparts. While the empirical results vary depending upon the "cohort" group based on year of arrival, three clear trends emerge.

First, immigrants tend to have a higher rate of participation in the paid labor force and tend to work longer hours. This reflects a smaller accumulation of savings or wealth or a relatively late entry into the labor market, often due to interruptions in their working lives caused by economic and political events. The relatively high rate of labor force participation is especially the case among women immigrants as the incidence of two-income families tends to be greater among immigrants than non-immigrants (Worswick, 1996, 1999).

Second, after adjusting for all measurable productivity characteristics (such as education, work experience, and language skills) immigrant workers face an "entry penalty" in terms of a lower initial wage relative to their native-born counterparts. Over time, however, the earnings of immigrants gradually "catch-up" with those of native-born workers who possess equivalent skills. Interpretations of this "economic integration" vary. On the one hand, it may reflect the acquisition of "unobservable skills" (such as greater English to French language proficiency or greater familiarity with Canadian cultural norms) it may reflect the gradual decline in discrimination faced by new immigrants, particularly visible minorities, as they acculturate.

Third, the rate of economic integration indeed, whether or not immigrants' incomes ever "catch up" to those of native born during their working lives has varied significantly among different cohort groups depending upon their year of arrival. Evidence from the 1981 and 1991 Census indicated that more recent immigrant cohorts experienced a higher initial entry penalty and a much slower rate of integration such that the prospect of ever catching up with the earnings of their native-born counterparts was unlikely (Bloom et al., 1995). More recently, an exhaustive examination of the 1991 Census suggests a break in the pattern. While the 1981-85 cohort had lower initial earnings than the previous cohort, the following group arriving in 1986-90 had earnings that were approximately equal to those of the 1981-85 cohort, pointing to the possibility that the decline in entry earnings of successive cohorts has stopped. As well, the integration rate of the 1981-85 cohort was found to be 17.2 per cent over the first five years in the country, compared to a 0 per cent integration rate over the first five years for those immigrants arriving between 1976-80 (Grant 1999).

A separate question, unaddressed in the literature, concerns the post-retirement incomes of immigrants. The simple life-cycle model implies that individuals will save during their working lives in order to accumulate sufficient wealth for their retirement years and during retirement, their assets gradually diminish as they dis-save (Modigliani and Brumberg, 1954). In effect, individuals seek to "smooth out" their life-time consumption when their annual income varies significantly over time. For the elderly, future income is known with reasonable certainty (notwithstanding variations in the rates of inflation and interest), but one's longevity may not be. With perfect fore-sight regarding longevity, wealth should fall to zero at the time of death or, under the more realistic assumption of uncertain longevity, wealth will gradually diminish as the retiree ages. Alternatively, if leaving a bequest is an important goal, the rate of dis-saving may be less acute.

Empirical investigation of life-cycle models finds that proxies for human capital (the level of education and years of work experience) as well as gender, marital status, ethnicity and cohort effects play a major role in explaining the heterogeneity in the saving behavior of American households (Hildebrand 2001). For the elderly with children, the "bequest motive" is also found to be a significant determinant of dis-saving. The overriding result, however, is that many individuals or households do not accumulate sufficient wealth for their retirement years, which results in a greater dependence on government transfers, a high incidence of low income, and a gradual decline in total income with age.

As insightful as this literature is, it has not considered the importance of immigration status on the age-earnings and age-wealth profiles. Even if the rate of economic integration is sufficiently high such that immigrants' earnings indeed catch up to those of non-immigrants, it is not clear whether their life-long employment earnings provide sufficient savings for their retirement years. This argument is stylized in Figure 4. Assume that an immigrant enters the country in age 'a' to begin his or her working life in Canada. After adjusting for all "observable" differences in productivity (education level, work experience and language skills), the immigrant faces an entry penalty 'e' in terms of a lower initial wage, but enjoys a faster increase in annual income with greater experience in the Canadian labor market. This more rapid rate of increase in income is attributed to the economic integration which occurs. The immigrant's annual income then catches up to the non-immigrants (with the same observable skills) at age 'c'. If, however, income catches up sufficiently late in the immigrant's working life, his or her lifetime earnings may be lower and, assuming similar rates of savings, the immigrant enjoys a lower income during retirement, starting at age 'r'.

It follows that if immigrants enter the Canadian labor market at a relatively late age, the age-earnings profile is attenuated and the likelihood of their incomes catching up to that of the native-born counterpart is reduced. Accordingly, their accumulated saving will be less and that income gap at retirement will be greater. Moreover, an important corollary is that incidence of poverty among the elderly at a point in time may reflect historical trends in the distribution of income in the general population. Of particular importance in this regard is the possibility that the relatively difficult economic circumstances faced by particular cohorts of immigrants – such as those arriving in the early 1980s – may eventually be reflected in poverty data among the elderly.

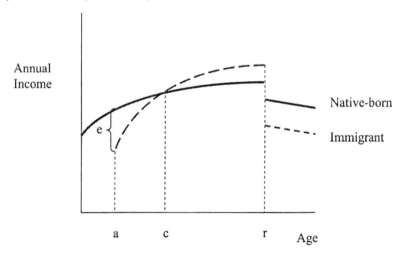

Figure 4. Hypothetical Income Paths of Imigrant and Native-born Canadians

The Incidence and Determinants of Poverty Among the Elderly

The 2006 Census (Statistics Canada, 2006) microdata file permits an examination of the incidence and determinants of low-income status for the elderly in Canada. Retaining only those individuals 65 years of age and older leaves a sample consisting of 778 515 individuals, representing 3 976 970 Canadians in this age group. In Table 1, we present the incidence of poverty for elderly men and women based on immigration status. For each group, we also present poverty rates by economic family status, educational attainment, official languages spoken, and where applicable, age of arrival to Canada and region of birth. An individual is classified as poor if the combined income of the individual's economic family in 2005 was below the appropriate Low Income Cut-off (LICO). All figures are computed using the sample weights provided with the Census and are representative of the population of seniors in Canada.

In 2005, the incidence of low income status among elderly immigrants (12.5% among men and 20.1% among women) was higher than that for native-born (8.0% among men and 17.6 % among women). Consistent with the results in Section 2, poverty is much higher among unattached individuals, with rates ranging from 26.7% for native-born men to a staggering 43.8% for immigrant women. High levels of poverty are also evident for immigrants originating from regions characterized by developing economies; for example, males from West Asia and the Middle East face poverty rates of 28.3%, while females from the same region face poverty rates of 35.7%. Poverty rates for male and female immigrants originating from regions of the world with "developed" countries have similar poverty rates to those of native-born Canadians. For immigrants, a later age of arrival is also associated with significantly higher rates of poverty. Immigrant males and females that arrived before turning 30 experience poverty rates similar to or below those of native-born Canadians. In contrast, those that arrived later in life face accentuated poverty rate.

For both men and women, greater educational attainment is associated with a decline in the probability of being poor, regardless of immigration status. This likely reflects the role of education as human capital; individuals with more education were able to earn more during their working life, and consequently they were also able to save more for retirement. Language also played a role in the probability of being poor. Individuals able to speak at least one official language faced a lower probability of being poor. If English was spoken, the probability was further reduced.

Although the overall rates of poverty are similar by gender for immigrants and the native born, this analysis shows a heightened incidence of poverty for immigrants arriving later in life and for immigrants that were born in certain regions of the world. Furthermore, the ability to speak at least one official language and higher levels of education reduce the probability of being poor.

	Male		Female	
Table 1 **Incidence of Poverty for the Elderly, by Gender and Immigrant Status,**				
	Native Born	Immigrant	Native Born	Immiigrant
All	8.0	12.5	17.6	20.1
Attached to an economic family				
Attached	3.1	9.2	3.6	9.4
Unattached	26.7	32.4	36.6	43.8
Age of Immigration				
Less than 20		7.2		15.5
20-29		7.6		14.1
30-39		9.7		18.6
40-49		15.3		25.9
50-59		25.2		31.2
60 and above		28.5		27.8
Place of Birth				
Canada	8.0		17.6	
USA, W. Europe, Oceania		7.6		15.4
Eastern Europe		11.8		24.4
W.Cent. Asia, Middle East		28.3		35.7
South Asia		14.8		15.4
East/South-East Asia		24.2		26.7
Africa		18.7		28.7
Central and South America		19.8		28.1
Educational Attainment				
Less than High School	11.0	14.7	24.0	23.2
High School Diploma	7.5	15.2	14.1	17.6
To College diploma	6.1	9.0	12.0	15.4
University Degree	3.7	12.1	7.2	15.5
Knowledge of Official Language				
English	6.5	10.3	14.1	17.6
French	12.2	20.0	26.7	31.4
Both	9.5	12.3	19.6	18.2
Neither	8.5	25.2	16.5	27.8
N	239 725	108 150	304 615	125 975
Notes: Authors' tabulations, 2006 Census microfile.				

Many of the characteristics examined above are likely to be correlated, making it difficult to assess the relative importance of any one factor in contributing to the probability that an individual will be poor. To isolate how particular characteristics are related to the probability of being under the poverty line, we use a logit model to estimate the probability of being poor conditional on the various characteristics outlined before. The methodology, described in detail in the appendix, involves establishing a reference group, which is defined by a set of characteristics commonly observed in the data set (e.g., English-speaking native-born men with a high school education, and examining how changes in each characteristic (e.g., a university degree) changes the probability of being poor. The change in probability is the "marginal" effect of the characteristic in question. The results are sensitive to the choice of reference group. By using a common "type" of individual, we provide some insight into the relative importance of various characteristics in accounting for differences in poverty groups across groups. In what follows, we identify the characteristics of the relevant reference group.

Figure 5 shows the role of birthplace on poverty. The comparison group is an individual that is 65–69 years old, attached to an economic family, speaks English, has completed a high school education, and is Canadian-born. (The fitted probability of being poor is .064 for men and .057 for women.) Certain regions are associated with a substantial increase in poverty, even after accounting for possible differences in levels of education attainment, family arrangements and so forth. These include West Central Asia and the Middle East, East and South-East Asia, Central and South America, and Africa. We report these results without attempting an explanation, except to note that poverty increases for immigrants from developing countries as opposed to Europe and the United States.

Figure 6 shows the effect of age of arrival. The comparison group is again 65 years old, attached to an economic family, speaks English, has not completed a high school education, and is Canadian-born. The results for age of arrival indicate that immigrants that arrived in the first twenty years of life from a developed country are no more likely to face poverty than native-born Canadians. This is not true for later arrivals; late arrival increases the probability of being poor and this effect is stronger for men. Immigrant men that arrived between ages 40-49 faced a 3.8% greater probability of being low income in retirement; for women, the probability is only 2.6% greater. For men arriving their fifties, the probability of being poor increases by 12.5%.

Figure 7 shows the effect on poverty of a number of characteristics not directly related to immigration status. This includes attachment to an economic family, languages spoken, and educational attainment. Results are organized around the same four groupings used in Table 1. In each case, the comparison group is 65-69 years of age, is attached to an economic family, speaks English, and has completed a high-

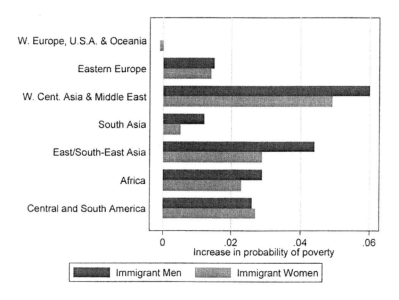

Figure 5. Marginal Effects of Birthplace on Poverty.

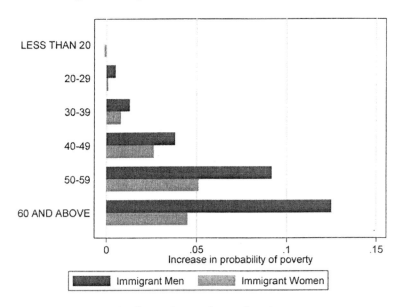

Figure 6. Marginal Effects of Age of Arrival on Poverty

school education; for immigrants, the comparison group arrived to Canada in the first 20 years of life and the place of birth was in Western Europe. Marginal effects are computed for those that differ from this group in one dimension. Individuals that are not attached to an economic family face a substantially increased risk of being low income. The effect is larger for woman than for men, regardless of immigration status. While this partly reflects the economic benefits of cohabitation and the sharing of income that occurs within families, the nature of government income policies for the elderly probably has a more direct bearing on this result. In the absence of personal savings, from both private pensions and otherwise, government transfer payments and pensions are simply too low to ensure an escape from poverty.

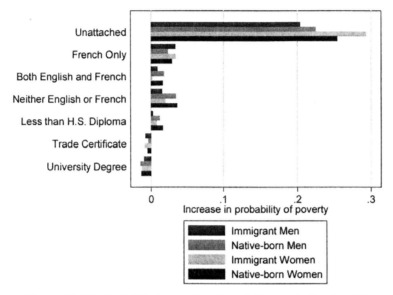

Figure 7. Marginal Effects on Poverty of Economic Family Status. Official Languaes Spoken and Educational Attainment

As expected, higher levels of educational attainment are associated with a lower probability of poverty. This holds for both genders, regardless of immigrant status. The magnitude of the marginal effect of having a university degree is smaller for immigrant males, which is consistent with the view that human capital is often country-specific, such that immigrants who acquire their education in their country of origin find their qualifications less portable or less appropriate to the Canadian labor market.

With respect to knowledge of an official language, our analysis replicates some ambiguous and curious results that previous studies on incomes, language and immigration status have found. Among immigrants, when compared to those who speak only English, knowing neither English or French increases the likelihood of being poor (by 1.5% for men and 2.0% for women); knowledge of French only leads to a somewhat greater increase (3.3% for men and 3.3% for women); while knowledge of both official languages results in a small increase for men (0.9%) and a negligible effect for women. The results are similar for the non-immigrant population; French speakers and those that speak neither official language suffer a much greater likelihood of poverty (There are a total of 96 native-born Canadians in our sample that reportedly speak neither languge.) One possible explanation for why a penalty exists for French speakers may be that that it reflects different labor market conditions inside and out-side of Quebec, as opposed to the actual return on language skills. (In this sample, 78% of French-speakers live in Canada.)

Taken together, the results suggest that the determinants of poverty among the immigrant and non-immigrant elderly population are similar: the effects of education, language and family status are of the same rough order of magnitude. This magnifies the importance of immigration status and, in particular, the age at arrival on the risk of poverty. While there is a statistically insignificant difference in the risk of poverty between non-immigrants and immigrants arriving before the age of 30 years, immi-grants arriving after this age suffer a large economic cost. This supports the contention that it is the years of experience in the Canadian labor market, and therefore the capacity to save for retirement, that determines one's risk of poverty after reaching the normal age of retirement. That the penalty of late arrival is less severe for immigrant women probably reflects the differing degrees of labor force attachment between men and women and their dependence on own-sources of income. In other words, its is immigrant men, more likely destined for the Canadian work force and less likely to be married to a spouse with higher income, that suffer the greatest economic penalty for arriving in Canada at a relatively late age.

Conclusion

Pension reform has led to a significant improvement in the economic lives of eld-erly Canadians, and this is apparent in the rising levels of average income and the declining incidence of poverty since 1960. This is a significant achievement and the cause for celebration. At the same time, however, much economic hardship persists and it is heavily concentrated among immigrants. This being the case, it is appropriate to rethink income maintenance policies for the elderly in Canada and, in particular, the intersection between poverty and immigration status.

Two observations are salient in this regard. First, as Myles argues, reliance upon past employment earnings to provide income upon retirement in the form of public pensions, private pensions and RRSPs tends to reproduce among the elderly the income inequality that existed during their working lives. Concurrently, government transfer payments (OAS and GIS) have contributed to sharply reducing in size the bot-tom tail of the income distribution. These initiatives, taken together, have significantly reduced the incidence of poverty among the elderly living in families; however, the high incidence of poverty among unattached individuals indicates the inadequacy of these initiatives.

Second, the intersection between an immigrant's age of arrival and risk of poverty has prompted calls for greater age-based discrimination in the selection of immigrants. A recent Canadian legislative review recommended a thorough revision of immigration policy with greater emphasis on limiting the costs to society, with a greater emphasis on the immigrant's age singled out as a factor in the selection process (Trempe et al., 1997). Over the past three decades, Canada's immigration policy has been directed towards three objectives: attracting skilled workers selected on the basis of the labor market conditions, accepting family class immigrants to meet the desirable social goal of reunifying families; and offering protection to refugees as a central aspect of Canada's international commitments. If Canada remains committed to the latter two goals of reunifying families, and providing protection to refugees, then it also has an obligation to provide adequate economic opportunities and mitigate their risk of living in poverty. If such a responsibility is acknowledged, then income-maintenance policies for the elderly must rely less upon past employment earnings.

Appendix - Logit Estimation

The determinants of an individual's current income is typically estimated using cross-sectional data and an equation which fits employment income to employment characteristics (such as education, work experience, language skills) and personal characteristics (including marital status, gender and age). Consider a conventional income function:

$$\log(Y) = \alpha_0 + Z_i \alpha_1 + P_i \alpha_2$$

where

$\log(Y)$ = the log of annual employment income;

Z_i = a vector of employment characteristics;

and P_i = a vector of personal characteristics.

Employment (as opposed to total) income is used as the dependent variable in order to capture differences in wages, hours of work, and unemployment rates. Employment characteristics include years of schooling, work experience and language skills as proxies for human capital endowment. Personal characteristics included as explanatory variables differ depending upon the hypothesis to be tested; some studies include marital status to control for expected differences in the choice of hours of work, while others include country of source or ethnicity.

This specification, however, can be expected to yield a poor fit when applied to the elderly since most of their current income is derived from past saving, or from previous as opposed to current employment earnings. Accordingly, we assume that an elderly individual's annual income (Yi) is derived from previous employment earnings which are, in turn, a function of past human capital endowments, personal characteristics and the duration of normal working life spent in Canada. For simplicity, assume that the individual derives a constant annual income derived from accumulated savings at the time of retirement.

$$Y_i = \lambda \sum^{65}(sY_t)(1 + r)^{65-t}$$

Where λ is the rate at which an individual draws down savings in retirement, *s* is the average propensity to save, *r* is the interest rate, *a* is the age of entry into the Canadian labor market, *r* is the interest rate, Y_t is the individual's income at age *t*, and the normal age of retirement is 65 years. The important factor in determining the impact of immigration status upon income is the age of arrival in the Canadian labor market. The conventional earnings function, therefore, can be modified in the following fashion. The standard proxies for human capital endowment (education and language ability) are included, but labor market experience is not explicitly considered since, applying Mincer's rule, it is assumed to be the same for all native-born individuals with the same number of years of education (Mincer's rule assumes that experience is equal to age minus 6 minus years of schooling. It is assumed that all years not spent in early childhood or school were spent working). Personal characteristics included are gender (to capture differences in past labor market attachment); current age (since it is expected that accumulated savings, and therefore current income, decline over time); and family status (to reflect the extent to which income sharing occurs). We do not test for marital status (a standard proxy for labor force attachment) because of the high correlation between marital status and family status. Finally, our analysis of immigration status is restricted to a consideration of the immigrants age of arrival for immigrants, expected to capture the years of potential experience in the Canadian labor force. We do not explicitly consider immigrant cohort effects for two reasons: a) given that one's age and age of arrival are included in the regression equation, year of arrival is redundant; and b) age of arrival and year of arrival are highly correlated when the analysis is restricted to those over the age of 65 years. This yields the following specification:

$$log(INCOME) = \alpha_0 + \alpha_1 EDUCATION + \alpha_2 LANGUAGE + \alpha_3 AGE$$

$$+\alpha_4 GENDER + \alpha_5 FSTATUS + \alpha_6 AGEARRIVAL$$

$$+\alpha_7 BIRTHPLACE + \epsilon$$

where
EDUCATION = educational attainment;
LANGUAGE = knowledge of English and/or French;

AGE = current age;

GENDER = a dummy variable for male or female;

FSTATUS = a dummy variable for whether unattached or living in an economic family;

AGEARRIVAL = for immigrants, their age of arrival in Canada;

BIRTHPLACE = for immigrants; their region of birth;

å = a random error term.

Our interest is not in Yi directly, but in whether total family income falls short of the appropriate LICO for that family. We wish to estimate the probability of this event occurring, conditional on the characteristics listed above. We estimate the probability of being poor by applying a binomial logistic model using 2001 Census data. For an individual with characteristics xi, the probability of being poor is given by

$$Pr(Y_i < LICO) = \frac{exp(x_i\beta)}{1 + exp(x_i\beta)}.$$

Data and description of variables used are summarized in Table A1. The model is estimated for the entire sample of elderly, and for immigrants and non-immigrants separately. Results are reported in Table A2.

Given the difficulty of interpreting the coefficients, (β), of a logit regression, we calculate the marginal effect of various characteristics on the probability of being poor. Results are presented in Table A3 for all characteristics except region of birth, which are presented in Table A4. To do this, we calculate the fitted probability of being low income for a representative "type": in columns (1) and (2) and columns (5) and (6) this type is a native-born English speaking individual aged 65-69 with less than a high school diploma that is attached to an economic family. In columns (3) and (4) the representative type is an English-speaking immigrant from the developed world aged 65-69 with a high school diploma that is attached to an economic family. We then consider how the various characteristics in our regression change the probability of being low income by looking at an individual that is identical to our representative type in all ways but for the characteristic under consideration. These are the "marginal" effects reported in Tables A3 and A4.

Table A-1 Description of Variables and Summary Statistics			
Variable	Description	Categories	Mean
Poor	Incidence of Poverty	Incidence of Poverty	14.3
Age	Current Age	65-69	30.2
		70-74	20.8
		75-79	17.3
		80-84	11.9
		85+	9.1
Immigrant	Immigrated to Canada, Permanent Resident		30.2
Language	Knowledge of an Official Language	English only	66.9
		French only	14.8
		both English and French	13.5
		neither English or French	4.7
Education	Highest degree/Certificate/Diploma	Non High School Graduate	42.4
		High School Graduate	21.4
		Obtained Certificat/Diploma	21.9
		Obtained University Degree	14.2
Male	Male or Female	1 if male; 0 female	44.7
Unattached	Economic Family Status		29.9
Arrival Age	Age of Arrival in Canada	0-19 years	4.2
		20-29 years	9.9
		30-39 years	6.6
		40-49 years	2.9
		50-59 years	3.1
		60+ years	3.5
Birthplace	Region of Birth	Western USA & Oceania	16.3
		Eastern Europe	4.3
		W. Central Asia, Middle East	0.7
		South Asia	1.9
		Africa	0.8
		South/Central America	1.9
n = 96 935			
Source: Authors' tabulations, 2006 Canadian Census Microdata			

Table A-2. Logit Results – Determinants of Poverty						
	All Elderly		Immigrants		Native Born	
	Men	Women	Men	Women	Men	Women
Age						
70-74	-0.17*	-0.14*	-0.08*	-0.07*	-0.23*	-0.17*
75-79	-.0.34*	0.17*	-0.25*	-0.17*	0.39*	-0.16*
80-84	-0.54*	0.15*	-0.46*	-0.28*	-0.59*	-0.08*
85 +	0.41*	0.17*	0.42*	-0.10*	-0.38*	0.28*
Economic Family Status						
Unattached	2.35*	2.75*	2.11*	2.66*	2.45*	2.79*
Age of immigration						
0-19	-0.02	-0.05				
20-29	0.17*	0.03	0.14*	0.01		
30-39	0.37*	0.27*	0.34*	0.28*		
40-49	0.84*	0.71*	0.78*	0.73*		
50-59	1.48*	1.14*	1.39*	1.15*		
60+	1.75*	1.05*	1.64*	1.08*		
Educational Attainment						
<H.S.	0.28*	0.46*	0.08*	0.22*	0.37*	0.55*
College	-.21*	-.28*	-0.27*	-0.33*	-0.18*	-0.26*
University	-0.52*	0.80*	-0.34*	-0.50*	-0.77*	-0.99*
Officia lLanguage						
French	0.62*	0.83*	0.7*	0.73*	0.61*	0.85*
Both	0.42*	0.47*	0.22*	0.06	0.50*	0.56*
Neither	0.29*	0.43*	0.36*	0.50*	0.82*	0.98*
Place of Birth						
E. Europe	0.42*	0.48*	0.40*	0.47*		
W. Central Asia	1.16*	1.17*	1.07*	1.09*		
s. Asia	0.35*	0.25*	0.26*	0.13*		
E./S.E. Asia	0.94*	0.83*	0.83*	0.70*		
Africa	0.71*	0.72*	0.66*	0.69*		
S. America	0.65*	0.80*	0.64*	0.72*		
Constant	-3.44*	-3.63*	-3.26*	-3.38*	-3.53*	-3.75*
n	347 925	430 590	108 150	125 975	239 775	304 615
Note: *Indicates coefficient is significant at .05 level						

Table A-3. Marginal Effects of Age, Educational Attainment, Official Language Spoken, Economic Family Status, and Age of arrival on Being Poor						
	All Elderly		Immigrants		Native Born	
	Men	Women	Men	Women	Men	Women
Age						
70-74	-0.005*	-0.003*	-0.003*	-0.002*	-0.006*	-0.004*
75-79	-0.009*	-0.004*	-0.008*	-0.005*	-0.009*	-0.003*
80-84	-0.013*	-0.003*	-0.013*	-0.008*	-0.012*	-0.002*
85+	-0.010*	0.005*	-0.012*	-0.003*	-0.009*	0.007*
Educational Attainment						
<H.S. Diploma	0.010*	0.014*	0.003*	0.008*	0.012*	0.016*
College	-0.006*	-0.006*	-0.008*	-0.009*	-0.004*	-0.005*
University	-0.012*	-0.014*	-0.010*	-0.013*	-0.015*	-0.014*
Official Languages Spoken						
French	0.025*	0.031*	0.033*	0.033*	0.023*	0.029*
Both	0.015*	0.015*	0.009*	0.002	0.018*	0.016*
Neither	0.010*	0.013*	0.015*	0.020*	0.034*	0.036*
Attachment to Economic Family						
Unattached	0.220*	0.267*	0.204*	0.293*	0.225*	0.254*
Age of Arrival						
0-19	-0.000	-0.001				
20-29	0.005*	0.001	0.005*	0.000		
30-39	0.013*	0.008*	0.014*	0.010*		
40-49	0.038*	0.026*	0.041*	0.033*		
50-59	0.092*	0.051*	0.097*	0.064*		
60+	0.125*	0.045*	0.129*	0.058*		
N	347 925	430 590	108 150	125 975	239 775	

References

Baker, M. & Benjamin, D. 1994. The performance of immigrants in the Canadian labour market. *Journal of Labour Economics 12* (3), 369–405.

Baker, M. & Benjamin, D.. 2002. *Are elderly immigrants a burden?* Paper presented at the conference Canadian Immigration Policy for the 21st Century, Kingston, ON, Oct.18/19, 2002.

Basavarajappa, K. 1999. *Distribution, inequality and concentration of income among older immigrants in Canada, 1990.* Research Paper Series 129, Statistics Canada, Analytical Studies Branch, Ottawa.

Bloom, D., Grenier, D. & Gunderson, M.O. 1995. The changing labour market position of Canadian immigrants. *Canadian Journal of Economics 28* (4b): 987–1005.

Boyd, M. 1989. Immigration and income security policies in Canada: Implications for elderly immigrant women. *Population Research and Policy Review 8* (1): 5–24.

Grant, M. 1999. Evidence of new immigrant assimilation in Canada. *Candian Journal of Economics 32* (4): 930–55.

Hagenaars, A. (1991). The definition and measurement of poverty. In L. Osberg, ed. *Economic Inequality and Poverty: international Perspectives,* 134–156. Armonk, New York: M. E. Sharpe Publishers.

Hildebrand, V. 2001. Wealth accumulation of US households: What do we learn from the SIPP data? *Social and Economic Dimensions of an Aging Population Research Papers 41*, McMaster University.

Modigliani, F. & R. Brumberg. 1954. Utility analysis and the consumption function: An interpretation of cross-section data. In K. Kurihara, ed. *Post-Keynesian Economics. New Brunswick*, NJ: Rutgers University Press.

Myles, J. 2000. The maturation of Canada's retirement income system: Income levels, income inequality and low income among the elderly. *Research Paper 147*, Statistics Canada, Analytical Studies Branch, Ottawa.

National Council of Welfare. 2002. Poverty profiles, 1999. *National council of welfare reports*, National Council of Welfare, Ottawa.

National Council of Welfare. 2006. Poverty profiles, 2002 and 2003. *National council of welfare reports,* National Council of Welfare, Ottawa.

Oja, G. & Love, R. 1988. Pensions and incomes of the elderly in Canada, 1971-1985. *Technical report,* Statistics Canada.

Osberg, L. 2000. Poverty in Canada and the USA: Measurement, trends and implications. *Canadian Journal of Economics 33* (4), 847–77.

Osberg, L. 2001. Poverty among senior citizens: A Canadian success story in international prospective. *Luxembourg Income Study Working Paper No. 274.*

Paquet, B 2001. Low income cutoffs from 1991 to 2000 and low income measures from 1990 to 1999. *Technical report,* Statistics Canada, Ottawa.

Phipps, S. & Burton, P.. 1995. Sharing within families: Implications for the measurement of poverty among individuals in Canada. *Canadian Journal of Economics 28:* 177–204.

Sen, A.K. 1976. Poverty: An ordinal approach to measurement. *Econometrica 44*: 219–231.

Statistics Canada. 2005. 2001 *Census Public Use Microdata File Individual Files* User Documentation. Ottawa: Industry Canada.

Statistics Canada. 2008. *Research Data Centres 2006 Census code book*. Ottawa: Industry Canada.

Statistics Canada (2008). Census of Canada, 2006. Individual File (microdata file). Statisitcs Canada (producer). Accesed at the Manitoba Data Resarch Centre.

Statistics Canada. No date. Table 202-0802 Persons in low income; Canada; Low income cut-offs before tax, 1992 base (table). CANSIM (database). Using E-STAT (distributor). Last updated June 1, 2009.http://estat.statcan.gc.ca/cgi-win/CNSMCGI.EXE?CANSIMFILE=EStat%5-CEnglish%5CCII_1_E.htm (accessed September 8, 2009).

Trempe, R.S., Davis, S. & Kunin, R.. 1997. *Not just numbers: A Canadian framework for future immigration.* Technical report, Advisory Group, Immigration Legislative Review, Ottawa.

Worswick, C. 1996. Immigrant families in the Canadian labour market. *Canadian Public Policy 22*(4):378–396.

Worswick, C. 1999. Credit constraints and the labour supply of immigrant families in Canada. *The Canadian Journal of Economics 32* (1):152–170.

We appreciate the assistance of Ian Clara and the staff of the Manitoba Data Research Centre in providing access to the Statistics Canada Census of Canada, 2006, individual microdata file. All computations, use and interpretations of these data are entirely those of the authors.

7

Restorative Justice Mediation for Elder Abuse Among Ethno-Racial Minority Older Women

Atsuko Matsuoka, Antoinette Clarke and Darlene Murphy, (York University)

The Advocacy Centre for the Elderly and Community Legal Education Ontario (Wahl & Purdy, 1991) refers to elder abuse as a "hidden crime." Agism in the justice system is part of the context in which few older victims dare to report incidents (Groh, 2003; Poirier & Poirier, 1999; Spencer, 2001). Other barriers in the justice system for older people are difficulties in obtaining evidence of elder abuse, values of older people, such as the importance of passing on money and property to offspring, and fear of damaging relationships and general lack of knowledge to identify elder abuse (Groh, 2003). Poirier and Poirier (1999), reporting to the Law Commission of Canada, found that one-third of randomly sampled seniors felt the legal system is too complex and anxiety-provoking and did not have the energy or time to spend on lawsuits. In Ontario, over 60% of older immigrants could not speak an official language (Ontario Human Rights Commission, 2001, p. 30-31). Not comprehending the language makes it even harder to understand and trust complex processes such as the justice system. Immigrant seniors, who are unfamiliar with or suspicious of the justice system and do not speak an official language, are understandably reluctant to report incidents of abuse.

Many definitions of elder abuse exist (National Centre on Elder Abuse, 2005; Health Canada, 2000). The National Advisory Council on Aging (2003/4, p.2) adopts the World Health Organization's definition that elder abuse is "a single or repeated act, or lack of appropriate action – occurring in any relationship where there is an expectation of trust – that causes harm or distress to an older person." Health and Welfare Canada (1993, p.4) defines it as "any action/inaction which jeopardizes the health or well-being of an older person." These definitions are adopted for this chapter. However, caution must be exercise about solely depending on mainstream definitions, as perceptions of ethno-racial minority seniors do not always correspond with widely accepted categories such as physical, emotional, sexual, and financial abuse and neglect (Moon, Tomita & Jung-Kamei, 2001; Moon & Williams, 1993; Tam & Neysmith, 2006; Tomita,

1998) and levels of tolerance also differ between American-born and immigrant ethno-racial minority seniors (Moon & Benton, 2000; Moon, Tomita & Jung-Kamei, 2001).

The Ontario Human Rights Commission (2001) observed that society had failed to build responsive structures for seniors, particularly ethno-racial minority seniors. Because of agism and their small numbers, ethno-racial minority seniors face various challenges, including structural, cultural and personal racism and oppression. In 2000, 65% of victims of family-related violence were women (Canadian Centre for Justice Statistics, 2005). Among family homicides of seniors, two-thirds of victims were killed by their husbands (Statistics Canada, 2003, p. 24). Thus elder abuse persists as a serious women's issue and alerts us that interventions must be informed by a framework that addresses not only structural, cultural and personal oppression based on age and race but also based on gender and issues of power and control within relationships.

When perpetrators are the immigrant senior's sole support, prosecution is not a viable option. Mediation has been suggested as an appropriate alternative to achieve justice for abused and neglected seniors (Craig, 1994, 1997; Spencer, 2001). Intervention based on restorative justice mediation and strengths-based critical social work seems useful. This chapter presents restorative justice mediation as an alternative intervention for addressing abuse and neglect of ethno-racial minority older women. Here we apply the model to two minority populations: Japanese-Canadian and African/Caribbean-Canadian older women.

A Strengths-based Critical Social Work Framework (SCSW) and Restorative Justice Mediation

Situations of abuse faced by ethno-racial minority older women must be examined in terms of structural, cultural and personal oppression and issues of power and control within relationships. Within this context, one promising avenue is a strengths-based critical social work framework based on a social constructionist perspective. This approach is anti-oppressive and includes nine areas to be examined: systemic and structural inequalities, values and ideologies, power/control relationships, oppression, strengths and resiliency, language and narratives (stories), hope, collaboration and resources. A strengths-based, critical, social work framework (SCSW) views reality as socially constructed. To understand complex reality, one must deconstruct it and help people reconstruct an anti-oppressive reality by addressing the nine areas.

Mediation is a paradigm shift in how disputants conceptualize resolving conflicts. Mediation refers to an intervention that uses an impartial and neutral third party to help participants voluntarily reach a mutually agreeable settlement of the dispute (Moore, 2003). However, in work with older survivors[1] of elder abuse, we have adopted restorative justice mediation based on a humanistic approach developed by Mark

Umbreit (1995). This involves shifting from a problem-solving paradigm to a healing paradigm that facilitates growth through dialog. Restorative justice mediation involves meeting four basic needs of victims of injustice. These are: having information on the offense, telling their stories, having control over the prosecutorial process and having restitution, either symbolic or actual (Waldman, 2003/4). Restorative justice mediation works toward rebuilding relationships after nurturing psychological healing by focusing on redress and repair, rather than revenge and retaliation (Umbreit, 1995; Waldman, 2003/4).

Various models exist in restorative justice practices and, in Canada, healing circle mediation has been tried to address elder abuse (Groh, 2003). The model presented here is victim-offender mediation (VOM). VOM is dialog-driven and allows for victim healing and offender accountability (Bellard, 2000; Waldman, 2003/4). VOM is defined as:

> a process which provides interested victims of primarily property crimes and minor assaults the opportunity to meet their offenders in a safe and structured setting with the goal of holding offenders directly accountable while providing important assistance and/or compensation to victims. (Umbreit, 1998, p.6)

VOM has been used successfully for minor and serious crimes by youths and adults, including intimate partner violence against women. Lund and Dodd (2002) concluded that restorative justice can contribute to healing victims, to the rehabilitation of offenders and to community safety. VOM participants re-offended at a rate 32% lower than non-participants (Nugent, Umbreit, Wiinamaki & Paddock, 2001).

Many victims felt re-victimized by the judicial system by not having their voices heard, by encountering officials who use dynamics similar to those of offenders and by finding outcomes that were not meaningful. As for offenders, they often stand mute for the sake of a legal defence and take no responsibility for their actions or their impact on victims. Another problem is that the justice system views crime as committed against the state, rather than against the person who was wronged. Restorative Justice programs (including VOM) overcome these shortcomings and offer meaningful experiences for both victims and offenders (Galaway & Hudson, 1996; Umbreit, 1998; Waldman, 2003/4). A noteworthy outcome is reduced fear among victims (Umbreit, 1999). Considering older adults who fear perpetrators and damaging relationships with them and who seek some control over the process, humanistic mediation, such as restorative justice mediation, is promising for bringing them sensitive alternative justice.

The restorative justice process should be incident-driven and guided by a set of principles (Groh 2003). However, a careful screening model on abusive behaviors and a theoretical approach must be incorporated (Edwards & Haslett 2003). Keeping this in mind, we modified six basic philosophical principles in restorative justice by Sharpe (1998, p. 48) to fit elder abuse situations and we identified five phase-restorative justice mediation processes for elder abuse and neglect by using strengths-based critical social work. The process is broad enough to use an incident-driven approach but provides a theoretical basis for accountable intervention. The six modified basic philosophical principles for restorative justice mediation for elder abuse and neglect include:

- Hold victim involvement as central;
- Make provision for all participants' safety;
- Facilitate dialog among persons involved;
- Ensure accountability to support reintegration;
- Have available adequate resources for reparation and reintegration; and
- Address systemic roots of elder abuse.

Before discussing the details of restorative justice mediation for elder abuse and neglect among ethno-racial minority older women, we present two case scenarios.

Case Scenarios

Mrs. C

Mrs. C is an African/Caribbean woman with four children. Her eldest son and daughter immigrated to Canada for educational opportunities and a better economic future. They married in Canada and had children. Mr. and Mrs. C raised these Canadian-born grandchildren in the Caribbean with little financial support from the children's parents as they tried to establish themselves in Canada. Mr. and Mrs. C considered it their way of assisting their adult children.

The grandchildren returned to Canada. Later, the daughter sponsored Mrs. C, who was then a widow. Mrs. C was "strong enough" to take a part-time job that brought income but allowed time to assist with the grandchildren. She saw this as helping the family. When her daughter purchased a home, she contributed some of her savings, which included her earned income, benefits from her husband's death and savings from her home country, yet she was not named on the property title. There was no written or verbal agreement about how or if Mrs. C would be compensated for her contribution to the purchase of the home. The remainder of her savings was put into a joint account with her daughter. Mrs. C lived with her daughter's family and contributed to paying the mortgage, because this is the "thing to do" for the family. She saw her future with the daughter's family since she and her daughter were close.

Ill health prevented her from working but she continued to assist in the household. Since she came to Canada at a late age, she qualified for a limited public pension and has no private pension. The grandchildren no longer need her help and are disrespectful of her. Her home is far away from other members of the ethnic community and the son who lives in Canada. The son has no interest in having her live with him because he feels she devoted all her time and money to the daughter's family. Although Mrs. C is capable of managing her financial matters, she no longer has access to her bank account without asking her daughter.

One day, Mrs. C confided to her friend that she wishes she could access her money without asking her daughter so she can manage health issues. She also wants a way to address this without upsetting the daughter and without the community finding out about her problems. She does not want to bring shame to the family and is afraid of repercussions from her daughter, as she loves her and wishes to live with her.

Mrs. J

Mrs. J is in her early 70s and came to Canada with her husband 45 years ago from Japan. She was a full-time homemaker for most of her life, raising two children while her husband had full-time employment. Since Mrs. J does not read and speak English well Mr. J manages family finances. When upset or stressed, he becomes verbally abusive, occasionally pushing her and throwing things at her. They now live on Mr. J's pension and their savings. Mrs. J knows Mr. J thinks this is his money, not hers. As Mr. J has become older, he has become more controlling over finances and verbally abusive.

Mrs. J could not envisage raising her children alone in Canada or Japan and did not find the latter option fair to her children, who are Canadian and feel little connection with Japan, so she endured his abuse. Now her children have their own families and live in different parts of Canada. After World War II, few Japanese immigrated to Canada and due to racism against Japanese-Canadians during the war, when Japanese-Canadians were forced to relocate east of British Columbia, they were dispersed and Mrs. J had no Japanese neighbors. Although, Mrs. J eventually became involved in the close-knit, pre-War, Japanese immigrants' community; Japanese-Canadians of her generation, who are typically Canadian-born, do not speak Japanese fluently while her English is limited. Although they were kind and helpful, Mrs. J could not help feeling different and isolated even among Japanese Canadians.

Mrs. J does not discuss "family problems" with friends and does not want anyone to talk about her family in the community. She has pride and does not want to be pitied or made to feel ashamed of her family. Her daughter, who does not want to be involved, worries about her. Her daughter explains her rights and encourages her to leave her husband if her situation worsens and settle in court. Mrs. J, however, feels she does not know the court system; rather, she wants something more amicable, that she can understand and over which she has some say. She feels she should understand English better after years in Canada and understands why her husband looks down upon her. Although she is ashamed, she feels she did all she could. While she is fearful of her husband, she insists that "he is not a monster." After all, he is her husband and the only person upon whom she has depended for many years.

Restorative Justice Mediation Process for Elder Abuse and Neglect

Adhering to the six philosophical principles, we propose the following five phases as elements of a restorative justice mediation process for elder abuse and neglect. We will discuss each phase and apply them to the cases. They are:
Phase 1: Preparation of mediators;

Phase 2: Entry phase of participants;

Phase 3: Case development;

Phase 4: Final preparation for joint/shuttle session; and

Phase 5: Joint session/shuttle session.

Phase 1: Preparation of the Mediators

Justice must do more than "restore" when people live with chronic injustice (Sharpe 1998, p 52). Several assumptions are made in mediation: parties coming to the table have equal levels of power; they are willing to participate in the process and to negotiate the issues; and they will act in good faith. Assumptions shift when mediation concerns relationships with abuse and neglect, imbalance of power and reluctance by one or both parties to participate. Because of this, the initial phase, of preparing mediators, becomes crucial for successful and meaningful mediation with elder abuse survivors. The key is **centring** of mediators. We identified three essential preparations to achieve this: a) continuous self-reflective and self-awareness practice, b) understanding neutrality and impartiality and c) gaining advocacy skills. Additionally, as mediation involving elder abuse situations is complex and requires higher skills and training, mediators should engage in continuous training and skill development.

a. Continuous self-reflective and self-awareness practice

Mediators working with elder abuse survivors must take self-reflective and self-awareness practice seriously so they do not unwittingly re-victimize survivors. When doing cross-ethno-racial mediations, they must reflect on their own biases, assumptions and stereotypes of particular ethno-racial groups. Even when mediators are from the same ethno-racial community, they must reflect on how differences in gender, generation, age, circumstances of migration, social economic class, religion, regions where they live now and where they are from, (dis)ability, sexual orientations, and so on, affect assumptions and expectations about participants.

b. Understanding neutrality and impartiality

Understanding neutrality is fundamental to successful and ethical mediation (Fuller, Kimsey & McKinney, 1992; McCorkle, 2005; Rifkin, Millen & Coff, 1991; Taylor, 1997) and critical to mediators' effectiveness. In mediation, self-determination of participants is critical. Outcomes must be decided by both participants, not by mediators. To ensure this, mediators must be neutral by not favoring any party or having a special interest in the outcome.

Two stances in "neutrality" are "strict neutrality" and "expanded neutrality" (Taylor, 1999; Weckstein, 1997; Solstad, 1999; Beck & Sales, 2001). "Strict neutrality" is influenced by a professional orientation and mediators with this stance do not intervene even when power imbalances exist between participants. Mediators who apply "expanded neutrality" are more active in the process and balance power through education or other techniques as required. Some see these two as distinct and others see them as existing on a continuum. How to exercise "neutrality" differs according to a mediator's values, ethics, experiences and the settings (Taylor, 1999). When seeing "neutrality" as existing on a continuum, mediators should recognize their influence in the process.

To understand neutrality, mediators must examine the concept of impartiality. Impartiality is defined as an unbiased relationship with each disputant (Cohen, et al. 1999) and as not having a special interest in the outcome (McCorkle, 2005). Taylor (1997, p. 405) says impartial means "not predisposed toward either of the parties" and, thus, mediators exercise either strict or expanded neutrality. Cobb and Rifkin (1991) see the mediation process as a discourse construction, where a mediator helps to deconstruct oppressive stories presented by either party, and reconstruct non-oppressive, mutually agreeable stories as an outcome. In elder abuse mediation, when we adopt Cobb and Rifkin's approach, mediators exercise impartiality and neutrality, as they closely examine how stories are constructed and then reconstruct them.

c. Gaining skills for advocacy

When mediation involves an inevitable imbalance of power, in approaches such as VOM, skills such as empowerment, emotional support, information giving, education and advocacy are essential. Under VOM, mediators are neutral to disputants, however mediators are not neutral to the wrong (Price, 2001). To make mediation fair, mediators must ensure both disputants participate fully by being heard and by expressing their positions, needs, ideas and priorities (Menzel 1991). Mediators' advocacy skills are crucial to a fair process where older survivor's stories are heard and non-oppressive stories emerge as mutually agreeable outcomes through mediation.

Phase 2: Entry Phase of Participants – Initial Contacts, Initial Screening and Assessment

For many, mediation is new and for some ethno-racial minority older women, it represents something different than what is discussed here. For example, mediation among South Asians suggests an intervention by elders that is not necessarily sensitive to women's needs (Peel Family Mediation, 2007). The Japanese use intermediaries to solve conflicts, and Japanese-Americans use them for elder maltreatment (Tomita, 1988). Unlike mediations discussed here, however, this may not respect self-determination and confidentiality. Therefore, mediators must provide a full picture of the process and the goal to ensure that participants do not have incorrect expectations.

Depending on complexity, the entry phase may last a few sessions: one to one and a half hours each. However many sessions it takes, some conditions must be met. We identified the following nine conditions for a successful outcome in restorative justice mediation for ethno-racial minority older women survivors of elder abuse, which clarify what mediators and participants must do:

1. Both participants must be fully informed of the process and options other than mediation and give consent to proceed;
2. Confidentiality must be respected;
3. Participants must be able to negotiate;
4. Participants must have a sincere will to negotiate;
5. Participants must explore perceptions on abuse and neglect;
6. Recognizing power differences is essential for the mediation process;
7. Voluntary determination by participants must take place;
8. Outcomes must be meaningful for participants; and
9. A safety plan must be in place throughout the mediation process.

This entry phase gives opportunities to answer participants' questions, to explain other available options and to obtain their fully informed consent to proceed. Mediators can provide community referral information if appropriate. Mediation involving abuse and neglect must address participants' safety. An effective screening and intake process is critical. We include points for screening and assessment for survivors and perpetrators based on the aforementioned eight conditions in this section.

We strongly recommend that the person doing the screening is the mediator who will be working with the participants. The mediator should have extensive training and experience in elder abuse. All screening should be **in person** and **the same medi-**

ator should screen both participants. The mediator must assess and screen survivors and have their safety plan in place before the mediator contacts perpetrators.

Initial assessment should verify basic demographic information (e.g., age, family/household composition) and general contact information (e.g., safest and sure way to get in touch with the individual). In the case of ethno-racial minority older women, information should be noted on migration, preferred language, religious affiliation, if it is important, and ethno-racial community affiliation. The screening tool must assess the following: history of abuse and neglect, mediation readiness, safety, social support, strengths and resiliencies, financial resources, and other noteworthy points.

The history of abuse and neglect should include assessing the existence of abuse and neglect and their severity.[2] It should also assess past and present violence. Physical, emotional and financial isolation should be included in the history of abuse and neglect. The fear and anger of survivors and perpetrators should be assessed. The mediator must explore participants' perceptions of "abuse" and gain their views on harmful and distressing situations.

Mediation readiness must be assessed carefully. The nine conditions listed above provide a helpful guide. Safety is essential for mediating cases involving abuse and neglect. The mediator addresses past and current safety concerns and issues. Identifying past and current social support, strengths and resiliencies and financial resources (or lack thereof) helps determine how safety concerns can be met. Other noteworthy information includes reoccurring themes throughout the assessment, for example, participants' beliefs, values and assumptions. Through initial screening and assessment, a mediator determines:

a. the level of the power imbalance (Is the imbalance too severe? Are abuse and neglect serious and unsafe for the survivor?);

b. if the survivor's safety can be assured;

c. participants' ability, readiness and willingness to negotiate;

d. participants' ability and understanding of needs to make decisions voluntarily;

e. if participants can respect confidentiality; and

f. if the mediator and the mediation program have the appropriate resources and skills to work safely and effectively to produce meaningful outcomes. By doing so, a mediator can decide if the case is appropriate for mediation.

When working with ethno-racial minority older women the program/agency and the mediator must have the resources to provide linguistically and culturally sensitive services and collaboratively work with other agencies without threatening confidentiality. We identified Mrs. C as an African/Caribbean without reference to a particular country in the region not only to protect her confidentiality, but also to reflect how she sees herself and the current community movement in Ontario shaping Black identities

(Gooden, 2008). Caribbean societies are considered matriarchal and in Mrs. C's case, this seems to emerge from her story. Her motherhood and identity seem linked to close family ties with her daughter. However, these relationships are not simply "cultural" and given. Mediators must understand their meanings and how such relationships are maintained/perpetuated and, sometimes, unappreciated and devalued by political, economic and social relations in Canada. Her experiences must be understood in the context of systemic racism within Canada, where African/Caribbean-Canadians "are fighting daily both for cultural survival and against anti-Black sentiment" (Gooden, 2008, p. 413).

As for Mrs. J, her story illustrates differences within ethnic groups and alerts us to social, economic and political factors. The mediator must recognize that these factors, rather than culturally determined views, might have influenced Mrs. J's expectations about marital relationships.

Also, the mediator must check the elder's comfort level in working in English. If she is not comfortable in English the mediator must determine if appropriate resources can be provided. This is a major barrier for non-English speaking older women; services may exist but are not accessible unless users have English language skills. When an interpreter is available, the program must ensure the interpreter understands her or his role and the importance of confidentiality. At this stage the mediator should have determined if Mrs. J feels comfortable speaking in English or through an interpreter.

With both Mrs. C and Mrs. J, the mediator must have clear safety plans. To make safety plans the mediator should not assume perceptions and manifestations of elder abuse and neglect are universal. Tomita (1998) identified how elder abuse manifests itself differently among Japanese-Americans. They do not fit commonly recognized categories of elder abuse. Thus, the mediator must be open-minded and willing to see the conflict situations from the point of view of ethno-racial minority older women.

In particular, because Mrs. J experiences physical violence, the mediator must engage in discussions about creating safety at home if she decides to stay with Mr. J, as well as an emergency escape plan and other safety plans.[3] Detailed plans for safety with the survivor's and abuser's commitment to a non-abusive relationship must be accomplished before moving to the next phase.

Phase 3: Case Development Stage

Once the safety of the survivor is ensured and both parties are ready and willing to undertake mediation, participants move to the next phase. We list seven main tasks for Phase 3:

1. On-going screening and assessment for power imbalance and safety;

2. Developing rapport with participants;

3. Developing appreciation of ethno-racial specific meanings of elder abuse;

4. Hearing stories (experiences) – Narratives;

5. Acknowledging strengths and resilience;

6. Developing self-awareness;

7. Deconstructing stories; and

8. Holding perpetrators accountable and honoring survivors.

Through several sessions, a mediator sees each participant separately. The purpose is to develop rapport and prepare participants for mediation. Ongoing screening throughout the entire mediation process is essential. Even with effective initial screening, ongoing screening and assessment are critical to participants' safety. As the mediator and participant develop their relationship, they may share more information or, simply, new information may become available.

The essential part of restorative justice mediation from a humanistic approach is "dialog" among participants. This does not necessarily mean face-to-face dialog but could mean dialog through the mediator. To stimulate dialog at this stage of mediation, the mediator encourages participants to tell their stories to him or her without the other participant present. Through listening to participants' stories, the mediator, by utilizing strengths-based, critical social work, identifies power differences, values and beliefs influencing the situation, assesses the availability of supports and resources, acknowledges participants' strengths and resilience and places stories within their socio-economic and political context. By doing so the mediator may notice forms of harm and distress not recognized in commonly recognized categories of elder abuse. Sharing this helps participants develop awareness that "taken-for-granted" conflict situations may be abuse. This in turn helps them deconstruct the narratives they shared and reconstruct narratives that empower them as survivors and hold perpetrators accountable. Gaining self-awareness helps survivors become effective negotiators and make their final decisions.

Deconstructing stories requires questioning "taken-for-granted" assumptions, values and beliefs. At this time, the mediator applies strengths-based, critical social work. For example, speaking to Mrs. C, the mediator gently questions if it is acceptable for her daughter's family to not acknowledge Mrs. C's love and contribution and to deny her control over her own finances. The mediator also effectively questions Mrs. C's expectations that "this is what family should do." Mrs. C chose mediation because she wants a positive relationship with her daughter. Knowing this, the mediator explores ways to build a mutually caring and loving relationship by deconstructing Mrs. C's stories with her. In working with Mrs. C's daughter, the mediator must act according to the purpose of restorative justice mediation. That is, to make perpetrators realize the consequences of wrongdoing and take appropriate actions to amend this. In this case, the mediator helps the daughter realize that she took her mother's financial contribution for granted and violated Mrs. C's trust by preventing Mrs. C from having access to her own money. The daughter may share her fear that Mrs. C is going to be a financial burden in the future as she does not receive a public pension. It is important for the mediator not to identify Mrs. C or her daughter as the problem, but financial control and needs as the problem.

Male dominance in marital relationships is common among Japanese of Mr. and Mrs. J's generation and they might have accepted it. In deconstructing their stories, the mediator explores how such beliefs might have shaped their current situation. If they express that, as an older couple, demanding him to change is out of line for an older Japanese woman, the mediator may explore the root of such oppressive assumptions and consequences. Being Japanese, Mr. and Mrs. J may use silence in various ways; silence can be used to shut out others and isolate them, to avoid escalating disputes or as a form of abuse (Tomita, 1998). Silence is used to control power relationships and the mediator must pay close attention to it. Throughout this process, the mediator reminds Mr. and Mrs. J that the problem is not Mrs. J nor Mr. J, but his physical and verbal violence and financial control.

Phase 4: Final Preparation for Joint/Shuttle Session

This is the final preparation stage through individual session(s) before participants have a joint session or shuttle session. A shuttle session means a survivor decides not to sit in the same room, but feels ready to negotiate with the other participant. In this case, each participant sits in a different room and the mediator moves back and forth between them. The mediator's key tasks include:

1. Developing a deeper trust in the mediator and the mediation process;
2. Reviewing stories to tell;
3. Ensuring a balance of power; and
4. Confirming consent to move forward.

The mediator helps survivors to acknowledge their own strengths and resilience, and helps perpetrators to acknowledge and be accountable for their actions. By nurturing a supportive, non-judgmental environment, where participants develop greater self-awareness, the mediator inspires trust in her/him and the mediation process. Through phases 3 and 4, participants explore all options and possible outcomes. This includes the possibility of bringing someone with them for support at the joint/shuttle session. If the participants wish to do so, the mediator prepares them and clarifies their roles in the joint/shuttle session. If Mrs. C wishes to bring her friend for support in the joint session, the mediator helps participants decide if the friend should be a silent participant or speak at the joint session. In this phase, participants decide who should enter the joint session room first, who should tell their story first, what they wish to discuss and what their priorities are. In the preparation stages, the mediator helps participants develop self-awareness and learn the use of language and stories to empower themselves. Participants may practice what to say and how to do so with the mediator and decide which stories to tell.

Since we adopt VOM throughout the mediation, "victim empowerment and offender accountability" takes place. Restorative justice mediation's humanistic approach allows the mediator to work with perpetrators acknowledging wrongs, empathizing with hurts and repairing relationships between victims and offenders (Umbreit, 1995; Waldman, 2003/4). This does not mean creating a friendly relationship. Rather, it means restoring an appropriate balance of power so that abusive relationships will not continue. The joint/shuttle session takes place within a balanced power environment that is safe for the survivor, and outcomes nurture a restored power balance. When power is balanced and participants are ready; the mediator must confirm and gain consent to move forward from both participants.

If Mrs. J is ready, but Mr. J is not, the mediator will work with Mr. J. Mr. J. may believe that he is being labelled as the problem. This may cause him to view the joint-session as a challenge to his identity and, as a result, he may find it shameful. The mediator must review with Mr. J the original incident(s) that brought them to mediation and Mr. J's stories and help him to identify his wrongdoing as the problem. The mediator can then reframe Mr. J's willingness to participate in the mediation process and amend the relationship as positive, rather than shameful.

Through this phase, both participants become more aware of their situations and identities. While preparing her stories for the joint session, Mrs. J may realize her contribution to her family and community in spite of systemic, cultural and personal oppressions. She may then see new possibilities for negotiating with her husband without dishonoring her family, thus giving her a positive identity. Mr. J may realize his wife's contribution to family assets and endurance against racial discrimination, which she would not have faced had they stayed in Japan. Similarly, by preparing her stories, Mrs. C may regain her identity as a "strong" African/Caribbean woman who supported her family and created close family ties, which could be the source of a positive ethnic identity (Campbell & McLean, 2002). Her daughter may realize the systemic barriers to economic success for which she immigrated but also understand that she violated Mrs. C's trust, and acknowledge the negative consequences of her actions. If the mediator is able to link their stories to the roots of elder abuse such as systemic racism, agism and sexism, the stories the participants reconstruct will be placed in a larger context.

Phase 5: Joint Session(s)/Shuttle Session(s)

Phase 5 begins, after thorough preparation, when both participants feel ready and consent to either a joint or shuttle session. The activities of phase 5 are as follows:

1. Mediator's opening statements;
2. Acknowledging strengths and resiliency;
3. Participants' storytelling;
4. Agenda development;
5. Deconstructing and reconstructing stories;
6. Developing agreement;
7. Written agreement;
8. Closing statement; and
9. Safety plan and information on resources.

The mediator opens the session by commending the participants' decision to work out the matter in a civil way and acknowledges their efforts and strengths. The mediator reconfirms their understanding of the process, such as who speaks first and how they will develop the agenda.

After this, participants begin their stories. The rule is that the other participant does not interrupt the speaker. Even when the other participant disagrees, s/he must listen respectfully. This helps balance power between participants and is a powerful experience for many survivors, whose actions have rarely been taken seriously and treated respectfully. Since safety should never be compromised, if either participant cannot act civilly, the mediator should not proceed until the rules are respected. Through telling stories, each participant presents his or her priorities and issues for discussion. The mediator helps finalize the agenda for the joint-session. By following a mutually agreed agenda, the mediator helps participants reflect on stories, deconstruct them, envision desirable situations and reconstruct stories with mutually agreeable outcomes. The mediator drafts agreements in writing. This is called a "memorandum of understanding (MOU)." This should be written in easily understood language. This agreement is not bound by law, but is a civil agreement that can be disregarded. Therefore, participants may wish to include what actions may be taken if the agreement is not honored. For example, in Ontario, the survivor may take the document to the complaint court within the Ontario Court of Justice if it is disregarded. In the closing statement, the mediator commends their efforts and achievement and notes that they may return to mediation for any reason if the need arises.

Mrs. C originally worried about upsetting her daughter and repercussions from her, but hoped to maintain their close relationship even after regaining financial control. If the mediator successfully utilizes restorative justice mediation, her daughter acknowledges wrongs, empathizes with hurts and intends to amend the relationship. Through envisioning desirable situations and reconstructing stories, Mrs. C's hopes will be integrated into the process and her concerns addressed. In cases of elder abuse and neglect, the MOU should be very specific and detailed with each step. For example, if the bank account will become solely for Mrs. C, the MOU should state when and how that will be done. Similarly, if her financial contribution will be recognized, it should specify when and how that will be done and by whom so survivors do not need to re-negotiate with perpetrators outside of the mediation.

Mr. and Mrs. J may want agreements written in Japanese. If the mediator does not understand Japanese, the mediator still writes the MOU in English and has it trans-lated, ideally in the joint session, so that any discrepancies will be resolved during the same session and participants have the same understanding of the MOU.

Because ethno-racial minority older women may believe the mediator knows how the MOU should best be written, the mediator must make sure the women themselves fully participate in the process of writing the MOU and explain differences in wording.

Although the joint/shuttle session is over, we recommend debriefing sessions with each participant separately immediately afterwards. The mediator ensures that the sur-vivor has a sound safety plan (which includes resources) in place and fully understands the outcome of the mediation. Participants may need further support, which can be included in the MOU. If it is not, however, a list of resources can be shared. The medi-ator should see if ethno-linguistic specific and anti-oppressive services are available. If not, this is worth advocating.

Concluding Remarks

In this chapter, mediation done by one mediator is described; however, commu-nity mediation (such as restorative justice mediation) often involves co-mediators. Community mediation tends to bring more participants for support. It is not the num-ber of participants, but mediators' skill and knowledge that are important factors. In other words, within the proposed model various formats exist. What we have present-ed here is one example of a complex process. Mediation may be shunned in cases of abusive relationships; however, skilled mediators can successfully mediate even abu-sive relationships. Careful preparation and on-going screening helps ensure the safety of survivors.

Studies now examine elder abuse among ethno-racial minority older people and unveil different meanings of abuse (Moon et al., 2001; Tam & Neysmith, 2006; Tomita, 1998). Mediators cannot assume mainstream analyses of elder abuse and neglect capture all conflict situations; they must see the situations through the eyes of ethno-racial minority older women by deconstructing their stories. Restorative justice mediation is dialog-driven and allows mediators to explore this and provides room for participants to narrate harmful and distressing situations.

Culture is not static and homogeneous, but fluid and socially constructed. Thus, even ethno-specific definitions of abuse and responses to such harm and distress are influenced by community dynamics and will evolve. One way to manage abuse among Japanese-Americans is an effective use of the community as a third party conflict management – "Disgruntlement is heard about indirectly" (Tomita, 1998, p. 50). Such conflict management is effective when the ethnic community is close and makes such communication active. However, in the case of Japanese-Canadian communities, such management tactics will soon become unavailable (or may already be non-existent) as the communities themselves are rapidly dissipating and "Japanese-Canadians' distinctive ethnic identity may fade away" because they are small in number, dispersed and rapidly entering inter-ethnic and racial marriages (Makabe, 2005, p.125). As a distinctive ethnic identity disappears unique resources for older generations also vanish and we may need to intentionally introduce alternative third party conflict management such as restorative justice mediation.

Disrespect is a key form of elder abuse among Chinese-Canadians in Toronto. A typical response by older people is to endure it as they protect themselves and their families from systemic racism in the social, health or criminal justice systems (Tam & Neysmith, 2006). Enduring abuse is not desirable, but is common where no appropriate resources exist, as our two case scenarios depicted. Systemic oppressions such as racism, agism and sexism must be challenged politically, but can also be challenged by adopting alternatives where people have more control over their situations and can respond to injustice.

Considering the limited resources available for ethno-racial minority older women, restorative justice mediation provides opportunities for them to address issues where they may gain control. Ultimately, this will help them realize their hopes of maintaining their existing support network while restoring their integrity and positive self-identities. Ways must be increased for ethno-racial minority elder abuse survivors to regain control over their lives and identities and to find resolutions that restore justice.

Endnotes

[1] In this chapter, we chose to refer to a woman who is abused as a survivor rather than as a victim. First, for some, the particular abuse is not the only one they endured; they might have survived multiple abuses throughout their lives. Second, from a strengths-based perspective, they are

survivors. Third, and most importantly, older women wished to identify themselves as survivors rather than victims.

[2]Although there are none specifically designed for ethno-racial older women, tools exist to assess safety such as violence/dangerous assessment for women: e.g., M. F. Shepard and J. A Campbell "Abusive Behaviour Inventory," and the Michigan Supreme Court has useful screening tools, Domestic Violence Risk Assessment by the Woman Abuse Council of Toronto, the Spousal Assault Risk Assessment (SARA) published by Multi-Health Systems. See http://www.mhs.com/ These require special training to fully utilize them. Safety is most important. If safety is doubtful, the mediator should involve specialists after gaining survivors' consent. For an assessment tool to identify caregiver's abuse see the Indicator of Abuse by Reis and Nahmiash (1995, 1998).

[3]The Peel Committee Against Woman Abuse (PCAWA) http://www.pcawa.org/index.htm has a good example for a safety plan in twelve different languages, although Japanese is not one of them and its focus is not on older women.

References

Beck, J.A & Sales, B. D, (2001). *Family mediation: Facts, myths and future prospects.* Washington: American Psychological Association.

Bellard, J. (2000). Victim offender mediation. *The Community Mediator. Fall,* 1-6

Bergeron, L.R. (2001). An elder abuse case study: Caregiver stress or domestic violence? You decide. *Journal of Gerontological Social Work, 34*(4).

Campbell, C. & McLean, C. (2002). Representations of ethnicity in people's accounts of local community participation in a multi-ethnic community in England. *Journal of Community & Applied Social Psychology, 12,* 13-29.

Choi, N.G. & Mayer, J. (2000). Elder abuse, neglect and exploitation: Risk factors and prevention strategies. *Journal of Gerontological Social Work, 33*(2), 3-25.

Cobb, S. and Rifkin, J. (1991). Practice and paradox: Deconstructing neutrality in mediation. *Journal of Social Inquiry, 16,* 201-227.

Cohen, O., Dattner, N. & Luxenburg, A.(1999). The limits of the mediator's neutrality. *Conflict resolution Journal, 16*(4).

Craig, Y. (1994). Elder mediation: Can it contribute to the prevention of elder abuse and the protection of the rights of elders and their careers? *Journal of Elder Abuse & Neglect, 6*(1), 83-96.

Craig, Y.J. (1997). *Elder Abuse and Mediation: Exploratory studies in America, Britain and Europe.* Aldershot, U.K.: Avebury.

Edwards, A. & Haslett, J. (2002). Domestic Violence and Restorative Justice: Advancing the Dialogue, Victim Offender Mediation Newsletter.

Fuller, R.M., Kimsey, W.D. & McKinney, B.C. (1992). Mediator neutrality and storytelling order. *Mediation Quarterly, 10*(2), 187-192.

Gooden, A. (2008). Community organizing by African Caribbean people in Toronto, Ontario. *Journal of Black Studies, 38*(3), 413-426.

Groh, A. (2003). *A healing approach to elder abuse and mistreatment: The restorative justice approach to elder abuse project.* Waterloo, On.: Community Access Centre of Waterloo.

Health and Welfare Canada. (1993). *Community awareness and response: Abuse and neglect of older adults.* Ottawa, ON: the Ministry of National Health and Welfare.

Health Canada. (1994). *Older Canadians and the abuse of seniors: A continuum from participation to empowerment.* Ottawa: Ministry of Supply and Services of Canada.

Health Canada. (2000). *Abuse and Neglect of Older Adults:* A discussion paper. Ottawa: Her Majesty the Queen in Right of Canada.

Canadian Centre for Justice Statistics. (2003). Family violence in Canada: Statistical profile 2005 Catalog no. 85-224-XIE. Retrieved from the World Wide Web: http://canada.justice. gc.ca/en/ps/fm/adultsfs.html

Canadian Centre for Justice Statistics (2005) *Family violence in Canada: Statistical profile 2005* Catalog no. 85-224-XIE.

Lai, D., Chappell, N., Chau, S. & Tsang, K.T. (2003). *Health and well-being of Chinese seniors in Canada: Report to community partners in Toronto.* Toronto: University of Toronto, Faculty of Social Work.

Lund, K. & Dodd, D. (2002). *The justice options for women who are victims of violence project. Final report.* Charlottetown, Prince Edward Island. Retrieved from World Wide Web: http://www.peitha.org/justiceoptions/finalreport.pdf

McCorkle, S. (2005). The murky world of mediation ethics: Neutrality, impartiality and conflict of interest in state codes of conduct. *Conflict Resolution Quarterly, 23*(2), 165-183.

Makabe, T. (2005). Intermarriage: Dream becomes reality for a visible minority? *Canadian Ethnic Studies, 37*(1), 121-126.

Menzel, Kent E. (1991). Judging the fairness of mediation: A critical framework, *Mediation Quarterly 9*(1), 3-20.

Moon, A. & Benton, D. (2000). Tolerance of elder abuse and attitudes toward third-party intervention among African American, Korean American, and White elderly. *Journal of Multicultural Social Work, 8*(3/4), 283-303.

Moon, A., Tomita, S.K. & Jung-Kamei, S. (2001). Elder mistreatment among four Asian American groups: An exploratory study on tolerance, victim blaming and attitudes toward third-party intervention, *Journal of Gerontological Social Work, 36*(1/2), 153-169.

Moon, A. & Williams, O. (1993). Perceptions of elder abuse and help-seeking patterns among African-American, Caucasian-American and Korean-American elderly women. *The Gerontologist, 33*(3), 386-395.

Moore, C. (2003). *The Mediation process: Practical strategies for resolving conflict (3rd edition).* San Francisco, CA: Jossey-Bass John Wiley & Sons.

National Advisory Council on Aging. (2003/4). *Expression, 17*(1), 1.

National Centre on Elder Abuse. (2005). Fact Sheet.

Nugent, W., Umbreit, M., Wiinamaki, L. & Paddock, J. (2001). Participation in Victim-Offender Mediation and reoffense: Successful replications? *Research on Social Work, 11*(1), 5-23.

Ontario Human Rights Commission. (2001). *Time for action: Advancing human rights for older Ontarians.* Toronto, ON: Ontario Human Rights Commission.

Peel Family Mediation (2007). *Peel Mediation Services- A symposium: A dialogue with the South Asian Communities of Peel.* Brampton, ON. Nov 23rd 2007

Poirier, D. & Poirier, N. (1999). *Older adults' personal relationships: Final report. Why is it so difficult to combat elder abuse and, in particular, financial exploitation of the elderly?* Law Commission of Canada.

Price, M. (2001). Personalizing crime: Mediation produces restorative justice for victims and offenders. Dispute Resolution Magazine. Retrieved from World Wide Web: http://www.vorp.com/articles/justice.html

Reis, M. & Nahmiash, D. (1995). *When seniors are abused: A guide to intervention.* North York, ON: Captus Press.

Reis, M. & Nahmiash, D. (1998).Validation of the Indicators of Abuse (IOA) Screen. *The Gerontologist 38*(4), 471-480.

Rifkin, J., Millen, J. & Coff, S. (1991). Toward a new discourse for mediation: A critique of neutrality. *Mediation Quarterly,* 151-164.

Sharpe, S. (1998). *Restorative Justice: A Vision for Healing and Change.* Edmonton, AB: Edmonton Victim Offender Mediation Society.

Statistics Canada (2003). Family violence against older adults. Catlog no. 85-224. Retrieved from World Wide Web: http://www.statcan.ca/english/IPS/Data/85-224-XIE.htm

Solstad, K. E. (1999). The role of the neutral in intra-organizational mediation: In support of active neutrality. *Mediation Quarterly, 17*, 67-84.

Taylor, A. (1997). Concepts of neutrality in family mediation: Contexts, ethics, influence and transformative process. *Conflict Resolution Quarterly, 14*(3), 215-236.

Taylor, A. (1999). Concepts of neutrality in family mediation. In J. MacFarlane (Ed.). *Dispute Resolution: Readings and Case Studies.* (pp.403-407).Toronto, ON: Emond Montgomery.

Tam, S. & Neysmith, S. (2006). Disrespect and isolation: Elder abuse in Chinese communities. *Canadian Journal on Aging, 25*(2), 141-151.

Tomita, S.K. (1998). The consequences of belonging: Conflict management techniques among Japanese Americans. *Journal of Elder Abuse & Neglect, 9*(3), 41-68.

Umbreit, M. (1995). The development and impact of victim offender mediation in the United States. *Mediation Quarterly, 12*(3), 263-276.

Umbreit, M. (1995). *Mediating interpersonal conflicts: A pathway to peace.* Concord, MN: CPI Publishing.

Umbreit, M. (1999). Victim-Offender mediation in Canada: The impact of an emerging social work intervention. *International Social Work, 42*(2), 215-227.

Umbreit, M. with Bradshow, W. & Greenwood, J. (1998). *Victim sensitive, victim offender mediation training manual.* Prepared for Office for Victims of Crime U.S. Department of Justice, Center for Restorative Justice & Mediation, School of Social Work, University of Minnesota.

Waldman, E.A. (2003/4). Healing hearts or righting wrongs?: A meditation on the goals of "Restorative Justice." *Journal of Public Law and Policy, 25,* 355-373.

Wahl, J. & Purdy, S. (1991). *Elder abuse: The hidden crime.* Toronto: the Advocacy Centre for the Elderly and Community Legal Education Ontario.

Weckstein, D. T. (1997). In praise of party: Empowerment and of mediator activism. *The Willamette Law Review, 33*, 501-560.

Zink, T., Regan, S., Jacobson, C J. & Pabst, S. (2003). Cohort, period, and aging effects: A qualitative study of older women's reasons for remaining in abusive relationships. *Violence Against Women, 9*(12), 1429-1441.

8

End-of-Life Care for Immigrant Seniors

Michael MacLean, Nuelle Novik, Kavita Ram and Allison Schmidt,
(University of Regina)

Introduction

The Canadian Multiculturalism Act, legislated in 1988, formally recognized the equality of all citizens and aims to ensure that all needs associated with culture are met (Majumdar, Browne, Roberts & Carpio, 2004). This policy was the result of generations of Canadians acknowledging that, apart from the First Nations Peoples of Canada, we are a country of immigrants that respects the cultural components and contributions of each ethno-cultural group in building the kind of nation that Canadians want to have. Even now, more than 140 years after Canada became a nation, Canada is still a country that is shaped by immigration, as Statistics Canada (2006) shows that presently one in five Canadians was born in another country. This fact contributes to the concept of Canada continuing to be a multicultural country and continuing to be guided by the *Canadian Multiculturalism Act.*

A significant component of Canadian society that is influenced by the multicultural nature of our country is the health care system. As Canada continues to become a more ethnically diverse nation, our health care system, and the providers who work within it, need to respond to the varied perspectives of the multicultural nature of health care. Cultural diversity in Canada requires that health care providers manage complex differences in attitudes, worldviews, expectations, and communication styles, as well as the reality of multiple languages (Ross, Dunning & Edwards, 2001). All components of our health care system are affected by different cultural perspectives of care and cure, but one that is growing in importance for many people in Canada but that has not received a great deal of attention from a multicultural perspective is palliative care or end-of-life care (Feser & Bon-Bernard, 2003).

There is a widely recognized need to improve cultural competence among palliative care teams that provide end-of-life care (Woo, 1999). Palliative care is a significant resource to people who are dying, and to their families and friends, because it provides a gentle and comfortable approach to the last stage of life and contributes to people dying with dignity. This health care resource can benefit all Canadians in this important stage of life (Feser & Bon-Bernard, 2003). However, despite efforts to include cultural competency in end-of-life care, people in ethno-cultural communities still make less use of palliative care services than expected (Payne, Chapman, Holloway, Seymour & Chau, 2005). Failure to use palliative care services by people from ethno-cultural communities should not be taken to mean that the services are not needed (Woo, 1999). Rather, the lack of use of these services may be directly related to the fact that they are culturally and linguistically limited to those in the majority populations of English and French-speaking Canadians (Feser & Bon-Bernard, 2003).

The purpose of this chapter on end-of-life issues for immigrant seniors is to present some of the issues that immigrant seniors and their family and community members face in receiving end-of-life care. Consideration is needed of these issues in the interests of contributing to a culturally-sensitive health care and social service system for this stage of life. Presented are some of the issues that social and health care practitioners have to consider in the provision of culturally-sensitive end-of-life care. First of all, definition of end-of-life care for seniors is presented in an attempt to establish a framework for considering this issue with immigrant seniors. Then briefly are presented some of the general issues that arise in the provision of end-of-life care for immigrant seniors. Then consideration will be given to the situation of some immigrants to Canada with respect to end-of-life care.

It is not possibnle to consider issues that all ethno-cultural communities have for this health care resource because there are many individual cultural considerations that would be beyond the scope of this chapter. However, consideration if given to the palliative care considerations from the perspective of Chinese-Canadians in a macro perspective and suggest that many immigrant seniors may experience some of the challenges that elderly Chinese-Canadians experience in the end-of-life stage. A theme from this information on Chinese-Canadians will be the importance of family and community considerations in end-of-life care. Focus is then made on a micro perspective by documenting the case of an elderly woman from Afghanistan in a long-term care setting in Canada to show some of the challenges that she, her family and the social service and health care providers met in dealing with end-of-life issues. Again, the theme of family and community will be a significant component of this care for this older Afghanistan woman. Finally, some insights are offered that two elderly Indo-Canadian individuals and two elderly Ukrainian-Canadian women gave about their expectations of end-of-life care in Canada.

From the examination of this material, the concept of family and community care in end-of-life situations may be changing is shown, and that these changes will have implications for immigrant seniors and health care teams that provide end-of-life care to them. These experiences will allow us to make some general statements about end-of-life care for immigrant seniors while, at the same time, being aware that these situations will not account for all the end-of-life care issues for all immigrant seniors. The conclusion of this chapter is a general statement about the importance of developing culturally-sensitive end-of-life care for immigrant seniors with special attention being paid to the family and community contributions to this care.

A Definition of End-of-Life Care for Seniors as Applied to Immigrant Seniors

In *A guide to end-of-life care for seniors* (Fisher, Ross & MacLean, 2000), the following definition has been proposed:

> End-of-life care for seniors requires an active, compassionate approach that treats, comforts and supports older individuals who are living with, or dying from, progressive or chronic life-threatening conditions. Such care is sensitive to personal, cultural and spiritual values, beliefs and practices and encompasses support for families and friends up to and including the period of bereavement. (p. 9)

This definition considers the cultural aspects of the end of life in a general way but it can be expanded to consider specific cultural aspects of end-of-life issues (Fisher et al., 2000). This definition leads to the cultural considerations of end-of-life care from the perspective of the philosophy of this care in that people in all cultures experience death in ways relevant to their philosophy of life and a philosophy of dying and death. How one evolves from life to death is inherently influenced by the values and beliefs that the culture holds dear. Therefore, the values and beliefs of a culture influence many aspects of dying and death such as the way that pain and pain control are understood. For example, is pain a meaningful experience that is accepted for significant benefit to the individual as a part of the life journey or is pain an unwanted aspect of life that must be eliminated by any means possible? Depending on which of these values (and many other interpretations in addition to these two with respect to pain) that people hold, the provision of physical care would be different in terms of the issues surrounding medication, privacy, dietary and nutritional needs, and the diversity of health care practices that we, in Canada, would call traditional, complementary or alternative, among others. Communication issues inherent in the dying and death stage of life are also strongly influenced by the cultural view of life and death. For example, in our western view of illness, we tend to want to know as much as possible about the illness we have and the prospects of the care we will receive. Many of us want to know this information directly from the health care practitioners (primarily doctors). However, in some cultures, there are values that suggest that the diagnosis and prognosis is not shared with the person who is in the last stage of life, but is shared with the family members instead and then they decide the amount of information that is conveyed to their loved one. How does this different communication perspective affect the provision of end-of-life care to some immigrant seniors? Another component that Fisher et al. (2000) suggest is important within the cultural context of end-of-life care is the ethics of decision making in this stage of life. An example is the do-not-resuscitate (DNR) statement that many institutions want to have on file that may be very difficult to accept for people in some cultures. Again, this aspect of care is often discussed with the person receiving care but the role of family and friends on this point may be more significant in some cultures than in others. It is important to be aware of cultural expectations in the process of considering the ethics of end-of-life care and decisions related to that care. Also, rituals and ceremonies, grief and mourning practices, spirituality and/or religious concerns may vary among different cultures so it is important to have a sense of expectations of various cultures with respect to these significant components of end-of-life care. And, finally, the influence of the family in end-of-life care for immigrant seniors may be much more significant and different for people from different cultural communities than in our western culture. We will first consider these general issues from the perspective of elderly Chinese-Canadians.

Chinese-Canadian Perspectives on End-of-Life Care

Many landed immigrants, refugees, and citizens of Canada are of Chinese descent. Recent numbers released by Statistics Canada (2006), indicate that the Chinese population is the fastest growing ethnic group in Canada. Currently, 18.6 per cent of immigrants to Canada are Chinese. Chinese people have come to Canada in many different ways. Some have immigrated to Canada from areas such as Hong Kong, Taiwan, or Singapore and some have come directly from mainland China. Some are landed immigrants, others as refugees, and some have lived in Canada all of their lives (Feser & Bon-Bernard, 2003). As the Chinese culture is comprehensive and complex, this presents a challenge to palliative-care professionals (Woo, 1999). Acquiring the necessary sensitivity to cultural beliefs and practices is required in order for health care providers to give optimal care to Chinese palliative care patients (Woo, 1999).

Palliative-care practitioners most often see older Chinese individuals. It is suggested that this group may reflect more traditional Chinese cultural beliefs and values (Feser & Bon-Bernard, 2003). Literacy levels in both written English and Chinese may be poor in less educated Chinese people (Sporoston, Pitson, Whitfield & Walker, 1999). The inability to access information and to communicate effectively may reduce their ability to seek appropriate health services (Payne et al., 2005). In addition, there may not be adequate words in the dialect to translate and express the type of illness that an individual is diagnosed with, and error is possible.

In Canada, the Chinese community is a heterogeneous population that draws upon many different influences reflected in their cultural beliefs (Guo, 1995). Religious philosophies including Confucianism, Taoism, Buddhism, and political philosophies like Communism have all had an effect on cultural values (Payne et al., 2005). Values embedded in the Chinese culture include filial piety, loyalty, the superiority of men over women, the collective well-being of the family, and the maintenance of a social order (Payne et al., 2005). These values reflect health behaviors of patients and have implications for palliative-care providers during care at the end of life (Payne et al., 2005).

Shared autonomy and collective decision-making tend to be regarded as the norm within Chinese culture (Payne et al., 2005). Gender specific roles are reflected with male members of a family usually entrusted to make medical decisions (Tang & Lee, 2004). Obligation to the family is of primary importance and the collective well-being of the family surpasses individual autonomy (Lapine et al., 2001). Older members of a Chinese family who are facing the end of life are typically reliant on their children to provide care and to communicate with health care professionals on their behalf (Lapine et al., 2001). Add to the mix the complexities of different levels of acculturation and it becomes even more difficult for palliative care providers to understand how their patients may experience illness (Bowman, 2000).

There is the potential for conflict between traditional Western principles of full disclosure and an individual's right to health care information at the end of life. These issues may collide with discussions that may not be appropriate to discuss in Chinese culture (Tang & Lee, 2004). Truth telling about the diagnosis and prognosis in end-of-life situations, and how this information is shared can be a sensitive issue for some members of the Chinese culture (Woo, 1999). For example, in traditional Chinese culture, the topic of death and dying is often avoided (Feser & Bon-Bernard, 2003). Some traditional Chinese families prefer that health care providers do not discuss the fact that the condition is terminal with a dying family member (Lapine et al., 2001).

A review of research was conducted which focused on major cities with a large Chinese population including Hong Kong (Fielding & Hung, 1996), New York City (Crain, 1996), and Sydney, Australia (Huang, Meiser, Butow & Goldstein, 1999). The results of these studies indicate that, contrary to traditional cultural beliefs, most patients do want to be informed of their diagnosis, prognosis, and also the treatment options available to them, at the same time as their family members. The conclusion drawn from this literature review is that it is important for health and social service professionals to check with family members about the extent of disclosure about the illness that will be made available to the person receiving end-of-life care.

The disclosure of information about the illness can also be influenced by the type of illness the person has. For example, the attitude toward the disclosure of the diagnosis for Chinese cancer patients is influenced by the exact stage of the disease. The opportunities for either disclosure or nondisclosure changed as the diagnosis of cancer changed between early-stage and terminal (Jiang et al., 2007). Even though open disclosure and truth telling was preferred, the older generations still preferred to receive less information and have minimal involvement in medical decision making (Payne et al., 2005). Results of research with the elderly Chinese people in Calgary (Feser & Bon-Bernard, 2003) revealed that thirty-six percent of participants indicated that some combination of medical information should be given to both the patient and the family. This is a research finding that may reflect an increasing Western influence of truth telling.

Physicians of Chinese descent seldom provide their patients with a direct diagnosis of terminal illness (Yu et al., 2007). Jiang et al. (2006) conducted research that reviewed the different attitudes of oncology physicians towards truth telling at different stages of cancer progression. They found that over 65 percent of Chinese doctors who preferred non-disclosure thought that this approach was helpful in maintaining a patient's quality of life and would reduce a patient's feelings of hopelessness and helplessness. Some Chinese physicians felt disclosure of diagnosis was necessary and advantageous as it enabled the patient to get their affairs in order (Jiang et al., 2006).

There are added complications that may cause problems with disclosure. Some individuals in the Chinese culture find negative displays of emotion as distasteful and embarrassing (Fielding, Wong & Ko, 1998). In cultures that are traditionally collectivist there is a strong emphasis on maintaining face for other family members (Smith & Bond, 1993). A challenge for a physician charged with disclosure of the terminal illness is that withholding the news may actually save face for their patient (Barclay, Blackhall & Tulsky, 2007). Therefore, in the Chinese culture, navigating what is appropriate can be a landmine of challenges. These landmines may also cause patients from collectivist cultures to suffer in silence and not seek the help that may be available to them. However, the desire to be treated with dignity, particularly at the end of one's life, seems to be a fairly universal principle found in most cultures.

Culture-specific beliefs about cancer causation can also influence psychosocial and help-seeking behavior (Yeo et al., 2005). Common to Chinese culture is the belief that family affairs are to be confined to the family (Yeo et al., 2005). It is considered shameful to discuss private matters such as cancer or illness with outsiders (Leung & Lee, 1996). Another issue that may affect help-seeking behavior is the traditional belief that getting cancer was one's destiny, fate, or karma (Facione, Giancarlo, Chan & Lillian, 2000). Accessing help or treatment may be seen as pointless and these beliefs may be hard to overcome. However, we must remain cognizant not to stereotype all Chinese people as homogenous.

Filial piety is a cultural obligation that includes the duty of children to care for, honor, and respect their parents (Barclay et al., 2007). This obligation may cause more complexity for end-of-life care providers. This obligation can be interpreted to mean that the children do all that is possible to keep their parent alive (Blackhall, Frank, Murphy & Michel, 1999). Removing a parent from life support may be seen as disregarding filial piety and seen as a disgrace on the family (Kagawa-Singer & Blackhall, 2001). Conflict can often occur during decisions concerning withdrawal of care at the end of life.

The concept of patient autonomy is a product of western culture (Tang & Lee, 2004). In Western medicine, making informed choices is the right of each individual patient. In Chinese culture, the principles of self-determination do not have the same priority as they do in Western cultures (Ross, Dunning & Edwards, 2001). If cultural tradition and problems with understanding prevent a frank discussion about the diagnosis, then a patient may not be fully informed as to the nature of their condition and the treatment that is available to them (Fielding et al., 1998). Moreover, some physicians may avoid informing their patient by informing the family as a substitute (Fielding & Hung, 1996).

In conclusion, it is apparent that family members of Chinese-Canadian seniors receiving end-of-life care are a significant resource to the older person and, therefore, an important resource for the health care team providing this care. There are so many ways that the family can be helpful to the senior and to the health care team in facilitating quality end-of-life care for older Chinese-Canadians. Thus, it is important for the health care team to call on family members of elderly Chinese-Canadians to ensure the provision of this care. It may also be important for the health care team to call on the family members of seniors from other ethno-cultural communities to help in the understanding of appropriate end-of-life care for other immigrant seniors. The next section of this chapter will examine a case study that focuses on a family of Afghani descent and their experiences with end-of-life care.

Senior Afghanistan Woman Receiving End-of-Life Care in Long-term Care

The past decade has shown an increasing awareness among health and social service providers and health consumers of the necessity for access to competent, holistic and respectful end-of-life care. As stated in the previous section, the success of this end-of-life care must consider the individual's socio-cultural needs, as well as spiritual and familial care needs, in addition to those related to their physical care and symptom management. A great deal of this end-of-life care is provided in long-term care settings because a large number of seniors spend their last stage of life in these settings. The complexities and challenges of such comprehensive cultural care are exceedingly evident when working with immigrant seniors in long-term care. In order to demonstrate some of these challenges, a case study of a senior Afghanistan woman is illustrated in the following discussion.

Mrs. K was admitted to a chronic care bed at a long-term care facility in a prairie city in 2005. She required extensive physical care following a series of heart attacks and strokes. Her illnesses had also left her with neurological deficits compromising her speech, memory and judgment. Mrs. K was a 60-year-old Islamic woman of Afghan origin whose first language was Farsi. She entered Canada as a political refugee with her daughter-in-law and several grandchildren. Both her husband and son were killed during the Afghan conflict forcing the family to flee to Iran and then to Canada. Shortly after her arrival in Canada, Mrs. K suffered the massive stroke and heart attack that eventually resulted in her admission to long-term care. Following her initial illness, she was transferred to a local rehabilitation hospital and, at the family's request, was eventually discharged to their home. The family managed her care for several months with extensive community home care assistance. Her continued physical deterioration eventually necessitated her admission to long-term care.

The impact of variations in language, culture and religion were evident throughout Mrs. K's stay in long-term care. Prior to her admission, her eldest grandson and his mother visited the nursing home. Although familiar with the acute care setting, they required information about the philosophy of long-term care in addition to the parameters of personal and medical care. They were informed that primary care and support was provided by a multidisciplinary health care team including a social worker, registered nurse and special care aide. An attending physician visited the facility on a bi-weekly basis and maintained regular contact with the charge nurse.

The pre-admission, admission and transition of Mrs. K into long-term care were marked by the exchange of cultural information, perceptions and expectations between the health care team and the senior's family. This occurred on both a formal and informal basis. For example, the family provided information regarding dietary requirements consistent with the Islamic tradition while the health care team worked to accommodate these needs within the parameters of the physician ordered diabetic, cardiac diet. Care staff was educated about the significance of the traditional *Hijab* (head scarf) and this resident requirement was documented on the nursing care plan. The resident and family became familiar with the facility care routines and functions, and they came to understand the individual roles of each multidisciplinary team member. The family was reassured that Mrs. K would receive excellent and compassionate medical and personal care during her stay in the facility. The health care team also became familiar with the traditional, Islamic family hierarchy. The primary family contact and substitute-decision maker was identified as the eldest male in the immediate family – the grandson. Mrs. K's daughter-in-law deferred all decision making to her twenty-year-old son.

Communication was a huge challenge throughout this time for many reasons centring on individual needs and policy concerns. The family initially received translation assistance from the only Immigrant and Refugee Settlement Agency in the city. However, as Mrs. K had been in Canada for more than twelve months, these services were no longer funded by the Federal Government and alternate assistance had to be obtained. The local Health Authority eventually funded translation services for formal meetings. The health care team developed, and became familiar with, a phonetic list of Farsi words used to assist in the provision of personal care (i.e., toilet; hungry; cold; pain; tired). A picture board was also used to aid in communication with Mrs. K, whose cognitive impairments further slowed this process. Occasionally, Farsi-speaking family and friends or community members provided translation assistance to the health care team. Unfortunately, the small size of the Afghan community in this city precluded anonymity or confidentiality and, as such, the family was often reluctant to use these informal resources. In this specific context, it appeared that contact with the local Afghan and Islamic communities did not function to enhance the quality of this family's social support network as much as had originally been hoped. Access to impartial translators and cultural educators would have greatly enhanced the efficacy of the care team's efforts when engaging the resident and her family. However, this was impossible in the context of care for Mrs. K.

Another challenge faced by the health care team was experienced when assisting the resident and family in accessing adequate funding to cover the costs of long-term care and the associated expenses (i.e., medications; nursing supplies; incontinent products; transport). The family was unaware of these costs as they were not required to pay for care previously received in the acute care setting. This was a great source of anxiety for the family who was unfamiliar with, and overwhelmed by, the process of pursuing such funding. The facility social worker worked with the provincial social service division and the family in order to secure funding and to educate the family about their financial responsibilities.

The complexities of Mrs. K's medical care continued to emerge as her condition deteriorated. She presented with increased confusion, agitation and exhibited disruptive behaviors related to vascular dementia. She would often call out for long periods of time and could be physically resistive to care. Attempts at reassurance only exacerbated these behaviors. Mrs. K would repeatedly strike herself and wail loudly. The health care team implemented various standard strategies used to manage behavioral issues such as pain management, toileting, redirection, reassurance and reduced stimulation. Unfortunately, all were unsuccessful. On various occasions, the family was summoned to the facility to provide Mrs. K with comfort and to assist staff with translation and understanding of her behavior. The family was equally perplexed and overwhelmed as they were unable to identify any obvious reason for these behaviors.

However, they indicated that this was a culturally acceptable way in which to express her immense grief and, therefore, the behavior continued. This created a unique situation where staff attempted to balance the disruption to the ward and other residents while allowing Mrs. K this cultural catharsis. Consultations were made to a psychiatrist and to the behavior management specialist within the health authority. Chemical restraints were suggested and used during the periods of Mrs. K's greatest distress. The health care team often felt frustrated and inadequate as their normal attempts at consoling and caring for this resident were largely ineffective. The combination of Mrs. K's cognitive deficits, language and cultural differences and limited informal support network created a challenging social milieu in which to provide end-of-life care.

Eventually the chronic nature of Mrs. K's health problems degenerated to the point of palliation as she entered the end-of-life stage. As with other residents in this situation, a formal multidisciplinary team meeting was held with the family to discuss Mrs. K's prognosis and the initiation of palliative care. The resident's poor cognitive and physical condition precluded her direct involvement in this process. Detailed explanations were provided elucidating the intent of comfort care measures including pain and symptom management, flexible personal care plans and support for the family. The Advanced Health Care Directive was discussed at length. Prior to this time, the family had requested "full code" status permitting all life sustaining measures including life support. However, following consultations with their family members who lived abroad and their former physician in Afghanistan, a decision was made to forgo further attempts to sustain life. In this context, the health care team became accustomed to the significance of the traditional extended family system that existed well beyond national boundaries.

It was at the request of family members living abroad that Mrs. K was transferred to acute care approximately 48 hours before her death. Her grandson and substitute-decision maker appeared to be pressured by senior members of the extended family to ensure that she was hospitalized, in spite of extensive efforts by the health care team to reaffirm their capacity to manage her care. The health care team were disappointed that they were unable to provide care to this resident during her final days of life. Mrs. K was moved to acute care where she died on the medical ward. Following Mrs. K's death, the family attended the facility with their Imam and received bereavement support. Assistance was provided to secure funding for the funeral and burial in the local Islamic cemetery.

There were many issues that arose in providing end-of-life care for Mrs. K. One of the most complex issues was the contribution of the family and community members. An unusual circumstance in this example was the reliance on the grandson as the primary decision maker in Mrs. K.'s care. Also, the fact that the family members and the community members from abroad played such a significant role created a new way of working for the health care team. A traditional understanding of community would denote a social network in close proximity and regular contact with the individual. In this example, the roles of the local Afghan and Islamic communities became secondary in influence to the family's community that existed overseas. This "global" concept of the extended family and community involvement was easy to accommodate once the health care team recognized and understood the significance of this resource. This concept of extended family and community involvement is one that health care teams in the future will have to engage with, in the provision of quality end-of-life care for immigrant seniors.

This case was characterized by mutual respect, compassion and the free exchange of cultural and spiritual mores. This health care team was challenged to consider previously unfamiliar gender roles, family structure, community involvement, language barriers and religious requirements while maintaining the provision of competent end-of-life care. The absence of parallel ethnic family support services in this city forced the team to engage in a problem-solving process that broadened their perceptions of family and community resources in the provision of end-of-life care for this senior from Afghanistan. Given the age and ethnic diversity of Canada's population, these skills will undoubtedly be utilized in the future to advance the integrity and breadth of end-of-life care in long-term care institutions. The theme of family and community support in end-of-life care is further illustrated in the next section that examines the perspectives of two elderly Indo-Canadian individuals, and two elderly Ukrainian-Canadian women.

Changing Family and Community Involvement in End-of-Life Care for Immigrant Seniors

Family issues with immigrant seniors, as those issues with others in Canada, are not static. The following material from interviews with two elderly East-Indian individuals and two elderly Ukrainian women show the complexity of family and community care at the end-of-life for those immigrant seniors that have lived in Canada for a considerable part of their lives.

Dr. A is a male, aged 77 years, from India. He left India in 1959 to complete postgraduate studies and immigrated to Canada in 1966 where he worked as a university professor. Mrs. B. is a recently retired acute care nurse, aged 67. She and her spouse immigrated to Canada in 1967. Mrs. B's primary reasons for immigration were the pursuit of educational and employment opportunities. Both individuals have resided in Canada for most of their adult lives but continue to strongly identify with their East Indian, Hindu heritage.

There is an expectation within traditional East Indian societal and familial structures that adult children care for their aging parents. Interestingly these interviews revealed that both participants recognized the difficulty of realizing this cultural norm within a Canadian context:

> Generally we as husband and wife talk that in India it is different and here is going to be different. We won't be children dependent. And even if the children want to look after ourselves, then we will say "no, you go and have your own busy life with your own little family." (Mrs. B)

> As I say the cultural context (Indian) does not apply here because in the cultural context you expect that when you are older, one of your children will live with you, his children and you would have at least a three generation family. Here it does not apply because I don't have any son. But even if I did, there would be no guarantee that the son would live close to me or with me. (Dr. A)

Mrs. B's concern for the well being of her children relinquished them from this significant and traditional responsibility:

> . . . but still we are thinking compassionately for them. That they should not be overburdened by the care that we have to go in their care. Especially staying with them in their houses. That is a no no. That we will say no, no matter what.

Given such profound shifts in the cultural expectations surrounding end-of-life care, it is probable that during this period both individuals will receive some degree of care from mainstream health care providers. As such the health care team must become accustomed to considering holistic strategies of care which meet the needs of immigrants in relation to their personal experiences and expectations rather than assuming the predominance of cultural or religious ideals.

Although of the same cultural and religious background, each participant expressed different perspectives of the future care they may receive as they near the end of their lives. Both discussed those habits that future caregivers would need to be aware of in order to ensure quality end-of-life care. Mrs. B described particular habits that were indicative of her personal spirituality:

> They (caregivers) would like to know something of my habits. Like you know, habits are grooves in the brain that imprints go and I believe in the rebirth of the soul, so I know that those habits are hard to remove. And I have some habits. And I would like them to know that I am a strict vegetarian and that I am a hygiene nut. Like you know I have to have a bath every day, no matter what happens a bath is a must. And I need to have some time to myself in silence. I am doing my own prayer in my own way. (Mrs. B)

Conversely, Dr. A expressed a more general attitude:

Watch me for a number of days. I am not a demanding person. I would like to
be left alone. I will not fuss over anything . . . I am almost vegetarian, but we are
not what you call strict vegetarians. If it is a well cooked dish with tender loving
care. I don't demand that it has to be Indian style or anything that is done well,
I'll go along with. (Dr. A)

Both participants also revealed differing opinions about comfort with physical
touch. While Dr. A expressed comfort with physical touch, Mrs. B. held a perspective
that was a reflection of her personal spiritual beliefs:

. . . somehow I feel that you can touch any part of my body but not my feet
because I am humbled here. Because feet would be touched to a great person or
we bow to the feet of deities. But you know, I don't want anybody to massage
or touch or anything. (Mrs. B)

These are just two brief examples of the complexities that continue to evolve
when considering the provision of end-of-life care to the immigrant senior. These comments suggest a very personalized and complex interpretation of culture and spirituality emanating from a vast source of life experience. Nothing can be assumed about any
senior simply based upon their purported cultural or religious affiliation. It is incumbent
upon the health care team to assist the immigrant senior and their family to identify
those elements of culture and spirituality that will be paramount in their individual
experience of end-of-life care. Such assessment and conversation between the immigrant senior and the health care team is intrinsic to the provision of excellent end-of-
life care.

Two Ukrainian-Canadian older women were also interviewed about their beliefs
regarding end-of-life issues. At the time of the interviews, both lived independently in
their own homes in a small rural town with a population of approximately 30 people.
Mrs. C is an 80-year-old woman who was six years old when her family immigrated to
Canada; Mrs. D is a 78-year-old woman who was seven years old when she immigrated to Canada with her family, so each of these women have lived in Canada for the
vast majority of their lives. Both of these women had provided end-of-life care to their
husbands within the two years prior to the interviews, as well as to their own mothers
earlier in their lives. Mrs. C had also provided end-of-life care to her mother-in-law.
Despite their own experiences with spousal and familial care-giving, neither of these
women expressed an expectation that their children would provide care for them at the
end of their lives. In fact, both adamantly expressed the desire to spare their children
the burden of having to provide such care. Mrs. C stated:

I don't know if I would want the children to worry about me . . . to take care of
me . . . It's not fair to the kids to take care of me that much. I don't know . . .

they're always saying, "We wouldn't let you go anyplace mom, to anything – a
Lodge. But I said, "It's not fair! You guys got your life." (Mrs. C)

While the role of care-giver for elderly parents and ailing spouses at the end of
life has traditionally been relegated to the Ukrainian female, there appears to have
been a distinct shift within the family structure of Ukrainian-Canadian families in
regards to such care-giving responsibilities. Although the assimilation process has
undoubtedly contributed to a movement of the care-giving responsibilities from the
private sphere into the public sphere, it appears that these two women have a concern about going into long-term care. Both of these Ukrainian-Canadian women
expressed their unwillingness to have to live out their final years in an institutional
facility. As stated by Mrs. C:

> My husband's mother was very scared to be given away to the Lodge. She
> always asked us . . . everyday . . . she asked us, "Please don't give me away."
> (Mrs. C)

While expressing her own unwillingness to move into an institutional setting,
Mrs. C also referred to a discussion about the possibility of moving her husband into
the Lodge when he was ill for the three and a half years that she cared for him at the
end of his life.

> I was just happy that I could take care of him. Really. Because if I would have
> give him away to a place, I would have died sooner because I couldn't be there
> and I don't drive. You know.[My son] said, "Mom there's no way. We'll never give
> him to the Lodge! Never." It's just one of those things. (Mrs. C)

Mrs. D also spoke about not wanting to have her children care for her at the end
of her life, and she also spoke about not wanting to live in an institution when she
could no longer care for herself.

> Well, to tell you the truth, I never want to go to the Lodge! Oh no. God, no. I
> said, "I'd rather die." I don't want no life supporters or anything whatever you
> call . . . I wouldn't want to go the Lodge. (Mrs. D)

It is clear that these older Ukrainian women have strong views about who will
provide end-of-life care to them. They do not want their children to provide this care
but, conversely, they do not want to go into an institution. This seems to be a significant contradiction as end-of-life care will undoubtedly have to be provided by family
members or a long-term care institution. This is a contradiction that health care teams
will have to consider in future work in end-of-life care with immigrant seniors. On the
other hand, the elderly Indian man and woman confirm that they do not want their
children to provide care at the end of life for them but they seem to accept that they
will go into long-term care as long as they had certain conditions satisfied. Again,
health care teams providing end-of-life care to immigrant seniors have to be aware of

the differences that these seniors will have with respect to receiving care at the end of their lives.

Conclusion

Individual concepts of wellness and illness are directly influenced by culture (Broome & McGuinness, 2007). Rust and colleagues (2006) have suggested that lack of cultural competence in palliative care has contributed to health disparities in this care. Therefore, when dealing with senior immigrants, it is vital that clinical practice be relevant and sensitive to the realities of the particular cultural situation with respect to end-of-life care.

Interacting with individuals who are at the end of their lives can be a very rewarding experience. People come to the end of their life within a cultural framework that will often influence their attitudes towards end-of-life care. With good communication, patients report improved understanding of their condition as well as enhanced treatment compliance (Robinson & Heritage, 2006). Therefore, an intervention in end-of-life care for immigrant seniors that may improve cultural awareness is cultural education for health care teams especially since few members of the health care team receive training on how they can ensure their care is culturally competent (Barclay et al., 2007). Empirical data on educational interventions showed improved health outcomes (Beach et al., 2005) as education is the key to preventing misunderstanding. Cultural-competence training impacts the knowledge and attitudes of health care providers and benefits patient satisfaction regarding the care they receive (Beach et al., 2005).

Significant conflict may occur when families are asked to consider limiting or withdrawing care at the end of life (Barclay et al., 2007). The root of the conflict is usually a breakdown in communication between the health care team and family members. A major factor in disagreements between clinical staff and family is often related to a lack of information (Barclay et al., 2007). Families require more information, the need for information to be free from medical jargon, and the need for the information to be consistent amongst providers (Norton, Tilden, Tolle, Nelson & Eggman, 2003). Good communication, while challenging, is especially difficult at the end of life but is key to building collaborative relationships and avoiding conflict.

Learning about an individual's culture requires close observation and a willingness to be open to the needs of all people involved in the process of end-of-life care within a cultural context. Cultural competence is about relationships and understanding that each individual is unique. A sensitive practitioner will be able to bridge the differences between cultures so that all sides of the care equation – the senior receiving end-of-life care, the family members, and the providers of care – are all respected and understood. In this way, we can foster an environment where cultural considerations are significant components of end-of-life care in Canada in order to ensure the provision of excellent end-of-life care for immigrant seniors in Canada.

References

Barclay, J., Blackhall, L. & Tulsky, J. (2007). Communication strategies and cultural issues in the delivery of bad news. *Journal of Palliative Medicine 10,* 958-977.

Beach, M., Price, E., Gary, T., Robinson, K., Gozu, A., Palacio, A., et al. (2005). Cultural competence: A systematic review of health care provider education interventions. *Medical Care, 43,* 356-373.

Blackhall, L., Frank, G., Murphy, S. & Michel, V. (2001). Bioethics in a different tongue: The case of truth-telling. *Journal of Urban Health. 78,* 59-71.

Bowman, K. (2000). Chinese seniors' perspectives on end-of-life decisions. *Social Science Medicine, 53,* 455-464.

Broome, B., & McGuinness, T. (2007). A CRASH Course in Cultural Competence for Nurses. *Urologic Nursing, 27,* 292-304.

Campbell M., & Guzman J. (2004). A proactive approach to improve end-of-life care in a medical intensive care unit for patients with terminal dementia. *Critical Care Medicine, 32,* 1839-1843.

Canadian Hospice and Palliative Care Association Website: www.chpca.net/home.html

Chan, K. (1995). Progress in traditional Chinese medicine. Trends. *Pharmocological Science, 16,* 182-187.

Crain, M. (1996). A cross-cultural study of beliefs, attitudes and values in Chinese-born American and non-Chinese frail homebound elderly. *Journal of Long Term Home Health Care, 15,* 9-18.

Dewar, A. (2000). Nurses' experiences in giving bad news to patients with spinal cord injuries. *Journal of Neuroscience Nursing, 32,*324-330.

Ebden, P., Carey, O., Bhatt, A. & Harrison, B. (1998). The bilingual consultation. *Lancet, 1,* 347.

Facione, N., Giancarlo, C. & Chan, L.M. (2000). Perceived risk and help-seeking behaviour for breast cancer: A Chinese-American perspective. *Cancer Nursing, 23,* 258-267.

Feser, L & Bon Bernard, C. (2003). Enhancing cultural competence in palliative care: Perspective of an elderly Chinese community in Calgary. *Journal of Palliative Care, 19,* 133-139.

Fielding, R. & Hung, J. (1996). Preferences for information and involvement in decisions during cancer care among a Hong Kong Chinese population. *Psycho-oncology, 5,* 321-329.

Fielding, R., Wong, L. & Ko, L. (1998). Strategies of information disclosure to Chinese cancer patients in an Asian community. *Psycho-oncology, ,7,* 240-251.

Flores, G. (2005). The impact of medical interpreter services on the quality of health care: A systemic review. *Medical Care Research Review,62,* 255-299.

Gervais, M. & Jovchelovitch, S. (1998). *The health beliefs of the Chinese community in England: A qualitative research study.* London, Health Education Authority.

Guo, Z. (1995). Chinese Confucian culture and the medical ethical tradition. *Journal of Medical Ethics, 21,* 239-246.

Hawker, S., Payne, S., Kerr, C., Hardey, M. & Powell, J. (2002). Appraising the evidence: reviewing disparate data systemically. *Qualitative Health Research, 12,* 1284-1299.

Ho, S., Ho, J., Chan, C, Chan, K.K. & Yenny, K.Y. (2003b). Decisional considerations of hereditary colon cancer genetic test results among Hong Kong Chinese adults. *Cancer Epidemiological Biomarkers Prevention, 12,* 426-432.

Huang, X., Meiser, B., Butow, P. & Goldstein, D. (1999). Attitudes and information needs of Chinese migrant cancer patients and their relatives. *Australia New Zealand Journal of Medicine, 29,* 207-213.

Jiang, Y., Li, J., Lui, C. et al.(2006). Different attitudes of oncology clinicians toward truth telling of different stages of cancer. *Support Care Cancer, 14,* 1119-1125.

Kagawa-Singer, M. & Blackhall, L. (2001). Negotiating cross-cultural issues at the end of life: "You got to go where he lives." *JAMA, 286,* 2993-3001.

Kagawa-Singer, M. & Kassim-Lakha, S. (2003). A strategy to reduce cross-cultural miscommunication and increase the likelihood of improving health outcomes. *Academic Medicine, 78,* 577-587.

Koo, L. (1987). Concepts of disease causation, treatment and prevention among Hong Kong Chinese: diversity and eclecticism. *Social Science Medicine, 25,* 405-417.

Lapine, A., Wang-Cheng, R., Goldstein, M., Nooney, A., Lamb, G. &, Derse, A.R. (2001). When cultures clash: physician, patient, and family wishes in truth disclosure for dying patients. *Journal of Palliative Medicine, 4,* 475-480.

Leung, P. & Lee, P. (1996). Psychotherapy with the Chinese, In M.H. Bond (Ed.) *The Handbook of Chinese Psychology* (441-456). New York: Oxford University Press.

Lin, C., Tsai, H., Chious, J., Lai, Y., Kao, C. & Tsou, T. (2003). Changes in levels of hope after diagnostic disclosure among Taiwanese patients with cancer. *Cancer Nursing, 26,*155-160.

Lin, C., & Tsay, H. (2005). Relationships among perceived diagnostic disclosure, health locus of control, and levels of hope in Taiwanese cancer patients. *Psycho-oncology, 14,* 376-385.

Majumdar, B., Browne, G., Roberts, J. & Carpio, B. (2004). Effects of cultural sensitivity training on health care provider attitudes and patient outcomes. *Journal of Nursing Scholarship, 36,* 161-166.

Muller, J. & Desmond B. (1992). Ethical dilemmas in cross-cultural context: a Chinese example. *Western Journal of Medicine, 157,* 323-327.

Norris, W., Wenrich, M., Nielsen, E., Treece, P., Jackson, J. & Curtis, J. (2005). Communication about end-of-life care between language-discordant patients and clinicians: Insights from medical interpreters. *Journal of Palliative Medicine, 8,* 1016-1024.

Norton, S., Tilden, B., Tolle, S., Nelson, C. & Eggman, S. (2003). Life support withdrawal: Communication and conflict. *American Journal of Critical Care, 12,* 548-555.

Payne, S., Chapman, A., Holloway, M., Seymour, J. & Chau, R. (2005). Chinese Community views: Promoting cultural competence in palliative care. *Journal of Palliative Care, 21,* 111-116.

Robinson, J. & Heritage, J. (2006). Physicians' opening questions and patients' satisfaction. *Patient Education Counselling, 60,* 279-285.

Ross, M., Dunning, J. & Edwards, M. (2001). Palliative care in China: Facilitating the process of development. *Journal of Palliative Care, 17,* 281-287.

Rust, G., Kondwani, K., Martinez, R., Dansie, R., Wong, W. & Fry-Johnson, Y. (2006). A crashcourse in cultural competency. *Ethnicity and Disease, 16,* 29-36.

Smith, P. & Bond, M. (1993). *Social psychology across cultures: Analysis and perspectives.* Hemel Hempstead: Harvester Wheatsheaf.

Sproston, K., Pitson, L., Whitfield, G. & Walker, E. (1999). *Health and lifestyles of the Chinese population in England. London:* Health Education Authority.

Statistics Canada. Statistics Canada 2006. Internet: www.statcan.ca/start.html

Tang, S. & Lee, S. (2004). Cancer diagnosis and prognosis in Taiwan: Patient preferences versus experiences. *Psycho-oncology, 13,* 1–13.

Tong, K. (1994). The Chinese palliative patient and family in North America: A cultural perspective. *Journal of Palliative Care, 10,* 26-28.

Wong-Kim, E., Sun, A. & DeMattos, M. (2003). Assessing cancer beliefs in a Chinese immigrant community. *Cancer Control, 10,* 22-28.

Woo, K. (1999). Care for Chinese palliative patients. *Journal of Palliative Care, 15,* 70-74.

Yeo, S., Meiser, B., Barlow-Stewart, K., Goldstein, D., Tucker, K. & Eisenbruch, M. (2005). Understanding community beliefs of Chinese-Australian about cancer: Initial insights using an ethnographic approach. *Psycho-oncology,14,* 174-186.

Yick, A. & Gupta, R. (2002). Chinese cultural dimensions of death, dying and bereavement: Focus group findings. *Journal of Cultural Diversity, 9,* 32-42.

Yu, J., Li, J.Y., Chang, L., Huang, M.J., Lin, Z., Mei, L., Yia, Z. & Wei, Y.Q. (2007). Different attitudes of Chinese patients and their families toward truth telling of different stages of cancer. *Pyscho-oncology, 16,* 928-936.

9

Cultural Diversity in Long-Term Care: Confusion with Cultural Tensions

Douglas Durst, (University of Regina).

There is probably no other seniors' issue that generates more fear and misunder-standings than the topic of long-term care. Unfortunately, the perceptions are often negative. The act of placing one's aging parent into the "old folks" home is viewed as the ultimate abandonment. Others view the adult child as callous and uncaring. After sacrificing a lifetime of love and care-giving, the adult child is viewed as shuffling the elder parent into a cold and depressing institution for reasons of personal convenience. Such views are grossly unfair to both the adult child and the health care service deliv-ered by the competent and dedicated professionals of long-term facilities.

This chapter examines long-term care in relation to immigrant and ethnic minori-ties. It is meant to inform the lay-person and ameliorate the guilt and misconceptions associated with long-term care. The health care field is a "culture unto its own" and this chapter will introduce the lay-person to the language and process of accessing quality and culturally appropriate services for their aging family member. The chapter will also inform those assisting immigrants/refugees and minority persons about the aging process and the need for increasing assistance in living. It is also hoped that those in the health care field and especially those in gerontology will find the chapter helpful in seeking ways to interface the access and integration of ethnic and minority persons in the mainstream social and health systems.

This chapter begins with an overview of the model of continuum of care, describ-ing the breadth and scope of health and social care for seniors. It describes long-term care, the process of admission into the system and the levels of care. Adult children with frail parents would find this information helpful in seeking appropriate care for their parents. The next section provides a summary of the current situation in Canada and the significance of the "industry" of long-term care. There is considerable provin-cial variance and some description of the resident population is provided along with a discussion of the cultural issues and tensions of long-term care for some ethnic groups.

The chapter concludes with a short discussion of integrated services and culturally specific homes.

Continuum of Care

Aging is about loss, it means the loss of physical abilities and can also include loss of emotional and intellectual abilities. As one ages, it means the need for increased support and care that represents a subtle "slope" rather than "steps" of care. The model of continuum of care can be quite confusing to the lay Canadian-born person and overwhelming to newcomers. Yet, all of these services offer immigrant families, with an aging member, possible options to sustain or improve the quality of life for the entire family. As to how the service can be delivered or accessed in a culturally appropriate context is open to consultation. The continuum of care model includes over 60 types of services that can be categorized into seven groups (Evashwick, 1987 in Dunkle, Kart & Luong, 2001). Following is a list and short summary of options that provide individuals and families with strategies:

- to delay illness and disease in healthy seniors,
- to maintain and maximize independence in culturally appropriate ways; and
- to improve the quality of life in the senior's later years.

1. **Extended inpatient care** is what is commonly referred to as *nursing homes* and derogatorily as *old folk's homes*. These formal institutions are for individuals who require constant nursing and support services because of limitations due to illness or disability. Most of this chapter focuses on this level of service.

2. **Acute inpatient care** includes hospitals and rehabilitation centres that provide health services on a short-term basis for serious but acute problems. Mental health services, physical rehabilitation and addiction services are also included. Normally, a treatment plan is established with goals leading to a discharge date.

3. **Ambulatory care** simply means "walking" care and includes all those health and social services where the client travels to the service. Examples include visiting the physician, outpatient services, counselling services, dialysis, and physiotherapy. These services can be preventive, diagnostic, rehabilitative, or aimed at maintenance..

4. **Home care** encompasses a broad spectrum of services provided in the home of the client who is limited in his/her ability to travel. It may include health-focused services such as nursing care or therapy, or support services for independent living such as respite care, "meals-on-wheels" domestic cleaning.

5. **Outreach programs** are designed to link clients to available programs and services, improving access. These may include transportation services such as para-transport for persons with disabilities, information services and referrals. Outreach programs can be highly effective in improving accessibility when offered by ethnic groups through volunteer associations.

6. **Wellness programs** are very popular in various ethnic communities. They are for those individuals who are healthy and wish to remain so, through health promotion, preventive and educational services. The programs are well suited to being provided by ethnic organizations. They can include exercise, and be recreational, social and educational in nature.

7. **Housing services** lend themselves to the ethnic community and are normally privately funded. They provide health and support services through the creation of a "home setting." They appear as independent senior apartments, retirement communities, assisted living homes with supervision and adult family homes.

The continuum of care model provides an overview of the breadth and scope of services and supports available to maintain independence and maximize physical, emotional and intellectual well-being (Hollander, 2002). These services can be provided on a short-term, intermittent or long term basis. There are vast opportunities for both inclusion and exclusion of culturally sensitive or culturally focused services. Who provides the services and how services are formulated and delivered can influence the success or failure of their ability to provide satisfying and welcoming programs for ethnically diverse communities. Critics of the model argue that it has been developed from the perspective of administrative and professional services of the care providers rather than the needs of the elder (Gubrium, 1991).

Under the Canada's Constitution (1982), health and health related services are mandated under the provincial/territorial governments. Policies and programs will differ slightly but the federal *Canada Health Act* ensures that services have uniformity under the principles of comprehensiveness, universality, portability and accessibility. However, long-term care is not included in the *Canada Health Act* and is not fully funded in any province or territory (Dignity Denied, 2007). While in the hospital, a senior may receive full medical services but in long-term care, he/she would be responsible as if in his or her own home. The study by *Dignity Denied* (2007) describes the system of continuing care as a "patchwork quilt" of complex and confusing services.

Long-term Care Homes

Long-term care homes are frequently referred to as "nursing homes" where 24-hour nursing care and supervision are provided in a secure environment. In Canada, there is no consistent nomenclature used to describe these homes (Neysmith, 1994; Havens, 2002). In Saskatchewan, the term "Special Care Homes" is used for "nursing homes" and "Personal Care Homes" is used for smaller private facilities without nursing care (Saskatchewan, 2008). Interestingly, in Quebec, the term "Centres d' Accueil" (meeting places) is used. In a continuum of care, long-term homes offer higher levels of personal care and support than retirement homes or personal care homes (supportive housing). The provision of long-term care is broader than only the provision of nursing homes. It includes a complicated matrix of health and related support services for individuals who have limiting abilities in order to maintain or maximize independent living. The health, social and personal care services include both informal and formal sectors. In recent years, the meaning of *long-term care* has broadened to include all those services to maximize the physical, psychological, emotional and social well-being of persons with compromised functioning (Barresi & Stull, 1993 in Dunkle, Kart & Luong, 2001). With this definition, family members provide the majority of health, social and personal care services in personal homes and it is estimated that 80-90% is provided and financed by relatives, mostly adult children (Dunkle, Kart & Luong, 2001). With differences in the language and terms, it can be equally confusing to both professionals and lay persons. When communicating with newcomers, it is important for professionals to carefully explain the terms and avoid "industry jargon."

Long-term care homes are mainly owned and operated by three types of organizations:

- Nursing homes that are owned and operated as for-profit private organizations that have their operating budget support through public funds;
- Municipal councils or regional health districts may be required to construct and operate a home in their area, sometimes in partnership with a local municipality; and
- Non-government homes operated by non-profit charitable corporations that may be community-based, faith-based or by ethnic/cultural groups.

It is these non-government homes that provide an opportunity to partner with government to own and operate ethnic specific homes. The Chinese-Canadian community has been one of the first visible minority groups to build and operate long-term homes for their aging population in communities where sufficient numbers of Chinese live. The Canadian Jewish community is another early provider of homes for their religious members.

There are mainly two types of accommodation. "Preferred Accommodation" is used to describe private or semi-private rooms with special features. "Basic or Standard Accommodation" is normally shared with 3 other residents. The term *resident* is the norm to describe the clients and avoids the connotation of illness/sickness in the term *patient.* The facility is meant to be a home and not a hospital. The features of each home vary depending upon depending upon when and how the home was built.

Each home has its own food services providing dining rooms and daily meals. Common rooms, lounges, and recreation services are also available and some larger homes may have beauty salons, gift shops, chapels and outdoor gardens. They are, in fact, a small community where the residents live, eat, socialize and sleep. At most homes, the staff work hard to create a *home-like* atmosphere, minimizing the institutional feel. In Regina, a visitor from the United States was shocked and complained that there was no security officer and *sign-in book* at the front entrance. Staff explained that such *security* would diminish the home environment. They asked the visitor, "Do you have security officers and sign-in books at your home?"

Along with 24-hour nursing care, personal care and supervision, the homes provide room furnishings, meals, laundry, housekeeping, social and recreational programs. Medication, physical therapy, personal hygiene supplies, and medical supplies and aids such as walkers and wheel chairs may be provided for a fee depending upon the income of the resident. Other optional services are offered for a fee such as cable TV, hairdressing, telephone and transportation.

A plan of care is developed for each resident that describes the necessary care and levels of service offered. In Ontario, the plan must be reviewed at least every three months and altered as the resident's needs change (Ontario, 2008b). Essentially, there are two kinds of "stay" – long stay and short stay. The terms for the stays may differ from province to province but they mainly fit under these two categories. Long stay is open-ended and for an indefinite period of time. In most cases, it means until end of life but could mean transfer to another type of care or transfer to another institution. For example, a home may transfer a resident with Alzheimer disease to another facility with a specialized unit that has closer supervision for persons with severe dementia. In Ontario, short stay is limited to a maximum of 90 days per year (Ontario, 2008b). In some cases, short stay is provided to give respite service to caregivers, freeing family members from daily caregiving duties. The break may be for a variety of reasons such as to rest and refresh or because of health issues of the caregiver. Supportive care, transition care or assessment care gives the resident an opportunity to recover from a hospital stay, accident or assessment to determine the resident's need. It can give the resident time to improve confidence and strength in order to return to his/her private home or some kind of assisted living. The service needs can be determined and implemented as the resident returns home or to another care level/facility. These transition and assessment services sometimes can prevent admission and enable the elder to return home to live independently for a little longer (Durst, 1998).

Since the homes need provincial funding to operate, each province has instituted legislation governing long-term homes. The provincial department responsible for carrying out the legislation sets standards for care and regularly inspects the homes. Homes have mission statements and service goals that recognize the rights of the residents to quality care, privacy and well-being. National standards are ensured through accreditation by the Canadian Council of Health Services Accreditation (CCHSA). Homes with this accreditation have completed a self-assessment and been thoroughly reviewed and evaluated by the Council (Young, 2002). In 1996, the Council implemented the Client-centred Accreditation Program (CCAP) with a emphasis on client-centred care and service (Young, 2002). Any resident, family member or prospective resident should ask for annual reports and evaluation reviews from the home supervisor or provincial authorities. Each home and province has a mechanism to handle complaints or requests for information such as toll-free telephone lines. Residents or family members from ethnic minorities may not be aware of helpful and constructive communication processes available to them.

Years ago, family members faced the daunting task of their parent's diminishing abilities alone. The decision to give up providing care in the home was a difficult one plagued with guilt and shame. As their parent required increasing levels of care, they sought admission to long-term care homes that were filled and holding long waiting lists. Today, the admission process is open and transparent with a single point of entry. Health districts or regions have strict policies and procedures regarding admissions and discharges. These are considered public documents and are available to all with most documents accessible on their respective webpage. In Regina, the System Wide Admission and Discharge Department (SWADD) accepts all applications, determine s need, and places the resident on a single waiting list for the first available home. The resident can refuse the first homes offered if he/she has a preference to wait for a specific home of his/her choice. There is no queue jumping and no direct opportunity for discrimination. In one case, a family member complained that it was taking too long to find a bed for her elderly mother. She was expressing frustration and implying discrimination until she was told that a resident would have to die before a bed would be available. She quietly realized that her "peace of mind" was dependent upon someone else's grief.

Before admission, a qualified social or health professional will complete a thorough assessment that includes demographic information, current living conditions, hospital stay, physical and mental health conditions and a list of daily activities to determine level of functioning. Usually, a case conference is held with professionals and family members. From the assessment, degree of risk is determined from minimal to high risk. The assessment determines the necessary services and the level of care. It is important that family members participate and provide input into the assessment. For ethnic/minority residents, cultural issues or concerns can be addressed before admission, thereby, preventing potential communication problems and concerns.

Regions vary as to language and definitions, but it is helpful to consider five levels of care. The following description is adapted from Saskatchewan Health (2007). In **Level 1, Supervisory Care,** clients may live at an assisted living apartment, their own home or with family members but require some moderate supervision and assistance with daily living.

Level 2, Personal Care is for clients who are ambulatory with or without walkers and aids or are independent with a wheelchair. They need supervision or assistance with hygiene and grooming. Normally, they are continent and capable of self-feeding. They may have some behavior problems.

At **Level 3, Intensive Person and/or Nursing Care,** the residents have advanced physical or mental illnesses that are stabilized and not likely to significantly deteriorate further in the near future. Most of the health care is provided by *special care aides* or nursing assistants under the supervision of a Registered Nurse and directed by the resident's physician. The resident may be completely ambulant, ambulant with a walker or aid, wheelchair restricted, or bed-fast.

Level 4, Extended Care includes residents who do not require acute hospital care and treatment but need constant advanced health/nursing care on a 24-hour basis. This care may include special medical procedures to achieve improvement or stabilize a condition. Almost all of these residents will be bed-fast, bed-chair-fast or severely limited in personal mobility. The exception will be residents with dementia who may be completely ambulant. Within Level 4 there are three subcategories. *Specialized Supervisory Care* focuses on the management of serious mental deterioration and the associated problems with care and safety. Along with the dementia, there may be physical health conditions that require medical attentions as well. *Supportive Care* is provided through nursing care to stop or slow health deterioration. *Restorative Care* is meant to improve the functional ability of the resident through gradual rehabilitation, physical therapy or medical treatment. The optimistic goal is to achieve a high level of functioning found in *Level 3 or 2.*

Level 5, Intensive Rehabilitation is not normally provided in long-term care facilities but in specialized rehabilitation centres. These centres provide aggressive rehabilitation for persons with physical disabilities from injuries including strokes, illnesses and congenital conditions. Under a team of rehabilitation specialists, a treatment plan is developed to restore or improve the resident's functioning. Results from intensive treatment are expected within approximately three months. Once the team has assessed that further improvements are unlikely, the resident will be assessed and discharged home, or to another facility. Depending upon the cause of the loss of functioning, the resident may move into a facility at *Level 3 or 4 Care.*

Because of the level of comprehensive care, long-term care homes need to be financially subsidized by provincial governments. The real costs would be prohibitive for all but the richest of residents. Residents are required to contribute to the partial costs and in Ontario it is called a "co-payment" (Ontario, 2008b). In 2008, Ontario residents pay about $1500 for basic accommodation, $1800 for semi-private and $2100 for private rooms. Indigent residents have Old Age Security and Guaranteed Income Supplement that will cover the basic payment and in some cases, other welfare/support programs make up the difference. In Saskatchewan, the standard resident fee was $948 plus 50% of their income between $1 151 and $2 855.

At the time of admission, a social worker or health professional will meet with the client and his/her family to calculate the resident's monthly fee. This income test normally only assesses income including all pensions, investments and interest from deposits. Personal assets such as private poverty and possessions are not considered in determining the monthly fee. There are considerations for married couples, separated couples and other circumstances. The process is open and transparent and potential residents are encouraged to ask questions. Unfortunately, the policies regarding the specifics of what services and products are covered depend upon provincial regulations. These services and benefits vary widely from province to province.

Usually, a short time after the admission, the staff will arrange a care conference with the family, doctor, senior nurses and other professional staff. A professional staff member will discuss with the admitting senior and his/her family *Advance Directives*. This is an opportunity for the senior to inform the doctor, the facility staff and family of his/her wishes as to the level of care when no longer able to speak for him or herself. The decision rests with the senior's wishes and takes considerable pressure off the family in times of emergency or end-of-life situations. In most provinces, there are four levels of care. Supportive or Comfort Care provides services to maximize comfort and normally does not include transferring to a hospital or cardiopulmonary resuscitation (CPR). For elderly persons with complicated health conditions or a terminal illness, CPR does little to save lives but only prolongs death. Limited Therapeutic Care may include hospital transfer for comfort reasons but not include CPR. Level Three involves emergency hospital transfer for treatment where an assessment is completed. The elder may be admitted for treatment or returned to the long term care home. Level Four includes CPR and full medical care, including admission to an intensive care unit.

In accordance with provincial legislation, a person must be identified to make substitute health care decisions. Soon after admission, a conference is held to determine the decision-maker. At this conference, the resident identifies a substitute decision maker who will make difficult decisions when the senior is no longer mentally or physically able. It is usually the person's spouse, adult child or sibling but may include other relatives. *Advance Directives* are reviewed annually and can be changed at the will of the resident.

Current Situation: Long-Term Care Homes in Canada

Long-term care for the aged is a significant health care industry and it has some unique features that separate it from most health care services. In Canada (outside of the Province of Quebec), there are 2 086 facilities with four or more beds that are funded, licensed or approved by provincial/territorial authorities, normally the departments of Health and/or Social Services. Since Quebec has a different method of data collection, their statistics are not included in this chapter; however, similar patterns can be expected.

In 2005/2006, these facilities provided 206 170 approved beds with 196 242 residents (95% occupancy rate). There are over 82 000 full time employees and 76 000 part-time employees working 335 million hours and earning close to seven billion dollars in salaries and wages (Canada, 2007). When comparing total expenses over total revenues ($11 billion), they operate with a profit margin of less than one percent.

It is an industry that is divided into three substantive sectors of the social and health service field based upon ownership: private (proprietary), government (federal, provincial, municipal) and non-profit (lay, cultural and religious operated). Although provincial standards establish quality and uniformity among the sectors, differing owners have different objectives based upon the purpose of their existence. In 2005/2006, there were 1 006 private facilities (81 085 beds); 420 government (42 448 beds) and 447 non-profit with 42 645 beds. Approximately 54% are for profit private facilities and almost half of the beds at 48.8%. On average, private facilities have 76.4 beds per facility; government have 89.1 beds per facility and non-profit have 95.1 beds per facility (Canada, 2007).

Although privately-owned facilities provide approximately half of the number of facilities and beds, they have only 43.4% of the full time employees, 37.2% of the part-time employees, 38.7% of the hours and only 36.2% of the wages. Private homes operate with lower employee-per-bed, hours-per-bed, and wages-per-bed than government and non-profit homes. Private homes provide less hours per bed and spend fewer dollars per bed than other owners. Private homes provided 1 154 hours per bed compared to government (1 598 hours) and non-profit (1 892 hours) and spent $39 001 per bed compared to government ($59 421) and non-profit ($52 845) facilities (Canada, 2006). Part of the explanation for the differing hours and expenses can be found in the type of care. Private facilities provide services to proportionately more residents at lower levels of care (higher functioning residents) than government facilities with higher levels of care requiring more employees, more hours, and higher skilled health workers. Therefore, government facilities have higher hours and operating expenses.

In 2005/2006, long-term homes spent $2 571 per person per month aged 65 or older but there is considerable variance among the provinces. For example, British Columbia spent a low of $1 874 per senior, Prince Edward Island spent $3 494 and a high of $6 530 per month in the Territories (Canada, 2007).

Table 1

**Characteristics of Long-term Care in Canada- Except Quebec
(Canada, 2007)**

	Private	Non Profit	Government	Total
Facilities	1 006	447	420	1 873
Approved Beds	81 085	42 645	42 448	166 178
Residents	75 837	40 910	40 751	157 498
Average Beds per Facilility	76	95.1	89.1	83.7
Full-time Employees	35 844	21 297	25 501	82 642
Part-time Employees	28 287	23 704	24 099	76 090
Paid Hours (x1000)	93 581	68 149	80 327	242 057
Wages & Salaries (x1000)	$1 841 283	$1 432 998	$1 806 979	$5 081 260
Total Expenditures (x1000)	$3 162 377	$2 253 585	$2 522 321	$7 938 283
Total Revenues (x 1000)	$3 347 388	$2 248 755	$2 484 689	$8 080 832

Resident Population

In Canada, the senior population in residential care has seen a steady growth in recent years. The population grew 5.5% in 2005 and another 3.6% in 2006. Within this growth, there are significant gender differences in resident populations. Reflective of women's longevity, women were more than twice as likely as men to live in long-term care for the aged. Of the total reporting population, 110 555 were women (70.2%) and only 46 943 were men (29.8%) (Canada, 2004, 2005, 2006).

Over 90% of residents lived in large facilities with at least 50 beds and about 70% lived in homes with 100 beds or more (Canada, 2006). The resident population is elderly with 71% over 80 years of age (59.3% of the men are over 80 and 75.9% of the women). It is not surprising that the chances of living in long-term care increase with age. In Canada, only 4.3 % of seniors 65 or older live in a home but increases dramatically to 12.5% for seniors aged 80 years and over. Women over the age of 85 years are much more likely to live in long-term care than men. About 18% of these women live in care compared to 12% of men. Since older men are close to twice as likely to be married or living common law, they have the benefits of supportive care that prevent or delay the need for residential services.

Table 2 provides the total number and percentage of residents over 65 years in long-term Care facilities in Canada and by provinces. Because the numbers are low, the three territories are totaled to protect the privacy of the individuals. It is clear that there is considerable variance among the provinces which demonstrate the "cultural" nature of long-term care. Of all adults 65 years or older, 4.3% of seniors are in long-term care with a high of 7.2% in Prince Edward Island and a low of 3.3% in British Columbia. Generally, the provinces of Atlantic Canada have higher rates of institution-alization. The progressive social programs of Quebec have broken the traditional pattern of institutions resulting in a low percentage of seniors in care (3.4%).

Table 2
Totals and Percentage of Residents Over 65 in Long-term

Province	Population of 65+	Total	Pop in LT 65+	Percentage
Canada	4 335 255	196 242	186 790	4.3
Newfoundland	70 265	4 246	3 974	5.7
Prince Edward Island	20 185	1 555	1 463	7.2
Nova Scotia	138 210	6 585	6 144	4.4
New Brunswick	107 635	6 333	5 561	5.2
Quebec	1 080 285	38 744	est 36 658	3.4
Ontario	1 649 180	84 365	79 823	4.8
Manitoba	161 890	9 541	9 032	5.6
Saskatchewan	149 305	7 873	7 353	4.9
Alberta	353 410	15 676	14 461	4.1
British Columbia	599 810	21 015	19 968	3.3
Territories	5 075	309	267	5.3
(Canada, 2007)				

There are no reliable statistics on ethnic diversity in long term care but it is understood that seniors of ethnic backgrounds have many barriers to accessing long-term care (MacLean & Klein, 2002). In a study of six special care homes including long-term homes in Regina, it was found that few residents were members of visible minorities (Wasylenka, 2004). However, one large home listed over seven percent as visible minorities which over represents the general population of senior visible minorities (2.4%). At the time, the city of Regina had a population of only 5.2% as visible minority but staff in the homes regularly exceeded the general population of minorities (Wasylenka, 2004). Among the six homes, 35.6% of staff members were visible minorities and the largest home with 390 residents had 47% visible minority staff (Wasylenka, 2004). In Regina, these staff members were located in all positions throughout the homes, from cleaning, kitchen, care-giver aids, nursing assistants, nurses and other professionals. Admittedly, the few higher level positions in the administration were not visible minorities. The professional care-givers are multicultural and it is generalized that this pattern exists in many homes across Canada and the United States (Morris, Caro & Hansen, 1998). Sadly, it is more common than admitted but many visible minority staff are subjected to racist slurs and comments from residents (MacLean & Klein, 2002).

Cultural Issues, Tensions and Conflicts

Historically and globally, the final years of the life cycle occurred in the home under the care of the extended family. People grew old and died at home surrounded by the extended family and multiple generations. Adult children automatically assumed filial piety – the care of their aging parents until death and everyone helped. In western societies, the responsibility of elder care has become shared with the family and the state with each taking on different roles. Among many ethnic groups, filial piety is the ideal and the expectation of family members from countries such as China, South Asia, the Philippines, and Latin America. However, life in Canada creates different pressures and many families need dual income earners in order to maintain the North American lifestyle. In addition, as the parent ages and demands for both physical and mental care increase, families do not have capacity to provide the level of care required. The realistic roles of the adult children may conflict with their wishes. Even though they want to provide care, the demands are just too great. These nuclear families may not have the larger extended family and its supports. There is no respite for them in their continuing care which can become 24 hours/seven days per week. In a study by Wong, Yoo and Stewart (2005), in situations where Chinese seniors were living independently, their preference was to utilize community and public services rather than family. Many foreign-born seniors are caught between two value systems – their traditional kinship oriented system versus the western value of independence and individuality. Clearly there is a role for formal assistance in maintaining and enhancing a sense of empowerment that strengthens family and community resources (Yang, Kim & Chiriboga, 2006).

Out of cultural guilt, these struggling families may delay accessing appropriate and timely care. Frequently, the elder enters care in very poor mental and physical health and has serious difficulty adjusting. In one case, a Lao grandmother came into care for about 2 weeks and returned home to die a week later. Had she entered the home in better mental and physical health she may have adjusted better and had an improved quality of life in her last months.

If the parent immigrated under the Family Class, the sponsoring adult children are responsible for all care and not able to access benefits afforded to seniors until ten years have passed. After ten years, the senior is eligible for Old Age Security, Guaranteed Income Supplement and related heath and social welfare benefits. The aging parent may have no choice but to stay with the family and be completely dependent for services like transportation, social and recreation activities, spending money, translation and information. Even though the family home may be quite luxurious, some seniors have described their lives as "living in a golden jail."

There are also differing expectations regarding filial piety. The parents may have one expectation and the adult children another. It can be difficult for the entire family, as in Chinese custom where the eldest son is expected to care for his parents but the weight of care falls on his wife – the daughter-in-law. If there is a poor relationship between the women, the situation can have some significant tensions. With feelings of guilt and tensions, the family may be reluctant to seek help, increasing the sense of burden on the caregiver. The appropriateness and support of homecare is lost.

There may also be stigma regarding mental illness, dementia and even physical conditions. All of these prevent the family from seeking outside supports. When the situation deteriorates to the level that the family cannot cope any longer, they seek long-term care. The elder enters the system in very poor physical and mental health.

On a more positive note, the family may be relieved and now has time to recover from the demands of constant care. Once in the home, they can participate in more engaging and personal ways as the aspects of physical care are mainly handled by the home. Regular visits, social outings and celebrations with food can enrich the parent's quality of life.

Staff of the home may encounter complicated family-based decision making. In many Asian cultures, there is heavy emphasis on preventing "losing face" so careful discussion and options are explored respecting the dignity of the parent and family. Some families will insist that all or important family members participate in the decision. It could complicate or delay the decision-making process when the eldest son is out of the city or lives in another city. Family decisions regarding important treatment may be delayed putting the elder at risk when all members are not available.

Cultural taboos about dying and death are not uncommon among many individuals and many cultural groups. Decisions around *Advance Directives*, including end of life care, may be avoided or complicated because of a reluctance to discuss or an inability to come to a family consensus. Among some cultures, the topic is taboo and very disturbing. This situation is common among mainstream families as well but the cultural context may further complicate the situation. Shortly after admission, the ethnic resident and his/her family will be confronted by professional staff openly talking and asking questions regarding the resident's wishes. Although the staff are sincere in following the resident's wishes, the family may find the experience deeply disturbing and shocking.

However, this is an excellent opportunity for the resident and family members to express their wishes regarding cultural and religious customs in care. Issues or concerns about recreation, social situations, diet, touching, modesty, and whatever is of concern should be raised at the earliest stage in the admission process. Confusion, disappointment and emotional hurt can be avoided through frank and open communication by both parties. However, it is recognized that there are structural barriers that can complicate the communication in this "foreign institution." Language limitations can put family members at a disadvantage when they are not able to understand the options available to them and able to express their wishes. Also, there are power relationships at work. After a cultural lifetime of deferring to authority and authority figures, it may be overwhelming difficult for elders and family members to assert their wishes and insist on special services or programs. Then the fear of having their wishes denying and the "loss of face" prevent some from pushing too hard.

In a private meeting and later in the resident's care, the family should discuss their specific wishes when the resident dies. If the family has cultural and religious customs regarding the deceased body and death rites, they should be clear. They should not assume that the staff will know their beliefs and customs. The family has a responsibility to inform staff and express their wishes at or near death. Good communication is essential at these times of stress and bereavement.

Finally, it is critical that professional staff at the home include and utilize the extensive support system many ethnic families have (Morris et al., 1998). The family members may be shy about their involvement, so staff should encourage and suggest their involvement, especially during special celebrations and religious holidays. Encourage the family to decorate the room and even common areas of the home with seasonal/cultural decorations and symbols. It will engage staff and other residents and make the elder feel comfortable and welcomed.

Staff members need to recognize each person's unique life experience and be careful not to generalize. Upon admission, a thorough assessment is normally done and it is here that a social history is documented. It is also an opportunity to assess the resident's degree of acculturation and note any special cultural considerations that should be undertaken. Some assessment of family involvement and degree of support should be documented and encourage their involvement in the resident's future care. It is helpful for professional staff to review the file and keep informed of culturally appropriate care. It is also helpful if professional staff members learn and document cultural practices and customs. There are important cultural differences regarding self-determination, trust, privacy and family care-giving responsibilities (Durst & Ram, 2003). An excellent and practical resource is the toolkit called *Diversity in Action: A Toolkit for Residential Settings for Seniors* (Ontario, 2008a). The report *Creating Welcoming Communities in Long-Term Care Homes* has numerous helpful tips for both professionals and members of ethno-cultural communities including a list of practical resources from across Canada (Christensen & Rajzman, 2007). The previous chapter (MacLean, et al.) provides interesting case studies that illustrate the issues raised in this chapter.

Future Issues

It is clear that our aging population is changing and changes are needed to address Canada's ethnic diversity. Specific to long-term care, there are two basic approaches to address the needs of frail seniors. Existing homes that have been created to provide services to the mainstream population need to respond with greater cultural sensitivity and appropriateness. These homes already have culturally diverse staff and the transition to increasing culturally appropriate services and programs should not be as difficult as it first appears. However, it does require recognition and commitment from the administration down through the entire staff of the home. It starts with leadership and serious effort to respect and develop sensitive services and programs.

The other strategy is the creation of long-term homes that are faith or ethnicity specific. This is not a new model as homes for Jewish seniors have been in existence for decades. There needs to be a large enough group of acculturated members in order to succeed in creating a home. Presently there are successful homes for Ukrainian, South Asian/Indo, Slovenian, Italian and many others across Canada. Homes that are specific to Chinese seniors are the fastest growing group of long-term homes. Many of these homes started with informal recreation and social programs for their aging seniors. Some groups developed day-care like programs and evolved into higher levels of care. One of the first steps in this process is the creation of a membership and Board of Directors leading to provincial incorporation. Provincial incorporation is necessary as no government or organization will grant or loan money to a non-incorporated body. Incorporation requires the group to have a level of sophistication and competency to deal with government and legal administrations. Hence, the group must be acculturated and "integrated" sufficiently into mainstream culture to be successful. They must be able to raise money through fund raising and grant applications. This spirit of volunteerism and altruism may be foreign to some groups where, if services are provided, they are provided through established institutions such as the government or religious bodies. The self-help strategy may be new to some groups. Many Chinese Canadians are highly successfully and possess significant resources; hence the creation of new homes in cities with sizable Chinese Canadian populations. Vancouver is also seeing the creation of specialized services and homes for Indo-Canadians (Chaudhury & Mahmood, 2005).

Often, there is an assumption that most ethnic seniors desire to live-in with adult children. For many years, they have lived independently and held successful careers and/or businesses. They have been sponsored to Canada in order to provide child care for their grandchildren, leaving behind their homes, businesses and family/friends. Times change and as the grandchildren mature and no longer require close supervision, many seniors are seeking independent living in retirement apartments and assisted living. They want to be on their own but being close to family and friends remains important (Chou & Chi, 2002).

In conclusion, the wish of most ethnic seniors is to age in their own homes but due to changes in their family's acculturation, it is anticipated that more of these aging seniors will seek long-term care. There are four needs to ensure the development and maintenance of quality care (Luh, 2003). First, there is a need for qualitative research to understand the meanings of quality of life, independence and values of older ethnic adults. Second, policy makers, service providers, and community workers need to be more informed about the importance and impact of ethnicity and culture. Third, there is a need for active recruitment of staff from diverse backgrounds for administrative and direct service provision. Fourth, there is a need for improved education and training both academically and in-service for staff on inter-cultural practice.

The solution to improving and maximizing the quality of life for frail ethnic seniors is communication and collaboration. If they work together, the resident, family members, staff of long-term care and members of the ethnic community can create warm and healthy environments for those in the last years of their life. Improved communication can go a long way in reducing confusion and healing the cultural tensions.

References

Bergman, H., Beland, F., Lebel, P., Contandrioopoulos, A., Tousignant, P., Brunelle, Y., et al. (2007). Care for Canada's frail elderly population: Fragmentation or integration? *Canadian Medical Association. 157* (8), 1116-1121.

Canada (2004, 2005, 2006). Statistics Canada. Census Reports. Population Demographics: Age and Province. Web pages. www12.statcan.ca.

Canada. (2007). Statistics Canada. Reports. Residential Care Facilities 83-237-XIE. Selected CANISM Tables. Web pages. www12.statcan.ca

Chaudbury, H. & Mahood, A. (2005). Seniors' housing in Vancouver's south Asian community. [Electronic version]. *Seniors' Housing Update. 14* (1), 1-3.

Chou, K. & Chi, I. (2002). Successful aging among young-old, old-old, and oldest-old Chinese. [Electronic version]. *International Journal of Aging and Human Development, 54* (1), 1-14.

Christensen, J. & Rajzman, E. (2007). *Creating welcoming communities in long-rerm care homes: support for ethno-cultural and spiritual diversity.* Toronto, ON: Concerned Friends of Ontario Citizens in Care Facilities.

Dignity denied: Long-term care and Canada's elderly. (2007). [Electronic version]. *National Union of Public and General Employees.* pp.1-52.

Dunkle, R., Kart, C. & Luong, V. (2001). Long-term care. In C.S. Kart & J.M. Kinney, (Editors). *The Realities of Aging: An Introduction to Gernotology* (pp. 454-484). Boston, Massachusetts: Allyn and Bacon.

Durst, J. (1998). Eldercare discharge planning: Listening to the voices of family caregivers. Unpublished Project Report, Master of Social Work. Regina: University of Regina.

Durst, J. & Ram, K. (2003). *Culturally sensitive practice with immigrant seniors in long term care, Regina, Saskatchewan, Canada.* International Metropolis Conference, Vienna, Austria. September 2003.

Gubrium, J. (1991). *The mosaic of care: Frail elderly and their families in the real world.* New York: Springer Publication Company.

Havens, Betty. (2002). Users of long-term continuing care. In Marion Stephenson & Eleanor Sawyer, (Eds.). *Continuing the care: The issues and challenges of long-term care. Revised edition.* Ottawa, ON: Canadian Healthcare Association. pp. 87-108.

Hollander, Marcus J. (2002). The continuum of care: An integrated system of service delivery. In Marion Stephenson & Eleanor Sawyer, (Eds.). *Continuing the care: The issues and challenges of long-term care. Revised edition.* Ottawa, ON: Canadian Healthcare Association. pp.57-70.

Luh, J. (2003). Ethnicity, older adults, and long-term care. *Innovations enhancing ability in dementia care. 2*(4), 1-2.

MacLean, Michael J. & Klein, Jennifer Greenwood. (2002). Accessibility to long-term care: The myth versus the reality. In Marion Stephenson & Eleanor Sawyer, (Eds.). *Continuing the care: The issues and challenges of long-term care. Revised edition.* Ottawa, ON: Canadian Healthcare Association. pp. 71-86.

Morris, R., Caro, F. & Hansan, J. (1998). *Personal assistance, The future of home care.* Baltimore, MD: The John Hopkins University Press.

Neysmith, S. (1994). Canadian long-term care: It's escalating cost for women. In L.Katz Olson (Ed.), *The graying of the world: who will care for the frail elderly?* (163-188). New York: The Haworth Press.

Ontario (2008a). *Diversity in action: A toolkit for residential settings for seniors.* Toronto ON: Queen's Printer of Ontario. www.ontarioseniors.ca

Ontario, (2008b). Ministry of Health and Long-Term Care. *Seniors' Care: Long-term care homes.* Web page. www.health.gov.on.ca.

Saskatchewan (2008). *Saskatchewan Health. Continuing Care.* Web page. www.health.gov.sk.ca.

Wasylenka, K. (2004). *Visible minority seniors in long term care: Not many and frail.* Unpublished Master of Social Work thesis. Regina: University of Regina.

Wong, S., Yoo, G. & Stewart, A. (2005). Examining the types of social support and the actual sources of support in older Chinese and Korean immigrants. [Electronic version]. *International Journal of Aging and Human Development, 60* (1), 105-121.

Yang, Y., Kim, G. & Chiriboga, D. (2006). Correlates of sense of control among older Korean-American immigrants; financial status, physical health constraints and environmental challenges. [Electronic version]. *International Journal of Aging and Human Development, 63*(6), 173-186.

Young, Sylvia. (2002). The quality factor in long-term care. In Marion Stephenson & Eleanor Sawyer, (Eds.). *Continuing the care: The issues and challenges of long-term care. Revised edition.* Ottawa, ON: Canadian Healthcare Association. pp. 291-312.

10

Senior Immigrants' Support Needs and Preferences of Support Intervention Programs

Edward Makwarimba, Miriam Stewart, Zhi Jones, and Knox Makumbe, (University of Alberta), Edward Shizha, (Wilfrid Laurier University), and Denise Spitzer, (University of Ottawa)

Introduction

In recent years, Canada has experienced an influx of immigrants. The 2001 Census (Canada, 2003) indicates that 18.2% or 5 448 480 individuals out of 30 000 094 people in the Canadian population were born outside of the country. Over thirteen percent or 3 983 845 of Canada's population were members of a visible minority group. In 2005, 13% of the Canadian population were 65 years of age or older. This proportion is expected to reach 23-25% in year 2032 and 25-30% in 2056 (Belanger, Martel & Caron-Malenfant, 2005). Similarly, Alberta is witnessing a steady increase of immigrant population, from 14 383 in 1995 to 16 468 in 2004 (National Advisory Council of Aging, 2005); Chinese immigrants account for 30% of all newcomers, Afro-Caribbean 9.5%, Spanish 3.8%, and 2.3% from the former Yugoslavi (Canada, 2005). While these groups represent collectively close to 50% of immigrants in the province, 18% of this population are seniors (Health, 1999).

Immigration leads to major changes to lifestyle and environment (Aroian, Tran & Balsam, 2001). The initial settlement is the most stressful stage for immigrants as they attempt to fit into new social networks and grapple with cultural shock (Ng, Wilkins, Gendron & Barthelot, 2005) which generates feelings of social isolation, exclusion, frustration, despair and helplessness (Au, 2003). Consequently, many immigrants find themselves faced with problems such as stress, change, loss, and trauma linked to acculturation (Lai, 2004). Others suffer from health-related problems such as depression, loneliness (Aroian, Tran & Balsam, 2001), psychological distress, and mental health concerns (Lai, 2004).

Although much evidence has revealed that inadequate official language skills, unaccepted foreign credentials, and unemployment (Leblanc, 2002) are often causes for emotional distress and depression for young and middle-aged adult immigrants (Au, 2003), the experiences of immigrant seniors are largely unexamined.

Our partners, Canadian Heritage and Multicultural Health Brokers Co-op, observe challenges faced by socially isolated immigrant seniors in accessing culturally-relevant health-related services in Edmonton. Yet the support needs and experiences of these socially isolated seniors have not been investigated. Most previous research, including our own (Stewart, Neufeld, et al., 2004), has emphasized the support needs and resources of young and middle aged adult immigrants or those of non-immigrant seniors, therefore neglecting to consider the support needs and resources, support seeking behavior, and support preferences of immigrant seniors. Moreover, the views of immigrant seniors on the influence of social support and ethnicity on health, health behavior, and use of health services have not been investigated. With support from Canadian Heritage, we undertook to address this gap in our knowledge. The objectives of this study were to:

1. assess and describe the social support resource needs and preferences of Chinese (Mandarin-speaking), Afro-Caribbean, Kurdish, former Yugoslavian and Spanish-origin senior immigrants in Edmonton;

2. identify personal coping strategies used by Chinese (Mandarin-speaking), Afro-Caribbean, Kurdish, former Yugoslavian and Spanish-origin seniors;

3. determine senior immigrants' preferences for support interventions in health and health-related sectors;

4. gather service providers' perspectives on support services available to immigrant seniors, services used by immigrant seniors, relevance and appropriateness of these formal support resources, and recommended support interventions;

5. compare support intervention preferences of senior immigrants from the Mandarin-speaking Chinese, Afro-Caribbean, Kurdish, former Yugoslavian and Spanish-speaking ethno-cultural backgrounds, and formal support intervention programs provided by service providers; and

6. recommend support interventions preferred by and appropriate to ethnic seniors in this study.

Review of Relevant Research

Immigration and Health

In Canada, older persons are most likely to suffer from chronic health conditions that restrict their activities (Eapen, Bajpai & Chiappa, 2002). Immigrant seniors suffer more negative experiences than their host-nation counterparts (Durst, 2005; Jang & Chiriboga, 2006). Although the needs of senior immigrants are similar to those of Canadian seniors (e.g., mobility, social contact, housing, affordable health services) (Yeh & Lo, 2004; Eapen, 2003; Walls, 2003), immigrant seniors encounter additional challenges pertaining to languages, literacy (Jang & Chiriboga, 2006), low self-esteem (Au, 2003), and a new socio-cultural context. Many seniors, who recently came to Canada under the family reunification program, do not speak English or French and are socially and economically dependent on their children (Durst, 2005; Ajrough, 2005). Their life experiences and subjective perspectives exert major influences on integration, life satisfaction, mental health and emotional stability (Hussain & Cochrane, 2004). Despite these problems that impact negatively on their health outcomes, immigrant seniors may embrace culturally-specific beliefs about illness and health behavior that influence their attitudes towards use of health services and supports (Lai & Surood, 2007).

Studies have documented immigrants' risks for poor health and reduced access to and use of health services, (Ajrough, 2005; Wong, 2006). Moreover migrants can be marginalized by systemic and institutional barriers in the health sector (Canada, 2005). Immigrant seniors have been institutionalized in culturally incongruent health care facilities created for Canadian seniors and few outreach programs for prevention and management of disease are targeted to their needsni. Adhering to their strong cultural values, immigrant elders may avoid mainstream services in favor of culturally congruent programs and may express difficulty accessing services that are culturally compatible with their unique needs (Lai & Surood, 2007). A study of seniors from Asian, Central American, South American and African backgrounds in Ontario revealed that home care services were used less by these seniors than by Canadian-born seniors because of language and cultural barriers (Yeh & Lo, 2004). In a similar study in British Columbia, 15% of immigrants had unmet health needs due to cost barriers, while almost half (48%) held negative perceptions of health care services which contributed to underutilization (Wu, 2004). Our previous studies, on immigrants and refugees (Eapen, 2003) and caregivers of seniors, (Au, 2009) in Alberta, document the effects of social and cultural barriers on mobilization of formal supports and services. However, deficiencies in social support and gaps in supportive programs and policies in Canada, which could have detrimental impacts on immigrant seniors' health and use of health services, need to be examined. These findings are supported by a study on health care use among elderly Mexicans in the United States (Wong, 2006).

Similarly, studies in Spain report that immigrant seniors under use health services due to inaccessibility of services, isolation, insufficient knowledge about available programs and services, low perceived efficacy of programs, and, perceptions of ethnic prejudice in health professionals (Hernandez-plaza & Alonso-Morillejo, 2004; Aroian, Wu & Tran, 2005). These problems contribute to negative health outcomes among immigrant seniors.

Research has shown that the acculturation process is more challenging for older immigrants who retain their traditional values, beliefs, and norms of their culture (Lai,

2004). Immigrant seniors are faced with a unique set of challenges when resettling in a new country including changing family dynamics, different or inadequate housing, language and communication difficulties, cultural shock and clash, loneliness, and barriers to integration (Pang, Jordan-Marah, Silverstein & Cody, 2003) that may lead to mental health problems such as psychological distress, anxiety, and trauma (Docum & Sharma, 2004). Depression may occur frequently among immigrant seniors due to limited resources, yet symptoms of depression often go unnoticed, undiagnosed, and untreated. While some studies suggest abundant negative effects of migration on mental health (Escobar, 1998), others report that immigrant possess mental health advantage compared to their Canadian-born counterparts (Flaskerud, 1999). Mental health problems over time among immigrant seniors were also reported in European Union countries. Research suggests that older immigrants are at a higher risk of depression than native-born seniors. Levels of acculturation have been hypothesized to relate both negatively and positively with mental health (Acevedo, 2000). Low acculturation due to lack of host country language skills has been associated with social isolation and low self-esteem; however, high acculturation may be linked to alienation from traditional supports, internalization of negative host-society beliefs, and increased exposure to alcohol and drug abuse. Minority group members who choose to maintain their cultural identity and, at the same time, become part of the larger societal networks in their host country have the best mental health outcomes Retention of cultural traditions may therefore contribute to positive health behaviors (e.g., better eating, less substance use) associated with good mental and physical health outcomes (Escobar, 1998).

Social Support and Health

Extensive research has revealed the positive effects of interpersonal relationships and social support on health outcomes (Wu & Hart, 2002). As well, the direct positive effect of social support networks on immigrants' adjustment is well documented (Shen & Takeucki, 2001). Epidemiological data confirm that social support (e.g., strong social networks, social contact) is related to longevity and decreased mortality (Seeman, 2000). Social support influences health behaviors and how individuals with health problems react to and recuperate from various diseases (Wu, 2004). Studies have demonstrated associations between increased levels of social support and reduced risk for physical disease, mental illness, and mortality (Seeman, 2000; Stroebe, 2000). Conversely, physical and mental health affects availability and quality of support (Wu & Hart, 2002). Chronic health problems erode social support and reduce social contact and participation (Aroian, Wu & Tran, 2005; Wu & Hart, 2002).

Successful aging has been linked to mental and physical functioning and social engagement (McReynolds & Rossen, 2004). Social support is an important factor in promoting and maintaining long-term health diminishing the impact of chronic disease and impairments on health status, maintaining ability to live independently, and, improving quality of life (McReynolds, 2004) for older adults. Whereas older adults' self-esteem and independence can be reduced through ineffective or undesired forms of support (McReyolds, 2004), social engagement of older adults is linked to greater cognitive vitality and active living (McReyonds, 2004). Seniors who engage in an active lifestyle report improvement in social relations (Eapen, 2003). Social interactions have an impact on healthy behaviors and optimal aging (Seeman, 2000). Social support from family and friends has been associated with long-term exercise adherence in older adults.

Despite challenges faced by immigrant seniors, those who have maintained cognitive abilities enjoy more social contact than those who have not (Wu & Hart, 2002). However, enduring health problems may cause chronic stress, which in turn results in disengagement from social support networks. Lack of social support generates emotional strain and psychological distress among elderly immigrants (Wu & Hart, 2002). Support provided by ethnic community members is associated with positive health outcomes (Hyman, 2001). Seniors with greater integration within the ethnic community enjoy more benefits For example, Chinese refugees in Canada, living in their own community, are reported to enjoy mental health advantage compared to non-Chinese refugees. However, immigrant seniors may not find accessible and trustworthy sources of formal or informal support when they migrate to new countries (Dominelli, 2004). Diversity in help-seeking behavior, support needs, and preferences for supportive interventions among immigrant seniors may emerge from differences in perceptions of health and illness, and attitudes toward the benefits of health services (Wu, 2004). An important dimension of unmet health needs for immigrant seniors is the social context of support-seeking behaviors, support needs, support intervention preferences, and health services (Wu, 2004; Perez, 2002) These issues were investigated in our study "Finding Firmer Ground: Support Intervention Preferences for Immigrant Seniors."

Social Support Intervention Programs

Although public and private organizations offer diverse types of social and health services and support resources for immigrants, some investigations show that newcomers' use of services is extremely low (Aroian, Wu & Tran, 2005). Research reveals that the main source of support for immigrants is their informal social network. Interpersonal contacts are an essential source of information about the receiving society. Interventions providing social support can promote health. Several intervention programs, encompassing social support, have been developed to promote the health and well-being of non-immigrant older adults (Saito, Sagawa & Kanagawa). Cultural customs and values should be recognized when planning support intervention programs for seniors from diverse cultural backgrounds (McReynolds, 2004). Dyadic, social network, group, and community-level support interventions have been suggested for migrant populations (Stewart, Reutter, Letourneau & Campbell, 2003). However, these interventions have not been designed for the unique needs and circumstances of immigrant seniors.

Research Gaps

In recent years, there has been a growing interest in research focused on aging and ethnicity, although language, cultural barriers and customs restrict access to immigrant seniors (Durst, 2005) and limit generalization (Durst, 2005). Moreover, most published research on immigrant seniors has focused on a single ethnic group (Olson, 2001). Little is known about how migrant elders from different countries of origin adapt following immigration late in life. Social support studies have either emphasized non-immigrant seniors or young to middle aged immigrants. Major gaps in relevant research include lack of attention to: immigrant seniors' perspectives on 1) support resources, support needs, support-seeking strategies, and preferences for supportive interventions, 2) the influence and intersection of social support and culture/ethnicity as health determinants, and 3) the influence of social support on access to health-related services. Consequently, in this initiative, we investigated the support resources and needs, support-seeking strategies, and support intervention preferences of immigrant seniors from five different ethnic groups. We also assessed immigrant seniors' perspectives on the influences of social support on health, health behavior and the use of health services. Finally, we sought service providers' views on support intervention(s) that could enable immigrant seniors to cope with challenges associated with aging and migration.

Theoretical Foundations of Study

The theoretical foundation underpinning this study is adapted from the theoretical framework developed by the Principal Investigator (Stewart, 2000) for this study and the Social Support Research Program. Social support is defined as ". . . interactions with family members, neighbors, friends, peers, and professionals that communicate information, esteem, aid, and emotional help" (Stewart, 2000). Social support is conceptualized in this study as interactions that can improve coping (e.g., support seeking), and reduce stressors (e.g., social isolation) associated with migration (Choi & Wodarski, 1996). When needs for belonging are not met, feelings of social isolation may develop. Different types of social support (emotional, instrumental, information, and affirmation) can be provided not only by the natural network of spouses/partners, family and friends, but also by service providers and health professionals (Carlson, 1999). Supportive persons can alter appraisal of stressors, sustain coping efforts, and influence choice of coping strategies (Carlson, 1999). The proposed study is based on a conceptualization of social support as a coping resource or coping assistance for stressful situations associated with immigration and settlement. Social support and coping have bi-directional effects on stressors. For example, the ways immigrant seniors cope provide clues to potential supporters about whether and what types of support are needed. Conversely, the amount and type of support received can influence immigrant seniors' choice of coping strategies. Similarly, support and stress have bi-directional effects. Appropriate support can lower stress (Carlson, 1999). However, immigrating as a senior may result in conflicted interactions, miscarried helping, and inadequate support that can increase stress. Indeed, the costs of providing support include over-involvement and burden (Carlson, 1999). Social network members may offer information and encouragement to maintain healthy behaviors, provide advice, act as role models, and, constrain people from inappropriate health behaviors. People who receive support experience a greater sense of belonging and enhanced health outcomes (Krause & Wulff, 2005).

Method

Phase 1
Sample and Recruitment

Purposive and snowball sampling was employed to select 48 immigrant seniors, 12 from each of four ethno-cultural groups – Chinese, Afro-Caribbean, former Yugoslavian, and Spanish – to participate as primary informants in the study. Respondents were selected to represent a balance of social characteristics (e.g., sex, education, years lived in Canada, living situation). Therefore, six men and six women were selected from each ethnic community.

Demographic data also indicated that the participants represented diverse demographic profiles. Immigrant seniors who participated in the study were 55 years old and more. Half of the participants were in the 61-70 age range. Only two of the seniors were aged more than 80 years. Strategies for recruiting immigrant seniors were guided by the Community Advisory Committee.

Data Collection

Qualitative data collection methods with participatory elements were employed in this phase to enhance understanding of meanings, perceptions, beliefs, values, and behaviors of immigrant seniors (Sptizer, Henry & Popp, 1998) to study sensitive issues and vulnerable groups (Tomblin-Murphy, Stewart, Ritchie & Weld, 2000). Four community brokers (one from each ethno-cultural community) were recruited as community research assistants (CRAs) and trained to conduct face-to-face interviews with immigrant seniors in the language of their choice. The interviewers came from the same ethnic communities as the immigrant seniors. These interviewers were able to overcome language and cultural barriers and foster confidence, trust, and disclosure.

The interviews elicited in-depth data from immigrant seniors about their support resources, support needs, support-seeking strategies, support intervention preferences and their perceptions of the influence of social support and ethnicity on health, health behavior, and use of health services.

The initial interview guide was reviewed by the Community Advisory Committee. Following the review and relevant revisions, the interview guide with open-ended questions and appropriate probes was translated into the languages of the immigrant seniors and later back-translated into English to ensure that all versions were consistent and accurate in meaning. The revised interview guide was pilot-tested with immigrant seniors – one from each ethnic group. Participants also completed a demographic data form which elicited information regarding age, sex, language, living arrangements, length of stay in Canada, and other factors relevant to support needs and preferences of immigrant seniors. All immigrant senior participants received a token of appreciation to compensate them for their time and expenses. The interviews were tape recorded and conducted at locations convenient for seniors and bus tickets were provided to seniors who needed this form of transportation. Five partner organizations offered space for these interviews. For example, some interviews with Chinese seniors were conducted at the ASSIST Community Services Centre. Field notes were generated by interviewers to document observations of the interview conditions and factors which might have influenced the individual interviews.

Phase 2
Sample and Recruitment

In the second phase of the study, group interviews were conducted with service providers and policy makers. Service providers (n=26) were selected from agencies/institutions/organizations in health and health-related sectors that provide services to immigrant seniors. Service providers were purposively sampled to represent different health-related disciplines (e.g., nurses, physicians, social workers, psychologists). Strategies for identifying service providers from health-related service organizations were guided by the Community Advisory Committee.

Data Collection

Group interviews with 26 service providers were facilitated by two research team members. The interview guide for the interviews was reviewed and revised by the Community Advisory Committee and investigators before it was used. The final interview guide, which included five questions, was used to solicit information regarding formal support services available to immigrant seniors, services used by immigrant seniors, relevance and appropriateness of these formal support resources, and recommended support interventions. The participants were divided into three groups comprised of nine, nine, and eight respectively.

Data Analysis for Phases 1 and 2

The individual and group interviews were taped and transcribed, and the qualitative data were subjected to thematic content analysis of social support for immigrant seniors and its influence on health, health behavior, and use of health services. Inductive analysis was used to create a coding framework and recurrent themes were systematically compared to identify substantive categories and potential theoretical codes. The coding framework was transferred to QSR N7™ qualitative data analysis software to enable data management and coding. The coding process entailed extraction of significant statements from transcripts and classification into appropriate categories.

Phases I and II Findings

In-depth qualitative data gathered from interviews from the four ethnic communities provided detailed accounts of immigrant seniors' and service providers' perceptions of support resources, support-seeking strategies, and support needs.

Social Support Needs of Immigrant Seniors

Most immigrant seniors described their social support needs along a continuum involving both formal and informal supports. Practical/instrumental support emerged as the major support need of immigrant seniors followed by informational support, emotional support, and affirmational support. Due to lack of English language proficiency, the majority of participants reported experiencing a major challenge in interacting with mainstream Canadians and people from outside their own ethnic communities. Consequently, some seniors did not know where and how to get the necessary information that could help them seek and access social services and programs.

> . . . Even though Canada provides very good service, since I don't understand the language, I don't feel they are very good. They are difficult for me . . . It's difficult for me to do something outside. (CH # 08, Chinese Mandarin)

> I need someone to translate for me. It contributes to me feeling good; it keeps me from feeling stressed when I go to the doctor. If I go by myself I won't know how to say it hurts here or there, but if I go with someone who speaks English he will translate for me. They will tell me if I need an exam for this or that, if I

need an x-ray for this or that, and he will explain everything, because he speaks
English. (Lat. #05, Spanish-speaking)

Social Support Intervention Preferences of Immigrant Seniors

Analysis of immigrant seniors' opinions for services and support reveals an over-arching theme of existing services were linguistically and culturally inappropriate. These seniors felt that services were either culturally insensitive or unavailable. Most emphasized the lack of communication and opportunities for seniors to get together and socialize. Seniors preferred services and programs that brought people together for social and cultural activities. They recommended the use of immigrants' languages by professionals, provision of services in different languages, and employment of immigrants to deal with immigrant issues.

Table 1

Social Support Needs of Senior Immigrants

Practical/Instrumental	Informational	Emotional	Affirmational
• Language translation • Learning English • Different language services • Transport • Medication • Ethnic doctors • Finance • Pension eligibility • Home and car repairs • Physical exercises • Social and cultural activities • Employment • Entertainment	• Directions • Legal issues • Health issues • Accessing services •Entitlement	• Listening • Counselling • Understanding • Sympathy	• Advice • Guidance • Sharing experiences • Affirming immigration status

I feel that, since Canada is a multicultural society, the TV program shouldn't just have English program. They should learn from Singapore. It has many programs. It has Malay program, English program, and Chinese program . . . you must have some program for the minorities. This is a real problem. (CH# 02, Chinese)

. . . no big problems, except language. For language, Canada is a multicultural society, services should be multicultural. (CH# 07, Chinese)

Preference was also given to programs that helped immigrant seniors to communicate among themselves and with other people in the mainstream Canadian society. "I would like most people speak English so I can learn English. If there are all Chinese, you always speak Chinese, you can't improve your English" (CH# 10, Chinese).

While some immigrant seniors prefer language programs, others especially those from the Afro-Caribbean community prefer programs that provide seniors with information.

> We need to know what the government has in place for us people from the islands you I think they should know what social support is there for seniors . . . they need to know about that. They don't know much about it. (AC # 10, Afro-Caribbean)

Preferred Sources of Support

Membership in groups was considered important for both the immigrant seniors' social life and their integration to the Canadian society. Most seniors preferred that support be provided by people of the same age, ethnic group, and of those speaking the same language. Immigrant seniors pointed out that language posed a barrier to their efforts to communicate with mainstream Canadians if they shared services/programs. Service providers agreed that seniors would prefer being part of a group with people who speak their language. To illustrate, immigrant seniors generally did not participate in tenant meetings due to language problems. In addition, attendance at social and recreational programs seemed to be dependent on the availability of other people who spoke the seniors' language. Gender mix did not matter to some participants.

In contrast, some seniors of Spanish and former Yugoslavian origins believed that the mixing of different people, particularly English speaking Canadians, not only helped them learn English much faster, but also enhanced their cultural understanding and improved their social integration.

> . . . People should be there in their own culture. It's not because I don't want to cross-culture. It's because you cannot understand me unless you know me . . . my background . . . (AC #02, Afro Caribbean)
>
> Well it would be people who speak the same language, if it is English I won't be able to understand. It is better to be the same language that you speak . . . (Lat.# 06, Spanish speaking)
>
> Mmmh . . . there you caught me . . . I would like to be where everyone speaks Spanish and also where some speak English so I can practice English. If it was mixed it would be nice because one would have two options. (Lat.# 04, Spanish speaking)

Another important source of support for immigrant seniors is their ethnic group. Service providers noted that even though they wanted to reach out to all people, at times seniors still were isolated and wanted to be served by someone who understood their culture, especially when it concerned sensitive information or personal problems. Immigrant seniors wanted to have their own cultural or ethnic group centres (e.g.,

Hindu, Sudanese or Indian) where they could meet, speak their own language, and cook their own food. One ethnic group, as an example, held meetings in their homes and preferred to have information dissemination sessions or health services provided at their own residence rather than going to the city hall.

> . . . they want a place of their own where they can go and meet with their own
> people, speak their own language, have their own place within, say, a long-term
> care facility where those seniors could be together, speak their own language,
> have someone cooking the appropriate food for them. So it is more of a segre-
> gated sort of model. (Service Provider)

Other seniors believed strongly in the benefit of mixing with people of different ages and backgrounds. Participation in new activities at seniors' centres was seen as an opportunity to learn from other cultures. In addition, some seniors believed that this would give them the opportunity to practice their English. Interfaith programs offered by some agencies were popular among seniors because they allowed them to practice their religions without any restriction. Through these multicultural and multi-faith programs, seniors are not only able to make friends with people from different parts of the world, but also to appreciate cultural differences.

Table 2.

Support preferred by immigrant seniors

Content of support intervention (What new interventions should provide)	Preferred support providers (Who should provide support to seniors in new intervention programs?)
• access to information • language classes • getting people together (socialization) • outdoor outings and cultural activities • physical activities and entertainment • creative arts including art display	• established immigrant seniors • professionals with organizational skills • volunteers (same language with seniors) • anyone willing to help
Ways to facilitate access to programs • transportation availability • use of cummunity brokers • use of translators • need financial support	Timing and duration of support • on arrival in Canada and as long as it is needed • at anytime and should be an on-going program • during periods of crisis and could be either short-term or of no fixed period

> I would like most people speak English so I can learn English. If there are all
> Chinese, you always speak Chinese, you can't improve your English. If you ask

Canadians, you can know how to say something in English, like children learn English. (CH.# 10, Chinese)

. . . there is a mixture; we are really a diverse group. I'm even surprised; you know, a woman just connected with another girl. She's from Libya and the other one is from Israel, and you think, "What? (Service Provider)

Preferred Level of Support

A combination of one-to-one and group support was preferred by most immigrant seniors. Interviewees pointed out that seniors needed help with different issues and that the nature of intervention should depend on issues at hand, immigrant seniors needed help with translations, accessing services, food, bill payments, and transportation. If seniors have problems with their families, for instance, they would prefer to talk to the social workers or counsellors individually. At times they could not disclose and discuss their personal problems in a group setting. Seniors would not like to discuss family issues in a group. Instead, they preferred to address and discuss issues that were common to all of them in a group setting. Service providers agreed that the level of intervention should depend on the situations and circumstances facing the individual.

The tactics need to be really individualized depending on the person's circumstances. And I would see that being very similar; you can't have one answer that meets everybody. But connecting them with services close to their home that will have transportation there is really critical. (Service Provider)

Both are helpful. I also think, um, it is better to have a place for seniors to have some activities together. We can discuss together. It is good. The one-to-one level is OK too. It is better to have different levels. The schedule can be flexible. (CH# 01, Chinese)

Preferred Mode of Support

Many seniors preferred face-to-face delivery of support to telephone contact only. This was particularly important to them because they experienced difficulty understanding service providers through the telephone due to language barriers. Face-to-face support delivery not only helped seniors receive emotional support because of their isolated nature, but also enabled them to access information they needed to navigate the complicated Canadian system.

Ah, face-to-face . . . Because personally speaking the senior people don't love talking, talking to a dumb telephone answering machine. (AC #02, African Caribbean)

It is OK to be one-to-one or group . . . The best way is to visit seniors, in their buildings where people older than 60 or 70 live. Sometimes they have problems with transport, communication, or with using simple things such as a wheelchair, those adjustable beds, or just having someone to talk to. To make groups where they can help other people, knitting gloves, there are many groups that do this at church. (Lat.# 11, Spanish speaking)

We need a person who would come out and visit us from time to time. This would ease our life here. We all have the need to open ourselves to somebody from time to time . . . . Sometimes we cannot discuss our personal problems in the group. (Yu # 04, former Yugoslavian)

Nonetheless, other immigrant seniors, in particular those from the Chinese community, suggested that the telephone mode of support may be convenient for seniors who could not participate in programs due to health or other barriers.

Preferred Location of Support Intervention

Although some immigrant seniors preferred convenient locations for support programs, others suggested that central sites would be acceptable if transportation was provided.

. . . I personally would prefer to have this centre near by as everyone else. The transportation is an issue again here. If I had transportation I do not care, the centre could be 100 kilometres away from me. (Yu# 06, former Yugoslavian)

I believe that the most suitable is in downtown Edmonton, so that all those people living in the periphery can have access. (Lat.# 00, Spanish speaking)

All respondents believed that providing services/ programs for seniors in established institutions (e.g., churches, community centres, community agencies) was cost-effective as they were "equipped" and knowledgeable to deliver support services. They emphasized desirable features including accessible locations of services, well-organized transportation systems, serving immigrant seniors in their own languages by service providers with the same ethnic backgrounds as seniors.

I think people who have knowledge, who want to support others and who are active in their communities. Experience and also knowledge is very important. Already existing programs have experienced and knowledgeable people. (Yu# 03, former Yugoslavian)

I would rather see already existing agencies delivering new programs. This is because every new agency and organization costs money. Having funds and a person capable of the task, for example, Catholic Social Services could organize new suitable programs for us. (Yu# 05, former Yugoslavian)

Support Providers

The immigrant seniors preferred support providers who spoke their languages. Some support providers could be seniors who have been part of community organizations or qualified peers with similar experiences. It was noted that peers and volunteers might need to be trained to work as intervention agents to effectively serve the seniors. Some service providers were already using this approach. For instance some Filipino seniors had been trained as community animators and were trusted by seniors. Another group that fostered the relationship between agencies and immigrant communities was the Multicultural Health Brokers Co-op which helped to deliver health services for immigrant seniors.

> Because I could stand up there and offer a program, and a lot of them will look at me and say: "Little white girl, what do you know about?" It just wouldn't be effective; it wouldn't be effective for me to stand up in front of a group of seniors who immigrated to this country. So I think that having a qualified peer is really key. (Service Provider)

Preferred Duration of Support Intervention

Seniors preferred prolonged intervention because they wanted consistency and did not have other venues for meeting in similar circumstances. For example, the ESL classes provided seniors with an opportunity to socialize and get away from homes where they might be experiencing problems. The key challenge to long-term intervention, as noted by service providers, was that funders wanted to fund new and or self sustaining programs.

> Just about some of that you talked about, too, the inconsistent like, the trend in funding over the last few years, I'd say maybe a couple of years. [Looking] at funding new stuff, which doesn't really help a lot, because some of the programs that need to be out there have to be at least a minimum of 3 years to kind of gain the momentum that it needs to take to be effective in the community. So with lack of funding, you might just have access to funding for a year for a 3-year program. (Service Provider)

Preferred Programs and Policies

Immigrant seniors recommended that major changes be adopted by the government of Canada, such as the introduction of a five-year waiting period for Canadian citizenship to access benefits from the government which could help them relieve financial burden of sponsors. Others pointed out that the lengthy process for citizenship application was a serious problem and recommended that the government reduce the length to two or three-year waiting period to reduce negative impacts on seniors' well-being. Participants believed that new immigration policies should enable them to acquire Canadian passports quickly so that they could maintain regular contact with their home countries and travel which would be psychologically and physically beneficial.

> Visiting my country and family will refresh and recharge my spiritual batteries . . . These batteries would last for a year and then I could go and recharge them again. This is the most important thing for us seniors . . . Visiting my country where my family, my parents, my sister, my husband have been buried is a part of my social life. You know, my sister passed away and I could not go to see her because I did not have a passport! Getting a passport along with a Canadian citizenship would be a nice gesture, a satisfaction for us seniors. It does not a matter of the cost for the process; it is more about the long wait. (Yu# 05, former Yugoslavian)

Some immigrant seniors expressed frustration regarding loss of recognition of their credentials in Canada despite their training, education, and employment experience in their homelands. They believed that if they could use their professional skills accumulated before coming to Canada, they could contribute positively to society and also experience self-satisfaction and well-being.

> Government policy towards immigrants should be changed. For example, many-immigrants were doctors in their home countries. They can't practice in Canada because they don't have the license. In fact, they are very good doctors. (CH# 02, Chinese)

> I think, if the seniors are in good healthy condition and they can contribute to the society, Canadian government should provide some supports. Language barriers can be overcome. For example, some engineering terms, you don't need to speak. You can show me blueprint, I can understand it. I can do it. Some seniors who come with their children have some skills and knowledge that they can share in Canada. (CH# 03, Chinese)

Other recommendations regarding programs included reduction in waiting time and cost of health services, and increased financial aid to alleviate poverty among immigrant seniors.

> Seniors have many diseases. They can't wait as usual, making an appointment, and then wait. They need to see the doctors as soon as possible. It is hard to do this in Canada. For other seniors with cardiovascular diseases, it is not good to wait for a long time. They need prompt treatment. If possible, it is better to have a hospital only for seniors to provide quick treatment to the seniors who are in need..(CH# 03, Chinese)

> Ah, yes, what I was telling you before the interview is about the dentist . . . that it is too expensive here. If I go to the dentist so he can check a tooth because

> it has a cavity it will cost me $500 and where am I going to get that? That is the most difficult thing I see because you don't have a choice but to pay . . . the medication, if you go to the doctor and he tells to buy this drug and well . . . you have to go and buy it. And it is very expensive. (Lat.# 05, Spanish speaking)

Although most seniors advocated accessible centres and resources for ethnic seniors, they supported multicultural services/programs that would allow them to share special occasions of cultural significance. Public transportation systems for excursions to inexpensive social, recreational and entertainment facilities such as community centres, museums, libraries, playgrounds, parks, and festivals could keep seniors active and healthy, and relieve their isolation.

> To us, we hope there are more information and more emotional support. Especially for seniors, the cultural activities are less. We don't have many entertainments. So there should be some emotional support. (CH# 07, Chinese)

> Canada has very different entertainment opportunities. However, I feel cut off from all of that. For example, in my neighborhood there is not one institution to gather us immigrant seniors who have language difficulties. (Yu# 06, former Yugoslavian)

Conclusion

In conclusion, immigrant seniors shared important insights regarding culturally sensitive services and supports that would enhance the well-being of these new members of Canadian society and foster their contribution to their own ethnic community and to Canada. From their personal and professional experiences, service providers concurred with immigrant seniors on the pressing need for support. They also agreed that meeting those needs requires accepting cultural diversity, and providing services and programs that are culturally sensitive. This includes involving providers who share immigrant seniors' culture, providing adequate human and financial resouces, and offering consistency new programs. Because of inadequate personal resources – among seniors – and financial and human resources in service organizations, service providers cannot be expected to provide self-sustaining programs without adequate or sustained funding. Working towards cultural diversity will also be aided by policies ensuring that major instituions (e.g., the city, community, health services) will recruit people from different ethnic and cultural backgrounds to help in the delivery of services. In addition, it is recommended that, if possible, immigrant seniors receive services in their preferred ways. For instance, some ethnic groups prefer information sharing sessions to take place in the seniors' residence as opposed to the city hall. Participants argued that such unorthodox methods not only are cost effective, but also enable service providers to reach people quickly.

This pilot study goes a long way towards facilitating the design of support programs that are culturally appropriate and sensitive because it is based on immigrant seniors' experiences of support needs and their support intervention/program preferences, an approach that has been largely lacking in the design of programs for immigrant seniors.

References

Acevedo M. (2000). The role of acculturation in explaining ethnic differences in the prenatal health-risk behaviors, mental health, and parenting beliefs of Mexican American and European Amercian at-risk women. *Child Abuse and Neglect, 24:*111-127.

Ajrough, K.J. (2005). Arab-American immigrant elders' views about social support. *Ageing & Society 25*: 655-673.

Aroian K.J, Khatusky, G., Tran, T.V. & Balsam, A.L. (2001). Health and Social Service utilization among elderly immigrants from the former Soviet Union. *Journal of Nursing Scholarship 33*: 265-271.

Aroian K, Wu B. & Tran T. (2005). Health care and social service use among Chinese immigrant elders. *Research in Nursing & Health, 28*: 95-105.

Au S. (2009). *Consultation with the Chinese community on inside/outside: A vision for black and ethnic minority mental health.* In: National Institute for Mental Health in England, Department of Health.

Beiser M. & Wickrama, K.A. (2004). Trauma, time, and mental health: A study of temporal reintegrationand depressive disorder among Southeast Asisan refugees. *Psychological Medicine,34*: 899-910.

Belanger A, Martel, L. & Caron-Malenfant, E. (2005). Population projections for Canada, provinces and territories. In: http://www.statcan.ca/bsolc/english/bsolc?catno=91-520-XIE.

Canada (2003). *Facts and figures: Immigration overview, permanent and temporary residents..* Ottawa: Citizenship and Immigration Canada.

Canada. (2005). *Seniors on the margin: Seniors from ethno cultural minorities.* Ottawa: National Advisory Council of Aging.

Carlson DSP, P.L. (1999). The role of social support in the stressor-strain relationship: An examination of work-family conflict. *Journal of Management, 25*: 513-541.

Choi N.G., Wodarski J.S. (1996). The relationship between social support and health status of elderly people: Does social support slow down physical and functional deterioration? *Social Work Research, 20*: 52-63.

Docum Document P., Sharma R. (2004). Latinos' Health Care Access: Financial and Cultural Barriers. *Journal of Immigrant Health, 6*: 5-13.

Dominelli L. (2004). *Social work: Theory and practice for a changing profession.* Cambridge: Polity Press. .

Durst D. (2005). Aging amongst immigrants in Canada: Policy and planning implications. In: 12th Biennial Canadian Social Welfare Policy Conference: "*Forging Social Futures.*"

Eapen S. (2003). Culturally appropriate best practice models for healthy aging. In: *Canadian Ethnocultural Council and Health Canada.*

Eapen S, Bajpai, S. & Chiappa, A. (2002). *Ethnic seniors and healthy aging: Perceptions, practices and needs.* Canadian Ethnocultural Council & Health Canada.

Escobar J.I. (1998). Immigration and Mental Health: Why Are Immigrants Better Off? *Arch Gen Psychiatry, 55*: 781-782.

Flaskerud J.KS. Health problems of Asian and Latino immigrants. (1999). *Emerging Nursing Care of Vulnerable Populations, 34*: 327 - 341.

Hernández-Plaza, C.P &. Alonso-Morillejo, E.. (2004). The role of informal social support in needs assessment: proposal and application of a model to assess immigrants' needs in the south of Spain. *Journal of Community & Applied Social Psychology, 14*: 284-298.

Hussain, F. & Cochrane, R. Depression in South Asian women living in the UK: (2004). A review of the literature with implications for service provision. *Transcultural Psychiatry, 41*: 253-270.

Hyman, I. (2001). Immigration and health. In: *Health policy working paper.*

Jang Y.K.G. & Chiriboga, D. (2006). Correlates of sense of control among older Korean-American immigrants: Financial status, physical health constrainst, and environmental challenges. *International Journal: Aging and Human Development 63*: 173-186.

Krause, N. (1991). Stress and isolation from close ties in later life. *Journal of Gerontology: Social Sciences, 46*: S183 -194.

Lai, D. (2004). Impact of culture on depressive symptoms of elderly Chinese immigrants. *Canadian Journal of Psychiatry, 49* :820-827

Lai, D. & Surood, S. (2007). Predictors of Depression in Aging South Asian Canadians. *Journal of Cult Gerontology.*

Leblanc, M. (2002). Career counseling East Asian Immigrants. In: *National Consultation on Career Development (NATCON).*

McReynolds, J.L.B.R., Rossen EKPRN.(2004). Importance of physical activity, nutrition, and social support for optimal aging. *Clinical Nurse Specialist July/August; 18*(4): 200-206

Narayanasamy, A. Mental health. Transcultural mental health nursing 1: benefits and limitations. *British Journal of Nursing (BJN) 5,8*: 664-668.

National Advisory Council of Aging (2005). *Seniors on the margin: Seniors from ethnocultural minorities.* Ottawa: National Advisory Council of Aging.

Ng, E, Wilkins, R., Gendron, F., & Barthelot, J.M. (2005). Health today, health tomorrow? Findings from the National Population Health Survey: Dynamics of immigrants' health in Canada. In: *Ottawa: Statistics Canada.*

Olson, L.K. (2001). *Aging through ethnic lenses: Caring for the elderly in a multicultural society.* Oxford, UK: Rowman & Littlefield Publishers, Inc.

Pang, E.C., Jordan-Marsh, M, Silverstein, M. & Cody, M. (2003). Health-Seeking Behaviors of Elderly Chinese Americans: Shifts in Expectations. *Gerontologist, 43*: 864-874.

Perez, C. (2002). Health status and health behavior among immigrants. *Health Reports,13* (supplement 0:98-109.

Russell, E. & Smith, C. (2003). Whose health is it anyway? Enabling participation. *J Epidemiol Community Health, 57*: 762-763.

Saito, E., Sagawa, Y. & Kanagawa, K. (2005). Social support as a predictor of health status among older adults living alone in Japan. *Nursing & Health Sciences, 7*:29-36.

Seeman, T.E. (2000). Health promoting effects of friends and family on health outcomes in older adults. *American Journal of Health Promotion, 14*: 362-370.

Shen, B.J. & Takeuchi, D.T. (2001). A structural model of acculturation and mental health status among Chinese Americans. *American Journal of Community Psychology, 29*: 387-418.

Stewart, M., Reutter, L., Letourneau, N. & Campbell, R. (2003). Support intervention for homeless youth project: Interim report. In: *Social support research program*.

Stroebe, W. (2000). Moderators of the stress-health relationship. In: *Social psychology and health.* Edited by Stroebe W. Philadelphia, PA: Open University Press 236-273.

Walls, P.S., S.P. (2003). *Real voices - survey findings from a series of community consultation events involving black and minority ethnic groups in England.* London: Department of Health.

Wong, R. (2006). Health care use among elderly Mexicans in the United States and Mexico: The role of insurance. *Research on Aging ,28*: 393-408.

Wu, Z & Hart, R. (2002). Social and health factors associated with support among elderly immigrants in Canada. *Research on Aging, 24*: 391-412.

Wu, Z.S., C.M. (2004). Immigrant status and unmet health care needs in British Columbia. In: Research on Immigration and Integration in the Metropolis. *Working paper series No. 04-18*: Vancouver Centre of Excellence; .

Yeh, S-CJ & Lo, S.K. (2004). Living Alone,Social Support, and Feeling Lonely Among the Elderly.. *Social Behavior & Personality: An International Journal. 32*: 129-138.

Part 2
Diversity and Identity of Immigrants and Refugees

11

Social Capital, Health and Well-Being of Elderly Chinese Immigrants in Canada

Daniel Lai, (University of Calgary) and Shirley Chau,
(University of British Columbia – Okanagan)

Introduction

Population aging and increasing cultural diversity in Canada are the key drivers behind this research. The shift toward receiving more immigrants from non-European countries further diversifies the ethno-cultural characteristics of Canada's population (Laroche, 2000). These changes mean that more people, including older adults, are from a wide variation of ethno-cultural backgrounds, making it important to understand aging in the unique context of culture (Lai, Tsang, Chappell, Lai & Chau, 2007). Previous research on relationships between culture and health, using the Chinese Canadian older adults as an example, has indicated that cultural uniqueness and specific cultural values and beliefs are related to health (Lai et al., 2007), access to services (Lai, 2006; Lai & Kalyniak, 2005), service barriers (Lai & Chau, 2007a), and the health disparities experienced by the aging Chinese (Lai, 2004). Cultural barriers are some reported key challenges, resulting access barriers (Lai & Chau, 2007a), and less favorable health status (Lai & Chau, 2007b).

In understanding healthy aging of immigrants, social capital is an emerging theme (Guista & Kambhampati, 2006; Li, 2004). Yet, research to understand the role of social capital on aging of older adults in an ethno-cultural context is limited. Although previous research has reported barriers and challenges faced by immigrants and minorities, there is a lack of research on the role of social capital in relation to healthy aging of immigrant and ethno-cultural minority older adults. In this study, an expansion is made of previous research on culture and health toward building a better understanding of how social capital of older immigrant adults drive healthy aging, using the elderly Chinese seniors as an example.

Literature Review

Healthy Aging as an Emerging Focus

With population aging comes more interest in research and policy to address seniors' health. "Healthy aging" is an emerging focus in government policies at the provincial (Alberta Community Development, 2000; British Columbia Ministry of Health, 2005) and federal levels (Healthy Aging and Wellness Working Group, 2006). Healthy aging can be understood as part of the concept of "good health," which refers to "not merely an absence of illnesses or infirmity, but a state of complete physical, mental and social well-being" (World Health Organization, 1946). One definition of healthy aging focuses on illness and impairment, wherein freedom from both becomes the hallmark of healthy aging (Bassett, Bourbonnais & McDowell, 2007; Ostbye et al., 2006; Reed et al., 1998). However, having illnesses and functional disability may not imply being unwell (Strawbridge, Wallhagen & Cohen, 2002). Many older adults consider themselves to be aging well despite having chronic conditions or disabilities (Strawbridge, Wallhagen & Cohen, 2002). Being able to adapt or manage physically and attitudinally to functional declines and maintaining functional autonomy are some aspects of healthy aging (Jang, Mortimer, Haley & Graves, 2004; Michael, Coditz, Coakley & Kawachi, 1999; Ostbye et al., 2006; Ryff, 1989). Healthy aging also means active participation, remaining socially engaged, maintaining positive interactions with others, taking part in activities, and having close personal relationships and social ties (Jang et al., 2004; Ryff, 1989; Knight & Ricciardelli, 2003). The spiritual aspect of healthy aging includes anticipating the future, having a sense of purpose, personal growth, an appreciation of life, and being able to have inner self-reflection (Fisher & Specht, 1999; Knight & Ricciardelli, 2003; Reed et al., 1998; Ryff, 1989). These different but related definitions have shown that "healthy aging" is a multi-dimensional concept, and it should be understood from a multiple perspective that includes consideration of the different socio-cultural contexts of the older adults.

Based on a recent review of healthy aging (Peel, Bartlett & McClure, 2004), it is clear that most studies adopted the "social determinants of health" and "population health" perspectives. Two major orientations can be identified, one taking an epidemiological approach to address specific health problems, focusing on factors predicting disease and disability. The prevalence of specific lifestyles or health behaviors of individuals has come under intense scrutiny (Laroche, 2000), with the assumption that if some seniors stay healthy, others should be also able to if certain preceding conditions are present. Research findings show that these conditions include a low fat diet, regular physical activity, volunteering, moderate alcohol consumption, and being a non-smoker (Almeida, Norman, Hankey, Jamrozik & Flicker, 2006; Byles, Young, Furuya & Parkinson, 2006; Herzog, Ofstedal & Wheeler, 2002; Michael Colditz, Coakley & Kawachi, 1999; Ostbye et al., 2006; Reed et al., 1998; Steptoe, Wright, Kunz-Ebrecht

& Iliffe, 2006; Thompson, Sierpina & Sierpina, 2001). Another approach these studies take aligns with the holistic perspective, and seeks to understand the role of external influences on healthy aging, including the role of public policy (Infeld & Whitelaw, 2002), the social determinants of health such as homelessness or poverty (Quine, Kendig, Russell & Touchard, 2004), and the effect of community characteristics (Harris & Grootjans, 2006; Masotti, Fick, Johnson-Masotti & McLeod, 2006).

These definitions and the research approaches on the topic of healthy aging are limited by the lack of attention to the role and influence of culture, resulting in the knowledge gaps that justify the need for this research. Firstly, most of these studies are focused on the mainstream aging population while little has been available on ethno-cultural minority seniors in Canada. For many seniors, their own definitions of healthy aging may differ from those of theoreticians (Ryff, 1989). Therefore, it is important to explore the conceptualization of healthy aging from the viewpoint of seniors as a way to identify appropriate healthy aging "markers" (Richard, LaForest, Dufresne & Sapinski, 2005). Despite attempts of researchers to address the self-perception of healthy aging (Knight & Ricciardelli, 2003), little research has examined the influence of culture on such conceptualization.

Secondly, most studies have failed to address culture and the effects of culture that affect values, beliefs, and behavioral norms in health service use, health outcomes, and attitude toward treatment (Day & Cohen, 2000; Evan & Cunningham, 1996). For elderly immigrants from a different culture, cultural values and beliefs influence their health status (Casado & Leung, 2001). Immigrants who were the most acculturated or bicultural reported being the healthiest (Shapiro et al., 1999). These findings demonstrate the role of culture in multifaceted forms, but little was done to incorporate such relationships in research on healthy aging.

Thirdly, healthy aging cannot be understood in isolation from the social and structural factors that shape it. Some researchers have identified the access barriers to health services (Biegel, Farkas & Song, 1997; Damron-Rodriguez, Wallace & Kingston, 1994). Previous research also identified the role of social inequity in terms of some social location factors such as gender (Gonyea & Hooyman, 2005), age (Evandrou, 2000), and socio-economic status (Huong, Van Minh., Janlert, Van & Byass, 2006; Newmann & Garner, 2005), as key factors affecting health outcomes. Yet, little research in healthy aging has investigated the intersections between cultural factors and these social location factors.

Social Capital and Health

In its simplest terms, social capital refers the to the "good" or resources developed and accumulated through social relations among individuals within groups, based on trust grown out of participation and social engagement with others within the conext of shared norms and expectations of reciprocity. This good is nurtured within the context of a social network that is ideally dense and vast. The greater the expansion of the network, the greater the likelihood of accumulating social capital that can be accessed and utilized when needed (Halpern, 2005). While many theorists from different disciplines have written and discussed the merits and problems of social capital, it is Putnam's theory of social capital that has gained considerable attention in academic circles in research and in policy development by governments and institutions from all over the world (e.g., the World Bank). The attractiveness of Putnam's theory of social capital lies in what it offers to address the perceived decline in community and the potential threat that declines in community may have on social cohesion, harmony, and economic prosperity. The strengthening of social relations has been viewed as a potentially important remedy; this idea has proliferated from political economics to health (Halpern, 2005). In particular, community is best maintained when individuals in the community relate well to each other based on trust, norms, and networks (Baron, Schuller & Field, 2000). It has been hypothesized that societies with high interpersonal trust are more likely to have less social inequalities (Campbell, 2007). Researchers have established that trust, at both individual and institutional levels, is beneficial to health (Putnam, 2000) and the promotion of policies and practices that increase trust and networks are important.

Debates about social capital in the production of health remain a highly complex arena of discussion in trying to figure out the conceptual definition of social capital, what it is, and how it exerts its effects on health. The link between social capital and health is about the "health-enabling community" (Campbell 2000), which is an environment that benefits health based on social associations between individuals and between individuals and social institutions, including the community in which one is a member. As well, the mechanism by which social capital benefits health is based on the density and proliferation of social ties to other individuals and groups, formally and informally, that make up a social network. A key component of the production of social networks leading to social capital is the element of trust that individuals have toward each other that facilitate behaviors to increase trust and future behaviors of support when needed. The implication of the link between social capital and health, usually discussed in terms of benefits, is that having social supports through one's network acts as a buffer against ill health (Berkman & Glass, 2000; Berkman & Syme, 1979; Cohen 2001; Cohen 2004; Kawachi, Kennedy, Lochner & Prothrow-Stith, 1997; Kritsotakis & Gamarnikow 2004).

Trust and networks are key ideas in social capital that give way to the development and production of social relations between individuals, between individuals and the community, and between individuals and institutions. Trust is important to establishing networks that in turn leads to support between agents. The idea of trust is to scholars such as Dasgupta (2003) and Fukuyama (1995) the facilitator of production and success in different areas of social and economic life. Scholars have pointed out that in understanding how trust works to mediate social relations and the production of social capital, it is important to consider trust in terms of intrinsic and instrumental trust (Dasgupta, 2003; as cited in Schuller, Baron, & Field, 2000). Trust is reciprocal. Trust is not only a personal attribute, but in the context of social capital, the presence and degree of trust among individuals and between individuals and institutions reflects the system in which trust is fostered, thereby shaping how individuals interact with others and with social institutions (Schuller, Baron & Field, 2000).

The concept of social capital and its relationship to health has garnered tremendous interest from policy makers locally (e.g., Health Canada) and internationally (e.g., World Bank, World Health Organization). This interest is fueled by the prospect of improving human health based on past and current research that have found positive associations between the presence and buffering effects of social support in promoting health (Cohen, 1992; Cohen, 2001; Cohen, 2004; Cohen & Hamrick, 2003; Cohen, Mermelstein, Kamarck & Hoberman, 1985; Cohen & Rodriguez, 1995; Cohen & Williamson, 1991; Kawachi, Kennedy, Lochne, & Prothrow-Stith, 1997; Kritsotakis & Gamarnikow, 2004). The body of research examining the relationship between social capital and health suggests, though still tentative, that individuals with vast social networks and the perception of access to social support from family, friends, and other helpers in the neighborhood appear to experience better health due to access to resources that provide support in the social, cultural, economic dimensions. Instrumental help by others to assist with chores, such as clearing the path for the elderly to safely walk on the street when it snows, contributes to the prevention of accidents and falls, thereby maintaining the health of the elderly person. In the area of chronic diseases, social networks that provide emotional support and other forms of support help individuals to cope and manage the emotional and social aspects of declining health. Social ties within the community are central in producing social capital. More recently, research have expanded on the topic of social capital to locate this social good within individuals. Attempts at capturing the essence of social capital and health has led to studies that focus on locating social capital in the individual, such as behaviors that build and accumulate social capital through civic engagement by attending church, voting, and volunteering in the community through involvement in community organizations. The implications of these studies' findings are that social capital is a construct that operates at multi-levels and is reciprocal in character because such capital is based on social relations that occur within a social, structural context.

However, the utility of these findings for policy in health has drawn criticism by scholars concerned with the problem of using social capital as the panacea to address health and wellness concerns without regard to the social inequalities, such as social structures, that produce health disparities (Campbell, 2000; Nakhaie, Smylie & Arnold, 2007). Research studies in the areas of public health and health psychology have also applied the concept of social capital to uncover how social capital may help improve population health (Nakhaie, Smylie & Arnold, 2007; Wilkinson, 1996; 1997). These studies have further reinforced the notion that social support, through availability and accessibility of social support benefits health, but these studies signal the need to look at how contextual factors, such as poverty, remain a factor in poor health and that social capital, not surprisingly, is low among individuals deprived of the social, cultural, and socioeconomic components important to achieve good health (Kawachi et al., 1997; Veenstra, 2002). The conditions of poverty undermine the building of social capital, as does systemic oppressions such as racism. Increasingly, the search for social capital in health requires an examination of individuals within the larger social, cultural context and a focus on social inequalities that undermine the building and accumulation of social capital. This is becoming an important area of focus as researchers and scholars engage in the debate about social capital and the criticism that social capital tends to be accumulated by those of higher socio-economic status. In other words, those who have more to begin with tend to get more.

The critiques of social capital as a useful concept for health also include questions about the appropriateness of applying social capital to everyone regardless of social location factors that play a role in determining health (Stephens, 2008). For instance, studies of social capital among visible, ethnic minorities have not yet produced findings that concur with existing research with non-visible, ethnic minorities where social capital was found of benefit to health. The fact that little research has been conducted to test social capital in socially marginalized populations leaves a considerable gap in understanding for appropriate application to these populations. One of many pressing issues at this time is the need to refine or develop policies that address the successful social integration of immigrants in host countries in order to avoid the problems that arise among immigrants living in poverty in the host country due to de-skilling, systemic barriers, cultural differences and conflict, social and political conflict, and the potential of accumulated deprivations that immigrants experience that could lead to failure in social cohesion in the host country's population.

An important sub-area of study with immigrants is the need to understand how social capital in visible, ethno-racial immigrant populations are produced and maintained in the host country. One question of interest is if social capital is equally distributed and accessed by immigrants versus non-immigrants? As well, is social capital, as conceived by Putnam, the same in immigrant populations? Given the limited research in this area it is important to study the relevance of social capital in these populations, at risk of experiencing deprivations across many life domains upon immigrating and settling in the host country, in order to fill the gap in this area for developing social and economic policies that enable health and social wellbeing in the life course of immigrants.

Currently, as many countries are faced with an increasingly diverse and aging population, services and policies need to be developed and refined to address the different and growing needs of aging individuals in the social and cultural realm. As the costs of health care are expected to continue to increase to meet the diverse needs of the elderly, more research is needed to examine the ramifications the interplay of aging, culture, ethno-racial identity, and social relations have in the maintenance and production of health from the individual to the macro-level. Social capital is currently heralded as an important concept that needs to be actualized to improve quality of life and population health. However, the application of social capital at the levels of policy and practice in social and health services requires more information and evidence, particularly with respect to how social capital works in different cultural and community contexts where social relations are dictated by different norms and expectations of relating between individuals. Therefore, to bridge the knowledge gap, this current study aims at answering the research question: "What are the effects of social capital variables on health and well being of the aging Chinese in Canada?"

Research Method

The data were collected as part of a cross-sectional survey on the health and well-being of older Chinese in Canada (Lai et al., 2007). The data were collected between summer 2001 and spring 2002 in seven major Canadian cities with a substantial concentration of Canadian-Chinese population and constitutes 89 percent of the entire Chinese-Canadian population in Canada (Statistics Canada, 2003). The target population was aging ethnic Chinese aged 55 years and older. Identifying Chinese surnames from telephone directories in each site formed the sampling frame, a method used in previous studies (Lauderdale & Kestenbaum, 2000; Tjam, 2001). From the local telephone directories, 297 064 Chinese surname listings were identified. Using the SPSS Version 11 random cases selection function, a sub-sample of telephone numbers was randomly selected, based upon the size of the Chinese-Canadian population and the estimated proportion of the population 55 years of age and older in each site. As a result, a total of 40 654 numbers listed under 876 Chinese surnames was randomly selected.

Trained telephone interviewers who were proficient in English and at least one other major Chinese dialect such as Cantonese, Mandarin, and Toishanese, made telephone contact to identify eligible participants (ethnic Chinese aged 55 years or older). The interviewers were mainly graduate students in social science or human service disciplines or community interviewers who had experience in conducting survey interviews with the Chinese community. All interviewers participated in a one-day structured training session conducted by the research team members. Eligible participants were then invited to take part in a face-to-face interview, either at the participant's home or at one of the community organizations that collaborated with the research project at the local site. For households with more than one eligible participant, only one was randomly selected through the "roll a dice" method. Bilingual interviewers using either English or a Chinese dialect spoken by the participants conducted the interviews. Subsequently, a total of 2 949 eligible participants were identified and a total of 2 272 completed the face-to-face interview in the original study, representing a response rate of 77 percent. For the purpose of this study, only participants (n = 1 537) at the age of 65 and older and who were born outside of Canada and came to this country as immigrants were included in the analysis (n = 1 537).

An orally administered structured questionnaire was used for data collection. Because most of the aging Chinese people in Canada are able to speak a Chinese dialect, the questions were initially constructed in written Chinese, except for the standardized instruments that have a Chinese language version. To attend to the language need of participants, an English version of the questionnaire was also prepared. A standard "forward-backward" translation process was used. First, the original questions in Chinese were translated into English, and then translated back into Chinese. This process would ensure that the English version is consistent with the Chinese version. In the interview, the participants could choose to answer either the Chinese or English version of the questionnaire.

As a large-scale study, the original questionnaire covered a wide range of health-related topics, including physical and mental health status, Chinese health beliefs, Chinese cultural values, and service utilization. The full questionnaire took about 45 minutes to an hour to complete. For the purpose of this study, only selected variables relevant to health and well-being and social capital were selected to be included in this study.

Measures of Health and Well Being

Health and well-being were the dependent variables represented by physical health, mental health, and life satisfaction. General physical health and mental health were measured by the Medical Outcomes Study 36-item Short Form (SF-36), a well-established standardized health assessment instrument that has been applied to people from various cultural backgrounds (Ware, Kosinski & Keller, 1994). This scale has also been adapted and translated for Chinese respondents. Psychometric evaluation confirms the reliability and validity of the instrument (Ren, Amick, Zhou & Gandek, 1998; Ren & Chang, 1998). This 36-item scale yielded scores for two dimensions, PCS (Physical Component Summary) and MCS (Mental Component Summary), representing the physical and mental health, with higher scores meaning better health status. When used with the elderly Chinese immigrant sample in this study, a Cronbach's alpha of .90 was reported for the PCS and .85 for the MCS.

Life satisfaction was measured by a single item measure asking the participants to rate, along a five-point Likert scale that ranged between very satisfied to very dissatisfied, their overall level of life satisfaction. A score between one and five was allocated to each answer provided, with a higher score indicating a higher level of life satisfaction.

Measures of Social Capital

Social capital was measured by a range of variables that are related to political participation in voting, citizenship status, informal social contacts, participation in organizations, and ties and connections with the Chinese community in Canada.

Political participation questions asked the participants to indicate whether one took part (i.e., yes or no) in voting in civic, provincial, and federal level election. Previous literature had used voting behaviors as one form of social capital (references) as voting indicates one's capacity to instil changes in higher-level policies and decision-making. On the other hand, the authors in this study understand that due to the citizenship requirement to become a registered voter, not all elderly Chinese immigrants were eligible to vote before they have acquired their citizenship status. However, from the perspective of political asset or capital, voting is an acquired behavior representing one's political capacity. For newer immigrants who are not yet eligible for voting, they have not yet had the political capacity to instil their political influence. Therefore, including voting behavior as a variable would delineate who has such political capacity and those who do not.

Similarly, citizenship represents eligibility to vote as well as entitlement to a Canadian passport and other social and political rights. Thus, citizenship can be treated as a form of political capacity. In this study, citizenship status of the participants was measured by asking the participants to self-declare whether they are a Canadian citizen (i.e., yes or no).

Informal social contacts referred to questions asking the participants to report the frequency of time spent with someone not living with them in the past week (i.e., none, once a week, twice to six times a week, and once a day or more), frequency of visiting with someone (i.e., none, once a week, twice to six times a week, and once a day or more), frequency of talking to someone on the phone (i.e., none, once, twice, once a day or more), whether one had someone to confide in and trust (i.e., yes or no), and whether one talked to friends in the past year (i.e. none, sometimes, or often).

Participation in formal organization was measured by a few questions asking the participants to indicate their frequency of visiting a senior centre (i.e., none, sometimes, or often), participating in celebrations or social functions (i.e., none, sometimes, or often), attending Chinese social functions organized by the Chinese community (i.e. ,none, sometimes, or often), and to indicate the strength of their tie with the Chinese organizations in Canada (i.e., not tight at all, not too tight, generally tight, or very tight).

Finally, questions were also asked regarding the participants' view toward whether as a Chinese person, one should vote for a Chinese political candidate, care about issues happening in the Chinese community, or donate to Chinese charities, along a five-point Likert scale ranged between strongly disagree to strongly agree.

Measures of Demographic Variables

To understand the demographic background of the participants, variables related to age, gender, marital status, living arrangement, education, self-rated financial adequacy, length of residency in Canada, and country of origin were included in the study.

These demographic variables were selected based upon their known effects on health and well-being as indicated in previous literature. For instance, being older in age has been found to be associated with less favorable health (Deimling, Sterns, Bowman, & Kahana, 2005; Femia, Zarit & Johansson, 2001; Gijsen et al., 2001). Gender is a significant correlate of health with older women often in poorer health than older men (Robert & Fawcett, 1998). Married elderly people often reported better health than those who are not married (Pettee et al., 2006). Older people living alone also reported poorer health than those living with someone (Gee, 2000; Kasper & Pearson, 1995). Finally, higher education level and better financial status are positively related to better health status (Plouffe, 2003).

Age referred to the chronological age of the participants. Gender was grouped into male and female. Marital status was grouped as unmarried or married. Living arrangement was grouped as either living alone or living with someone. Education level of the participants was grouped into four ordinal groups ranging from no formal education to post-secondary level or above, with a higher score indicating a higher level of education. Self-rated financial adequacy was measured by asking the participants to indicate how well their income and investments satisfied their financial needs. Participants rated their financial adequacy as "very inadequate," "not very well," "adequate," or "very well," with corresponding scores of 1, 2, 3, or 4 respectively. A higher score represented a higher level of financial adequacy. The length of residency referred to the total number of years that the participants had lived in Canada. The country of origin referred to the country from which the participants immigrated.

Based upon the answers provided by the participants in the survey and their distribution, country of origin was grouped into three groups including Mainland China, Hong Kong, and Taiwan and other countries.

Data Analysis

SPSS (version 16) was the statistical software used for data analysis. Descriptive statistics, including frequency distributions and means, were used to analyze the demographic information. Exploratory factor analysis using principal component analysis was conducted to examine the factor structure of the social capital variables, as a way to reduce and consolidate the number of variables used to represent the construct. Based upon the factors identified, hierarchical multiple stepwise regression analysis was performed to examine the effect of the social capital factors on each of health and well-being variables. The statistical assumptions of multiple regression analysis were checked and bivariate correlation coefficients were calculated to check for potential multi-collinearity problems among the independent variables. Missing values were minimal in the variables with only a maximum of one or two percent of the cases. They were replaced using the expectation-maximization (EM) method in which EM algorithm method was used to estimate missing values by an iterative process. In the regression models, the socio-demographic variables were entered first, followed by the social capital factors. This method served to identify the changes in the proportion of variance in the health and well-being variables explained, when the social capital factors were added to the regression models.

Results

Detailed demographic information on the older Chinese in this study is presented in Table 1. As a diverse group, the older Chinese vary by age, gender, marital status, education, and other socio-economic factors. The average age of the participants took part in this study was 74.1 years. In the sample, over half of the participants were female (55.8%). Most of participants were married (57.1%). Only 18% reported living alone. More than a third (34.2%) of the participants reported an elementary education level. Close to a third (31.4%) reported secondary education. A similar proportion of the participants reported no formal education (17.4%) and post secondary and above education (17%). In terms of self-rated financial adequacy, the participants reported a mean score of 2.8 (sd=0.6) along a four-point scale. Over half of the participants (52.2%) migrated from Hong Kong, followed by those from Mainland China (28.9%), and Taiwan and other locations (18.9%). The average length of residency in Canada for this sample was 18.5 years (sd=12.1).

Table 1
Demographic Variables and Health and Well Variables of Participants
(n=1 537)

Age in years, mean (sd)	74.1 (6.6)
Gender (%)	
Male	44.2
Female	55.8
Marital status (%)	
Married	57.1
Not married	42.9
Living Alone (%)	18.0
Education (%)	
No formal education	17.4
Elementary	34.2
Secondary	31.4
Post secondary and above	17.0
Financial adequacy, mean (sd), range 1-4	2.8 (0.6)
Length of residency in years, mean (sd)	18.5 (12.1)
Country of origin (%)	
Mainland China	28.9
Hong Kong	52.2
Taiwan and other locations	18.9
Health and Well-Being Variables	
General physical health (PCS) (mean, sd)	50.8 (8.9)
General mental health (MCS) (mean, sd)	48.2 (10.3)
Life satisfaction (mean, sd), range: 1-5	4.1 (0.7)

Principal component analysis was used to explore the factor structure of the 16 variables used for measuring the social capital of the elderly Chinese immigrants. The findings revealed that the 16 items used for measuring social capital were loaded to four unrotated factors with eignevalues greater than one, accounting for 58.9% of the variance in the scale. What it meant was that four significant preliminary factors could be extracted among the items used for measuring social capital and each of these four

Table 2
Factor Analysis of Social Capital Variable

	Political Asset	Organizational Asset	Informal Social Tie	Attitudinal Tie
Voted in provincial election	0.91			
Voted in federal election	0.90			
Voted in municipal election	0.86			
Canadian citizenship	0.47			
Attended Chinese social functions organized by Chinese community		0.89		
Participated in celebrations/social functions		0.76		
Closeness of ties with Chinese community		0.71		
Frequented senior centres		0.68		
Spent time with someone not living with you			0.80	
Visited with someone live here or people visited you here			0.76	
Talked to someone on phone			0.72	
Have someone to confide and trust in			0.52	
Talked to friends			0.43	
One should donate to Chinese political candiates				0.86
One should vote for Chinese political candidates				0.78
One should care about issues in the Chinese community				0.77
Extraction Method: Principal Component Analysis. Rotation Method: Varimax with Kaiser Normalization, rotation converged in 5 iterations				

factors at least explained a significant amount of the total variance of the concept of social capital. Among them, the first factor accounted for 16.6% while the second and third factors accounted for additional variability of 15.3% and 14.7% respectively. The fourth factor accounted for 12.3% of the variance. The factor loadings after the varimax rotation are presented in Table 2. These four factors are related to: (1) political asset, (2) organizational asset, (3) informal social tie, and (4) attitudinal tie.

Table 3
Regression analysis of health and well-being and social capital variable

	Block 1	Block 2	Block 1	Block 2	Block 1	Block 2
			Mental health (MCS)		Life Satisfaction	
	Standardized Beta		Standarized Beta		Standardized Beta	
Age	-.09**	-.08**	-.04	-.04	.00	.01
Gender[a] – Male	.11**	.11**	.03	.04	.05	.06*
Being married[b]	.07*	.07*	.04	.04	.03	.02
Living alone[c]	-.01	-.02	-.06*	-.08**	.00	-.05
Education	.04	.03	.02	.01	-.01	-.05
Financial adequacy (Range 1-4)	.11**	.11**	.14**	.13**	.20**	.17**
Length of residency in Canada	-.03	-.02	.01	.02	-.04	-.03
Country of origin[d]						
Hong Kong	-.02	-.03	.00	-.01	.04	.03
Taiwan and other locations	-.03	-.04	-.02	-.02	.00	-.00
Social Capital Variable						
Political asset	–	-.03	–	-.02	–	.01
Organizational asset	–	.05	–	.06*	–	.07**
Informal social tie	–	.04	–	.08**	–	.26**
Attitudinal tie	–	-.06*	–	.02	–	.09**

$*p<.05, **p<.01$ Reference groups: female;[a] not married;[b] living with someone;[c] Mainland China[d]

Based upon the four-factor model, four social capital factors were computed using the items loaded into each of the factors. Due to the fact that the scaling format of the items may be different, standardized scores were used. The mean of the standardized scores for the items loaded in each of the social capital factors was computed, thus resulting in four composite social capital factors representing political asset, organizational asset, informal social tie, and attitudinal tie. The Cronbach's alphas that indicated the internal consistency of items within each factor were quite acceptable at .81 for the factor of political asset, .76 for the factor of organizational asset, .71 for informal social tie, and .73 for attitudinal tie.

Hierarchical multiple regression analysis was used to examine the effects of the social capital factors on health and well being of the elderly Chinese immigrants. Separate analysis was conducted with each of the health and well being variables. Demographic variables were entered as a variable block, followed by the four social capital variables.

Results of the regression analysis are presented in Table 3. When adjusted for the demographic variables, stronger attitudinal tie was significantly related to less favorable general physical health. However, stronger organizational asset, stronger informal social tie were both significantly correlated with better general mental health. Finally, when life satisfaction was treated as the dependent variable, stronger organizational asset, stronger informal tie, and stronger attitudinal tie were all positively related to a higher level of life satisfaction.

Discussion

A few limitations of this study should be noted. First, although a random sample was used for this study, the self-reporting format used in measuring health status and well-being may not necessarily capture the actual health condition or severity of the illnesses that the participants may have. Second, as the data for this study on social capital were drawn from a previously conducted survey, the choice of social capital variables was limited by the availability of variables included in the original survey. There could be other social capital variables that are related to health and well-being of elderly immigrants but were not included in this study. Finally, as a study using secondary data, the conceptualization of social capital by the elderly Chinese immigrants was unable to be captured. Future research, probably using qualitative methods, may further enrich our understanding of social capital and its effects in the cultural context of the elderly Chinese immigrants as well as other elderly immigrant groups.

The effects of four types of social capital variables on health and well being of elderly Chinese immigrants were examined in this study. Three of the four types of social capital factors were found to be significantly related to health status and well-being of the participants. Informal social tie appears to have the strongest effect on mental health and life satisfaction.

Organizational asset is important to one's mental health and life satisfaction as well. On the other hand, attitudinal tie related significantly to one's physical health and life satisfaction. These findings indicate the importance of social capital to the elderly Chinese immigrants. As noted by other researchers, the presence of informal social networks provides benefits to health through perceived and actual access to social support (Berkman, 1984; Berkman & Syme, 1979; Cairney, Corna, Veldhuize, Kurdyak & Streiner, 2008; Cohen, 2004; Fitzpatrick, Gitelson, Andereck & Mesbur, 2005). This effect has been well demonstrated by the finding in this study that a stronger social tie is associated with better health and well-being of the elderly Chinese immigrants.

Organization asset allows one to be affiliated with formal groups and organizations through which resources can be better access and social connections can be better developed (Fitzpatrick et al., 2005; Takhar, 2006). However, it is not merely the number of organizations that one has contact with that produces this effect, but rather that organizations, particularly those specifically established to serve the needs of the group or community are hubs of information exchange to meet needs shared by the members. While this may seem to suggest the concerns of group insularity among ethno-racial visible minority members in preventing the development of bridging capital with communities outside of their own (Aizlewood & Pendakur, 2005), it is important to recognize the significant utility of ethno-specific organizations that meet in whole or in part cultural and identity needs that the broader, mainstream community and institutional structures may not adequately provide.

Attitudinal tie reflects the trust and strengths of connection with the Chinese community by the Chinese elderly immigrants. A higher level of identification and trust may result in a better sense of security, stability, and belonging, which may be a more meaningful indicator of trust between equal individuals who are members of the same group or community than trust between "unequal" individuals due to differential power based on differences in social location in the broader community context. Assuming the former is true, the findings of higher attitudinal ties can be interpreted in the Chinese cultural context and belief system as peace and harmony within a person (Zhang & Yu, 1998). As a result, it is not surprising to see the significant effect of stronger attitudinal tie on better health and well-being of the elderly Chinese immigrants. In addition, this traditional cultural value of interpersonal harmony could also be a driving force behind this for the elderly Chinese immigrant, a topic that deserves further examination in future research.

Political asset was not a significant factor of health and well being of the elderly Chinese immigrants in this study. Generally, this means that whether or not an elderly Chinese immigrant has become a Canadian citizen, or has taken part in voting, did not affect their health status and well-being. This finding goes against some literature on social capital in which political participation was considered as an important social capital (Putnam, 1995; Veenstra, 2007). On the other hand, the finding may have indicated the fact that political participation, specifically in voting, is not a good indicator of social capital in light of the barriers posed by eligibility requirements or other logistical matters that prevented these individuals from voting.

Other than the social capital variables, gender and financial adequacy were the two key factors contributing to physical health and life satisfaction. Being male was associated with better physical health and a higher level of life satisfaction. It also means that to reduce the gender gap in health and well being, services and adequate support for elderly Chinese immigrant women would be important. On the other hand, the longer one resided in Canada, the better one's physical health and mental health, and the higher one's life satisfaction level. In addition, living with someone (i.e., not living alone) was significantly related to better mental health. Financial support for elderly immigrants is also crucial to their health and well-being and relevant policies and programs to strengthen assistance in this aspect should be developed.

The effects of social capital identified in this study further reveal the directions that service providers and policy makers could take to address health and well being of the elderly Chinese immigrants in Canada. This study took the elderly Chinese immigrants as a case example to demonstrate the positive effects of social capital. While there are cultural differences between the elderly Chinese immigrants and elderly immigrants from other cultural backgrounds, the barriers and challenges faced by other elderly immigrants (Yamaoka, 2008) could be similar. Therefore, we believe that the positive effects of social capital may prevail within other elderly immigrant groups. The findings from this study could form the basis for identifying strategies and approach for improving health and well being of other elderly immigrants.

Specifically, based upon the significant social capital factors identified, programs and policies are needed to facilitate elderly immigrants to develop strong informal social ties with their peers and other support networks. For elderly immigrants, one difficulty they face is losing their friends and support networks due to death. Many may have social support networks well established in their home country. Due to immigration, many would have to leave their informal social ties behind. As immigrants, many would have to make new friends and build new social support networks in the host country. For elderly immigrants, cultural shock, acculturation stress, and other language and cultural barriers may further limit their social circle. As informal social tie was found to be an important social capital, service providers should develop services that suit the elderly immigrants' need to re-establish their social networks, so that their informal social tie can be further strengthened.

In additional to better health and well being, the benefits of organizational involvement include opportunities for information exchange on important matters such as finding a good and trusted physician, sharing of culture-based practices in health and daily living activities, and the building of trust and social networks towards the accumulation of social capital (Fitzpatrick et al., 2005; Takhar, 2006). Therefore, community groups and organizations could develop strategies to expand membership to include elderly immigrants. Through taking part in these organized activities, elderly immigrants would not only benefit from having the opportunity to expand their social networks, they would learn new knowledge and perspectives associated with the activities provided by these groups and organizations. In addition, it would also increase their opportunities for accessing resources and services through these organized groups.

The attitudinal tie as a social capital in this study referred specifically to identification with values and beliefs within the Chinese community by the elderly Chinese immigrants. In other words, maintaining stronger identification with one's own culture and ethno-cultural community is important to the elderly Chinese immigrants. While previous literature has placed strong emphasis on the importance of acculturation to immigrants' adjustment (Tran, Fitzpatrick, Berg & Wright, 1996), for the elderly immigrants, as noted in this study, maintaining a bicultural connection may serve them the best (Jang, Kim, Chiriboga & King-Kallimanis, 2007). Such findings further reinforce the importance of Canada maintaining the policy of multiculturalism, recognizing the values and importance of immigrants to keep close cultural tie with their own ethnic and cultural identity. Services and programs that celebrate cultural values, contributions, and ethnic diversity of different immigrant communities should continue to be developed, particularly for the elderly immigrants. For many elderly immigrants, cultural and ethnic identity is often tightly connected to their own personal identity. Being immigrant means one has to uproot from another culture to start a new life and to face with various forms of barriers (Lai & Chau, 2007a). Services and programs that facilitate elderly immigrants to keep a strong tie with their own cultural identity are recommended as a strategy for preventing or recovering a loss that many elderly immigrants risk suffering in the immigration process.

To conclude, this study examines the effects of social capital on the health and well being of elderly Chinese immigrants in Canada. Similar to previous research on social capital and health (Cairney, Corna, Veldhuizen, Kurdyak & Streiner, 2008; Kawachi, Kennedy, Lochner & Prothrow-Stith, 1997; Yamaoka, 2008), social capital also affects the health and well-being of the elderly Chinese in Canada. Based upon the significant social capital variables identified, policy makers and practitioners should integrate these factors in planning of services, programs, and policies that facilitate the developing and building of the favorable social capital factors as strategies for enhancing health and well being of the elderly immigrants.

References

Aizlewood, A. & Pendakur, R. (2005). Ethnicity and social capital in Canada. *Canadian Ethnic Studies, 37*(2), 77-102.

Alberta Community Development. (2000). *Alberta for all ages: Directions for the future.* Edmonton, Alberta: Government of Alberta.

Almeida, O., Norman, P., Hankey, G., Jamrozik, K. & Flicker, L. (2006). Successful mental health aging: results from a longitudinal study of older Australian men. *American Journal of Geriatric Psychiatry, 14*(1), 28-35.

Bassett, R., Bourbonnais, V. & McDowell, I. (2007). Living long and keeping well: Elderly Canadians account for success in aging. *Canadian Journal of Aging, 26*(2), 113-126.

Berkamn, L. & Syme, S. (1979). Social networks, host resistance, and mortality: A nine year follow-up study of Almeda County residents. *American Journal of Epidemiology, 109*, 186-284.

Berkman, L., Glass, T., Brissette, I. & Seeman, T. (2000). From social integration to health: Durkheim in the new millennium. *Social Science and Medicine, 51*, 843-57.

Biegel, D., Farkas, K. & Song, L. (1997). Barriers to the use of mental health services by African-American and Hispanic elderly persons. *Journal of Gerontological Social Work, 2*(1), 23–44.

British Columbia Ministry of Health. (2005). *Healthy aging through healthy living: toward a comprehensive policy and planning framework for seniors in B.C.: A discussion paper.* Victoria, British Columbia: British Columbia Ministry of Health.

Byles, J., Young, A., Furuya, H. & Parkinson, L. (2006). A drink to healthy aging: The association between older women's use of alcohol and their health-related quality of life. *Journal of the American Geriatrics Society, 54*, 1341-1347.

Cairney, J., Corna, L., Veldhuizen, S., Kurdyak, P. & Streiner, D. (2008). The social epidemiology of affective and anxiety disorders in later life in Canada. *Canadian Journal of Psychiatry, 53*(2), 104-111.

Campbell, C. (2000). Social capital and health: Contextualizing health promotion within local community networks. In S. Baron, T. Schuller & J. Field (Eds.), *Social capital: Critical perspectives.* (pp. 182-196). Oxford: Oxford University Press.

Casado, B. & Leung, P. (2001). Migratory grief and depression among elderly Chinese American immigrants. *Journal of Gerontological Social Work, 36*(1/2), 5–26.

Cohen, S. (1992). Stress, social support, and disorder. In H.O.F. Veiel and U. Baumann. (Eds.). *The meaning and measurement of social support.* (pp. 109-124). New York, Hemisphere Press.

Cohen, S. (2001). Social relationships and health: Berkman & Syme (1979). *Advances in Mind-Body Medicine, 17*, 5-7.

Cohen, S. (2004). Social relationships and health. *American Psychologist, 59*(November): 676-684.

Cohen, S. & Hamrick, N. (2003). Stable individual differences in physiological response to stressors: implications for stress-elicited changes in immune related health. *Brain, Behavior, and Immunity, 17*, 407-414.

Cohen, S., Mermelstein, R., Kamarck, T. & Hoberman, H. (1985). Measuring the functional components of social support. In I.G. Sarason & B.R. Sarason (Eds.), *Social support: Theory, research, and application.* (pp. 73-94). The Hague, Holland: Martinus Nijhoff.

Cohen, S. & Rodriguez, M. (1995). Pathways linking affective disturbances and physical disorders. *Health Psychology, 14*(5), 374-380.

Cohen, S. & Williamson, G. (1991). Stress and infectious disease in humans. *Psychological Bulletin, 109*(1), 5-24.

Damron-Rodriguez, J., Wallace, S. & Kington, R. (1994). Service utilization and minority elderly: Appropriateness, accessibility and acceptability. *Gerontology & Geriatrics Education, 15*(1), 45–63.

Dasgupta, P. (2003). Social Capital and Economic Performance: Analytics. In E. Ostrom & T.K. Ahn (Eds.), *Foundations of Social Capital* (pp. 238-257) Cheltenham, United Kingdom: Edward Elgar.

Day, K. & Cohen, U. (2000). The role of culture in designing environments for people with dementia: A study of Russian Jewish immigrants. *Environment and Behavior, 32*(3), 361-399.

Deimling, G., Sterns, S., Bowman, K. & Kahana, B. (2005). The health of older adults, long-term cancer survivors. *Cancer Nursing, 28*(6), 415-424.

Evan, C. & Cunningham, B. (1996). Caring for the ethnic elder. *Geriatric Nursing, 17*(3), 105-110.

Evandrou, M. (2000). Social inequalities in later life: The socio-economic position of older people from ethnic minority groups in Britain. *Population Trends, 101*, 11-18.

Femia, E., Zarit, S. & Johansson, B. (2001). The disablement process in very late life: A study of the oldest-old in Sweden. *Journal of Gerontology: Psychological Science, 56B*, 12-13.

Fisher, B. & Specht, D. (1999). Successful aging and creativity in later life. *Journal of Aging Studies, 13*, 457-472.

Fitzpatrick, T., Gitelson, R., Andereck, K. & Mesbur, E. (2005). Social support factors and health among a senior center population in Southern Ontario, Canada. *Social Work in Health Care, 40*(3), 15-37.

Fukuyama, F. (1995). *Trust: The social virtues and the creation of prosperity.* New York: Free Press.

Gee, E. (2000). Living arrangements and quality of life among Chinese Canadian elders. *Social Indicators Research, 51*(3), 309-329.

Gijsen, R., Hoeymans, N., Schellevis, E., Ruwaard, D., Satariano, W. & Van den Bos, G. (2001). Causes and consequences of comorbidity: A review. *Journal of Clinical Epidemiology, 54*, 661-674.

Giusta, M, Kambhampati, U. (2006). Women migrant workers in the UK: social capital, well-being and integration. *Journal of International Development, 18*(6), 819-833.

Gonyea, J. & Hooyman, N. (2005). Reducing poverty among older women: Social security reform and gender equity. *Families in Society, 86*(3), 338-346.

Halpern, D. (2005). *Social capital.* Cambridge: Polity Press.

Harris, N. & Grootjans, J. (2006). The potential role of ecological health promotion in progressing healthy ageing. *Ageing International, 31*(4), 276-282.

Health Canada. (2001). *The population health template working tool.* Ottawa, ON: Health Canada. Retrieved on September 25, 2006, from http://www.hc-sc.gc.ca/hppb/phdd/pdf/template_tool.pdf

Healthy Aging and Wellness Working Group (2006). *Healthy aging in Canada. A new vision, a vital investment from evidence to action.* Ottawa, Ontario: Public Health Agency of Canada. Available at: http://www.phac-aspc.gc.ca/seniors-aines/pubs/haging_newvision/pdf/vision-rpt_e.pdf

Herzog, R , Ofstedal, M. & Wheeler, L. (2002). Social engagement and its relationship to health. *Clinics in Geriatic Medicine*, 593-609.

Huong, D., Van Minh, H., Janlert, U., Van, D. & Byass, P. (2006). Socio-economic status inequality and major causes of death in adults: A 5-year follow-up study in rural Vietnam. *Public Health, 120,* 497-504.

Infeld, D., & Whitelaw, N. (2002). Policy initiatives to promote healthy aging. *Clinics in Geriatic Medicine, 18,* 627-642.

Jang, Y., Kim, G., Chiriboga, D. & King-Kallimanis, B. (2006). A bidimensional model of accultur-ation for Korean American older adults. *Journal of Aging Studies, 21*(3), 267-275.

Jang, Y., Mortimer, J., Haley, W. & Graves, A. (2004). The role of social engagement in life satisfac-tion: Its significance among older individuals with disease and disability. *Journal of Applied Gerontology, 23,* 266-278.

Kasper, J. & Pearson, J. (1995). Living arrangements, social integration, and personal control: corre-lates of life satisfaction among older people. *Journal of Mental Health and Aging, 1*(1), 21-34.

Kawachi, I., Kennedy, B., Lochner, K. & Prothrow-Stith, D. (1997). Social capital, income inequal-ity, and mortality. *American Journal of Public Health, 87*(9), 1491-1498.

Knight, T. & Ricciardelli, L. (2003). Successful aging: Perceptions of adults aged between 70 and 101 years. *International Journal of Aging and Human Development, 56,* 223-245.

Kritsotakis, G. and Gamarnikow, E. (2004). What is social capital and how does it relate to health? *International Journal of Nursing Studies 41*, 43-50.

Lai, D. (2004). Health status of older Chinese in Canada: Findings from the SF-36 health survey. *Canadian Journal of Public Health, 95*(3), 193-197.

Lai, D. (2006). Predictors of use of senior centers by elderly Chinese immigrants. *Journal of Ethnic & Cultural Diversity in Social Work, 15*(1/2), 97-121.

Lai, D. & Chau, S. (2007a). Predictors of health service barriers for older Chinese immigrants in Canada. *Health and Social Work. 32*(1), 57-65.

Lai, D. & Chau, S. (2007b). Effects of service barriers on health status of older Chinese immigrants in Canada. *Social Work, 52*(3), 261-269.

Lai, D. & Kalyniak, S. (2005). Use of annual physical examinations by aging Chinese-Canadians. *Journal of Aging and Health, 17*(5), 573-591.

Lai, D. Tsang, K., Chappell, N., Lai, D.C.Y., Chau, S. (2007). Relationships between culture and health status: A multi-site study on older Chinese in Canada. *Canadian Journal on Aging, 26*(3), 171-184.

Laroche, M. (2000). Health status and health services utilization of Canada's immigrant and Non-Immigrant populations. *Canadian Public Policy, 26* (1), 51-73.

Lauderdale, D. & Kestenbaum, B. (2000). Asian American ethnic identification by surname. *Population Research and Policy Review, 19*, 283-300.

Li, P. (2004). Social capital and economic outcomes for immigrants and ethnic minorities. *Journal of International Migration and Integration. 5*(2), 171-190.

Masotti, P., Fick, R., Johnson-Masotti, A. & MacLeod, S. (2006). Healthy naturally occurring retire-ment communities: A low-cost approach to facilitating healthy aging. *American Journal of Public Health, 96*(7), 1164-1170.

Michael, Y., Colditz, G. , Coakley, E. & Kawachi, I. (1999). Health behaviors, social networks, and healthy aging: Cross-sectional evidence from the Nurses' Health Study. *Quality of Life Research,* 8, 711-722.

Nakhaie, M., Smylie, L. & Arnold, R. (2007). Social inequalities, social capital, and health of Canadians. *Review of Radical Political Economics, 39,* 562-85.

Newmann, S. & Garner, E. (2005). Social inequities along the cervical cancer continuum: A structured review. *Cancer Causes and Control, 16,* 63-70.

Ostbye, T., Krause, K., Norton, M., Tschanz, J., Sanders, L., Hayden, K., et al. (2006). Ten dimensions of health and their relationships with overall self-reported health and survival in a predominantly religiously active elderly population: The cache country memory study. *Journal of the American Geriatrics Society, 54,* 199-209.

Peel, N., Bartlett, H. & McClure, R. (2004). Healthy aging: how is it defined and measured? *Australasian Journal on Aging, 23*(3), 115-119.

Pettee, K., Brach, J., Kriska, A., Boudreau, R., Richardson, C., Colbert, L., et al. (2006). Influence of marital status on physical activity levels among older adults. *Medicine & Science in Sports & Exercise. 38*(3), 541-6, 2006.

Plouffe, L. (2003). Addressing social and gender inequalities in health among seniors in Canada. *Canadian Saúde Pública, 19*(3), 855-860.

Putnam, R. (1995). Bowling alone: America's declining social capital. *Journal of Democracy, 6*(1), 65-78.

Quine, S., Kendig, H., Russell, C. & Touchard, D. (2004). Health promotion for socially disadvantaged groups: The case of homeless older men in Australia. *Health Promotion International, 19*(2), 157-165.

Reed, D., Foley, D., White, L., Heimovitz, H., Burchfiel, C. & Masaki, K. (1998) Predictors of healthy aging in men with high life expectancies.. *American Journal of Public Health, 88*(10), 1463-1468.

Ren, X., Amick, B., Zhou, L. & Gandek, B. (1998). Translation and psychometric evaluation of a Chinese version of the SF-36 Health Survey in the United States. *Journal of Clinical Epidemiology, 51,* 1129-1138.

Ren, X. & Chang, K. (1998). Evaluating health status of elderly Chinese in Boston. *Journal of Clinical Epidemiology, 51,* 429-435.

Richard, L., LaForest, S., Dufresne, F. & Sapinski, J. (2005). The quality of life of older adults living in an urban environment: Professional and lay perspectives. *Canadian Journal on Aging, 24*(1), 19-30.

Robert, P. & Fawcett, G. (1998). *At risk: A socio-economic analysis of health and literacy among seniors.* Ottawa. Ontario: Statistics Canada.

Ryff, C. (1989). In the eyes of the beholder: views of psychological well-being among middle-aged and older adults. *Psychology and Aging, 4,* 195-210.

Schuller, T., Baron, S. & Field, J. (2000). Social capital: A review and critique. In S. Baron, J. Field & T. Schuller. (Eds.), *Social capital: Critical perspectives* (pp. 1-38). Oxford: Oxford, University Press.

Shapiro, J., Douglas, K., de la Rocha, O., Radecki, S., Vu, C. & Dinh, T. (1999). Generational differences in psychosocial adaptation and predictors of psychological distress in a population of recent Vietnamese immigrants. *Journal of Community Health, 24,* 95-113.

Statistics Canada. (2003). *Canada's ethnocultural portrait: the changing mosaic.* Ottawa, Ontario: Statistics Canada. Retrieved on September 25, 2006, from http://www12.statcan.ca/english/census01/products/highlight/Ethnicity/Index.cfm

Stephens, C. (2008). Social capital in its place: Using social theory to understand social capital and inequalities in health. *Social Science & Medicine 66,* 1174-1184.

Steptoe, A., Wright, C., Kunz-Ebrecht, S. & Iliffe, S. (2006). Dispositional optimism and health behaviour in community-dwelling older people: Associations with healthy ageing. *British Journal of Health Psychology, 11,* 71-84.

Strawbridge, W., Wallhagen, M. & Cohen, R. (2002). Successful aging and well-being: Self-rated compared with Rowe and Kahn. *Gerontologist, 42,* 727-733.

Takhar, S. (2006) South Asian women, social capital and multicultural (mis)understandings. *Community, Work and Family, 9*(3), 291-307.

Thompson, B., Sierpina, V. & Sierpina, M. (2001). What is healthy aging? Family physicians look at conventional and alternative approaches. *Generations, 25*(4), 50-53.

Tjam, E. (2001). How to find Chinese research participants: use of a phonologically based surname search method. *Canadian Journal of Public Health, 92,* 138-142.

Tran, T., Fitzpatrick, T., Berg, W. & Wright, R. (1996). Acculturation, health, stress, and psychological distress among elderly Hispanics. *Journal of Cross-Cultural Gerontology, 1*1(2), 149-165.

Veenstra, G. (2002). Social capital and health (plus wealth, income inequality, and regional health governance. *Social Science and Medicine, 54,* 849-58.

Veenstra, G. (2007). Social capital and health in Canada: (Compositional) Effects of trust, participation in networks, and civic activity on self-rated health. In F.M. Kay, & R. Johnston (Eds.), *Social capital, diversity, and the welfare state* (pp. 251-277). Vancouver: UBC Press.

Ware, J., Kosinski, M. & Keller, S. (1994). *SF-36 physical & mental health summary scales: A user's manual.* Boston: The Health Institute, New England Medical Centre.

Wilkinson, R. (1996). *Unhealthy societies: The afflictions of inequality.* London and New York: Routledge.

Wilkinson, R. (1997). Socioeconomic determinants of health: Health inequalities: Relative or absolute material standards. *British Medical Journal, 314,* 591-595.

World Health Organization. (1946). *Preamble to the Constitution of the World Health Organization as adopted by the International Health Conference, New York, 19-22 June, 1946;* signed on 22 July 1946 by the representatives of 61 States (Official Records of the World Health Organization, no. 2, p.100) and entered into force on 7 April, 1948. Available at: http://www.searo.who.int/.

Wu, D. & Tseng, W. (1985). *Introduction: The characteristics of Chinese culture.* Orlando: Academic Press.

Yamaoka, K. (2008). Social capital and health and well-being in East Asia: A population-based study. *Social Science & Medicine, 66*(4), 885-889.

Zhang, A. & Yu, L. (1998). Life satisfaction among Chinese elderly in Beijing. *Journal of Cross-Cultural Gerontology, 13*(2), 109-125.

12

Elder Abuse: Perspectives in the Chinese-Canadian Community

Christine A. Walsh and Shelina Hassanali (University of Calgary)

The population of older adults in Canada is rising. It is estimated that by the year 2021 there will be 6.7 million Canadians aged 65 or older, which will increase to approximately 9.2 million by 2041 (Health Canada, 2002). The Canadian elder population is also becoming increasingly ethno culturally diverse (Citizenship and Immigration Canada, 2002; Statistics Canada, 2003). A relatively large proportion of seniors in Canada are immigrants. In 2001, 28.6% of persons aged 65 to 74 and 28% of those aged 75 to 84 were immigrants (Statistics Canada, 2006). These demographic shifts mean that issues affecting seniors should become more salient. Elder abuse is one such issue. It has been suggested that with the growing number of elderly persons, there will most likely be a concomitant rise in all forms of abuse (Fulmer, Paveza, Abraham, & Fairchild, 2000). Health disparities among older ethno-cultural populations have also been observed (Lai, 2005; Lai & Chau, 2007a, 2007b; McDonald, et al., 2006). Indeed more health care practitioners will be working with these culturally diverse seniors as population aging continues. These factors highlight the importance of increased understanding of elder abuse across the Canadian cultural mosaic.

The abuse of older persons was identified as one of two emerging areas requiring urgent action by *The International Plan of Action on Ageing* (World Health Organization [WHO], 2000). Elder abuse is recognized internationally as a pervasive and growing problem, warranting the attention of clinicians, epidemiologists, health services researchers and the general public (Lachs & Pillemer, 2004).

Elder abuse is a complex phenomenon. The Toronto Declaration on the Global Prevention of Elder Abuse (WH0, 2002) defines elder abuse as "a single or repeated act, or lack of appropriate action, occurring within any relationships where there is an expectation of trust which causes harm or distress to an older person. It can be of various forms: physical, psychological/emotional, sexual, financial, or simply reflect intentional or unintentional neglect" (p. 3). In 2002, the WHO and the International Network for the Prevention of Elder Abuse (INPEA) collaborated on an international study to gather the views of older persons and primary health care providers on elder abuse. Definitions of elder abuse were derived from information obtained from eight focus groups conducted in developed and developing countries including: Argentina, Austria, Brazil, Canada, India, Kenya, Lebanon, and Sweden. The definitions that emerged within these cross-cultural samples were more broadly framed than those previously identified in the published literature. Six key categories of abuse were found including: (a) structural and societal abuse (e.g., inadequate government policies, cuts in health care, inadequate pensions); (b) neglect and abandonment (including social exclusion); (c) disrespect and agist attitudes; (d) legal and financial abuse (e.g., violation of human, legal, and medical rights); (e) psychological, emotional, and verbal abuse; and (f) physical abuse.

Cultural Differences

Elder abuse is not intrinsic to one particular culture; rather it is experienced by members of various ethnicities and cultural backgrounds. One identified gap in the research within the literature is delineating the nature of elder abuse among specific cultural sub-groups as the focus has been primarily on the experience of Caucasian seniors in Western societies. Much of the available research tends to either treat elder abuse as a culturally benign phenomenon, by applying concepts derived from a Western cultural perspective to understand elder abuse in other cultures (Tam & Neysmith, 2006) or culturally muted by combining various cultural sub-groups such as "Asians" (Chan & Leong, 1994), rather than examining their experiences independently. The importance of studying culture as it relates to elder abuse is articulated by Tam and Neysmith (2006) who recommend that "researchers be cautious about applying elder abuse categories derived from a Western cultural perspective to understand or account for abuse in other cultures" (p. 149). In cases where research has been conducted on ethno-cultural groups such as African Americans, Hispanics, Aboriginal persons, Asian Indians and Asians, the vast differences within ethnic or the cultural groups has been negated (Buchwald et al., 2000; Parra-Cardona, Meyer, Schiamberg & Post, 2007; Rittman, Kuzmeskus & Flum, 1998). This is problematic as for example, Moon, Tomita and Jung-Kamei (2001) found very different experiences with and perceptions of elder abuse among four Asian-American groups (Chinese, Japanese, Korean, and Taiwanese); 5 percent of the Taiwanese, 8 percent of the Korean, 21 percent of the Japanese and 30 percent of the Chinese participants endorsed the statement that they would tolerate occasional yelling from their children. Nurenberg (1998) describes a conference held to explore elder abuse in Asian communities in which there were participants from Chinese, Japanese, Vietnamese, Filipino and Korean communities. The author concludes that although some commonalities were found, "each community represented was distinct in terms of its history, experiences, economic status, conventions and many other factors" (p. 207). Thus cultural factors must be examined and articulated to inform culturally-sensitive practice (American Geriatrics Society, 2002, 2006; Potocky-Tripodi, 2002).

This chapter discusses the experience of elder abuse among Chinese elders, members of the largest visible minority population in Canada (Statistics Canada, 2005). According to the 2001 Census there were 1 029 395 Chinese living in Canada, accounting for 3.5% of the total population in 2001 (Canadian Social Trends, 2005). The Chinese Canadian population is likely underestimated in the official census data due to the number of new immigrants who prefer to remain undocumented for legal, financial, and other reasons (Midlarsky, Venkataramani-Kothara & Plante, 2006).

This chapter explores cultural variables which make this experience similar to, and different than, that of elders from other ethnic backgrounds drawing on available literature and findings from the Elder Abuse Study. The Elder Abuse Study is an original investigation employing qualitative focus group methodology with older Chinese immigrant women and other marginalized elders and their caregivers in Alberta and Ontario (Walsh et al., 2007).

Elements of Chinese Culture Related to Elder Abuse

According to Chan and Leong (1994), Chinese elders have "experienced cultural change, cultural shock and cultural conflicts similar to those experienced by the immigrants of the past." (p. 264). Acculturation of Chinese immigrants is further impacted by important differences between the Chinese and Western cultures in time orientation, religious beliefs and perhaps most importantly, familial relationships (Chan & Leong, 1994). Traditional Chinese culture emphasizes the past, whereas, North American culture focuses on the present and future (Chan & Leong, 1994). The religious beliefs of Chinese elders also play a role in their perception of elder abuse. For example, Buddhist and Confucian teachings preach that one should expect suffering to be a part of life and "elders may view suffering as their fate and may think it cannot or should not be changed but simply endured" (Rittman, Kuzmeskus & Flum, 1998, p. 232-233).

Chinese culture focuses on lineal relationships, for example, the father-son relationship and responsibilities which come with it whereas Western society is more individualistic in nature, with each member striving to take care of him/herself (Chan & Leong, 1994). Family relationships and how they are manifested are prescribed by the Confucian philosophical construct of filial piety. Filial piety is a concept that "encompasses a broad range of behaviors, including children's respect, obedience, loyalty, material provision, and physical care to parents. It applies even after the death of a child's parents, mandating that children sacrifice for parents and not change the ways of their parents" (Zhan, 2003, p. 210-211).

Wu Lun is a Chinese construct which decrees the amount of power each person has, their role in the relationship and their respective responsibilities within the five major dyadic relationships (ruler-subject, father-son, husband-wife, elder brother-younger brother, and friend-friend) (Hwang, 2006). Relationships are circular in which parents care for their children when they are young and subsequently children take care of their parents in old age (Tam & Neysmith, 2006; Yan & So-Kum Tang, 2001). Within the Chinese family system young people are taught to respect and take care of older family members who are attributed with having life experience, wisdom, knowledge, power and status.

Chinese elders are more likely to live with relatives than non-Chinese seniors. In 2001 approximately 16 percent of Chinese aged 65 and older in Canada lived with relatives; four times higher than among the same age group in the general population and only 10 percent of senior Chinese Canadians lived alone compared with more than 30 percent of non-Chinese seniors (Canadian Social Trends, 2005). Although almost 70 percent of elderly Canadian Chinese endorsed the statement that having a senior in the home should be considered a treasure for the family (Lai, 2003), the reduction in multigenerational families (Tam & Neysmith, 2006) has been documented. Social and economic factors also contribute to the move towards nuclear families among Chinese (Martin, 1990; Zhang & Goza, 2006). As well, values about family among the younger generations (Yan & So-Kum Tang, 2001) seem to be changing along with the decline in filial piety observed both in Hong Kong (Yan, So-Kum & Yeung, 2002) and in Canada (Tam & Neysmith, 2006). Chinese elders who had moved to Canada and faced different norms and values reported expecting the same type of care from their children as they received in their country of origin; failure to do so was equated to a "type of mental abuse where clients feel lonely and depressed" (Tam & Neysmith, 2006, p. 147). Tam and Neysmith (2006) suggest that with the decline in filial piety "elderly people experience negative emotional effects and an increased risk of abuse" (p. 143).

Dependency

According to Tam and Neysmith (2006), older Chinese immigrants are dependent on their children both financially and as a result of language barriers. Everyday tasks such as using public transportation, going to appointments or attending social programs are compromised as many immigrant elders do not speak English. The language barrier serves to not only isolate the elder within the community, but it also separates them from their own families in the case of elders who cannot communicate with grandchildren, for example. It is also argued that the language barrier is also greater for Chinese immigrants in relation to other immigrants from European countries because English and Chinese are very different linguistically. Thus it might be easier for elderly Europeans to learn the English language than Chinese-speaking elders (Chan & Leong, 1994). A study of Chinese elders in Canada, reported that 41 percent of respondents stated that they did not understand any English at all and 20 percent stated that they did not speak any English (Lai, 2003).

The inability to communicate in English has profound effects on elders resulting in social isolation and heightened distress which in turn are major factors in both the occurrence and non-disclosure of elder abuse (Carefirst Seniors & Community Services Association, 2002). Tam and Neysmith (2006) suggest that, "socially isolated older victims have fewer opportunities to disclose what is happening to them" (p. 149). A socially isolated victim may encounter more emotional distress as a result of the abuse rather than a victim who has a strong social network (Tam & Neysmith, 2006). Further, Chinese elders are not only isolated within their own families, the family itself may also be isolated in society because they are a racial minority in the workforce (Tam & Neysmith, 2006) which may result in less access to supports to prevent abuse. Additionally newcomers are isolated because of their status in the new country which is compounded for elders because of their age. Social isolation is not only caused by the language barriers, but also by cultural expectations of the grandparents to stay home during the day and take care of the grandchildren and other household responsibilities which restrict their access to social supports (Rittman, Kuzmeskus & Flum, 1998).

Elderly Chinese immigrants in Canada are also often financially dependent on their children as they tend to be poor (Brotman, 1998). They have extremely low total income, which was only $4 321, or just 17 per cent of that for all seniors in the general population (Wang & Lo, 2005).

Disrespect as a Form of Abuse

Disrespect is viewed as key component related to elder abuse and this is articulated by the fact that when WHO researchers asked older adults in ethnically mixed focus groups to describe their experiences of abuse, examples of disrespect were more "pervasive and all-encompassing" than other forms of abuse and disrespect was attributed to agist attitudes; therefore, it was seen as both a cause of abuse and a form of abuse itself. Also, in their investigation of the Chinese-Canadian community, Tam and Neysmith (2006) state that "disrespect was a significant form of elder abuse that emerged in our findings" (p. 145). Focus group participants noted that respect in Chinese culture included the use of respectful language, respect for the elders' preferences (i.e., food), and spatial respect (i.e., giving the elder seats of honor). Sung (2000) noted that while in the presence of elders, young people should be "dressed plainly and neatly, to have their hairdos and make-up neat and moderate, and to maintain a posture that is polite and deferent" (p. 199). A study of Chinese homecare workers in Toronto reported that disrespect consisting of verbal threats and humiliation, movement and space restrictions and the provision of just the basic necessities was the most prevalent form of abuse (Carefirst Seniors & Community Services Association, 2002). Tam and Neysmith (2006) propose that disrespect is a culturally specific form of abuse, and that it is a powerful form of abuse in the Chinese context. The impact of disrespect on Chinese elders is highlighted by the fact that for some, disrespect attacked their sense of self-identity and belonging, in certain cases causing depression and leading to suicidal tendencies (Carefirst Seniors & Community Services Association, 2002). Although many elders may perceive that the respect which was once shown to them by their children is slowly diminishing, it has been suggested that the expressions of respect are simply shifting from subservient forms to reciprocal/egalitarian forms (Sung, 2000).

"Silencing" Family Problems

Another important element of Chinese culture found in the literature is that of "silencing" family problems. Intrinsic to Chinese culture is the notion that one should not meddle in other persons' family affairs and that individuals should not talk about their problems to outsiders (Manigbas, 2002; Yan & So-Kum Tang, 2001). The Chinese community holds family honor to the highest degree and; therefore, situations of elder abuse may be underreported in order to preserve family honor (Manigbas, 2002). "Silence" is also tied into the communist ideal that upholds that the welfare of the group is more important than the individual well-being (Wolf, Bennett & Daichman, 2003). Consequently, elders may not disclose abuse because of the perceived need to suffer in order to preserve the well-being of the family unit. Underreporting of elder abuse is not unique to the Chinese community. Factors related to underreporting include "low self-esteem, shame, fear of retaliation, dependency, fear of placement in a long-term care facility, and fear of reprisal from the perpetrator" (Simpson, 2005, p. 360).

Other Factors to Consider

Although culture plays a major role in defining abuse, the reactions to and perceptions of elder abuse, many concepts related to elder abuse transcend culture. For example, Tam and Neysmith (2006) argue that cultural factors alone are not sufficient to explain the nature of elder abuse in Chinese populations. A study of caregivers of elderly Chinese found that many caregivers identified being caught in a caring dilemma in which they would like to be freed from the burden of caring; however, they feel obligated to continue to provide care (Yan, So-Kum Tang & Yeung, 2002). The "burden" on the family is articulated by members of a focus group of care recipients who stated that "they would rather die than be sent to a nursing home or institution" (Tam & Neysmith, 2006, p. 147). In this case there would be an overwhelming burden on family members to care for the elder person regardless of the fact that they may not have the time, knowledge and resources to do so. In addition, the caregiver may also feel that they are being forced to provide care for the elder and this may cause anger, stress and perhaps even guilt, creating an environment which could lead to elder abuse. Litwin and Zoabi (2004) propose four explanations of the emergence of elder abuse in populations moving from traditional to modern culture using data drawn from abused (n=120) and non-abused (n=120) elderly Arab Israelis. The explanations are related to socio-demographic status, dependency, modernization and social integration. These risk factors may be of relevance to other cultures in transition such as the Chinese.

The importance of studying this elder abuse among Chinese families is articulated by Yan, So-Kum Tang and Yeung (2002) who state that as the traditional family values are eroded by rapid social changes and thus elder abuse may become a fact of life for the Chinese. It is imperative that we are aware of the experiences and perceptions of elder abuse and this education should not only be obtained by conducting reviews of previous research or speaking to caregivers. In this study, information collected from focus groups comes directly from the Chinese elders themselves.

Methods

A descriptive qualitative study was conducted using data from a focus group interview (Brown, 1999; Drabenstott, 1992). Part of a larger study, nine Chinese-speaking older immigrant women were interviewed who had been identified by a resettlement agency. Inclusion criteria were that the participants were older female members of the Chinese community. Participants conveyed their views through a certified translator who was a staff member of a local immigrant-serving agency. Focus group members were all able to give informed consent to participate.

Participants filled out brief demographic questionnaires and received CAD $20 as compensation for their time. The interview was conducted by two trained facilitators in a private setting within the community in the spring of 2003. A semi-structured interview guide was used. The areas of inquiry included the definitions and scope of elder abuse, indicators or risk factors associated with elder abuse, consequences of elder abuse and interventions. The interview was audio-taped and lasted approximately ninety minutes. Ethics approval was received from the research ethics board of

McMaster University (Hamilton, Ontario). Audiotapes were transcribed by a professional typist and all identifying information was removed. Codes were developed by
two or more researchers who each read a transcript independently, identified themes
and sub-themes in the text, and then compared their findings until consensus was
reached (Denzin & Lincoln, 2000; Guba, 1981; Patton, 1990). The composite version
of their codes was given to a member of the research team, who entered the codes
and later retrieved coded sections of text into a software program to assist qualitative
data analysis (NVivo). Codes and themes were validated through discussion in larger
team meetings in which consensus was reached for each theme and linked to transcript excerpts that best exemplified the theme. Illustrative quotes are presented for
each theme.

Findings

Chinese elderly women in the study described various types of abuse within their
community, however, neither physical abuse nor sexual abuse was considered to be
prevalent. One participant suggested that the Chinese culture considers it very important to teach the children not to physically abuse their parents. She stated that, "it
could be emotional or financial, but not physical." When asked specifically about experiences of sexual abuse among Chinese elders, the participants laughed and offered
examples of indecent exposure which they had witnessed. *Emotional abuse* and *disrespect* emerged as major themes related to significant types of elder abuse within
the Chinese elder community. While participants did not describe situations of financial abuse per se, they described how *financial dependency and feelings of indebtedness* were associated with vulnerability to emotional abuse and disrespect. Women
participants in this study felt that that they were often to *blame* for the abuse and
described having to *endure* the abuse while *suffering in silence.* Feelings of loneliness
and sadness related to the social isolation created by *language barriers* were also
highlighted by focus group members. Each of these themes with illustrative quotes will
be presented in the following section.

Types of Abuse

Emotional Abuse

Participants articulated that many Chinese elders suffer emotional abuse by
being disregarded by their children, as one participant articulated:

> You have to live with the family. At first it seems to be okay, but then after a lit-
> tle while, like the children have their own family and everything becomes so

inconvenienced. They would go in and out; they are pretending that you aren't there, they just totally ignoring them. There are a lot of pressures, like mentally.

Another concurred adding that the seniors' children "are pretending that you aren't there, they just totally ignoring them . . . also when they go out they won't take you and when they come home they don't say "Hi" or "Hello." So basically, totally being ignored. Participants were unanimous in stating that "the majority of the sponsored elderly in Canada are experiencing that kind of situation."

Disrespect as Abuse

Although in many Western cultures disrespect is not readily identified as a form of abuse, participants in this study articulated that it can be (and often is) considered to be so in Chinese culture. One participant actually moved out of her children's house because of this perceived disrespect:

She was saying that her daughter married a non-Chinese person and she felt very uncomfortable. Basically from the Chinese culture, they are brought up with respect and politeness. So, when her daughter first got married, her son-in-law called her by her first name. So she feels there's no respect, we don't call our mother-in-law or father-in-law by their first name. So she feels that the respect is no longer there . . . so she moved out.

Another participant spoke of the perceived disrespect when she was not included in family discussions:

In China, where she came from, normally the elder in the family has a place where when there's a conversation or when a decision is being made. But when they come here they lose that. They cannot speak, there's no respect so they have lost that important role that they used to have.

Financial Dependency and Indebtedness

Focus group participants indicated that financial dependency and a feeling of indebtedness arising from immigrant sponsorship increased the risk for abuse and often resulted in prolonged suffering. Participants shared that often elders were unable to gain employment due to age, disability, language barriers, retirement and responsibilities for providing domestic labor in their home. This meant that seniors had little if any personal income. Elders identified that they wished to be financially self-sufficient so that they would not have to ask their children for money or so that they could afford to live independently. As one women explained:

Sometimes you want to move out on their own but financially it's a problem because they are under their family's sponsorships and during that ten years they are not eligible for any government assistance. So, they can't do anything for ten years. They'll have to endure the abuse, financially, emotional.

As a consequence of the feelings of indebtedness elders described long hours of "cooking, cleaning; they take care of the children, grandchildren to repay the children for bringing them here." Another added that Chinese elders "feel like it is their obligation to do something for them [their children]. Related to feelings of indebtedness participants noted that many children continually remind their parents of how much they have done for them and this causes the elders to feel that maybe they should continue to endure the abuse. The children say things such as, "when the children brought them here, like the husband and wife, it's like, I already bring you over here so what else do you want? I already give you a place to live, I feed you; I brought you here."

In turn, many elderly parents feel indebted to their children who have spent considerable resources to sponsor their parents into the new country, so they stay silent and endure the abuse as a way to "repay" this debt. This idea was articulated by many group members. As the translator explained, "they are all saying that because most of them are under sponsorship. They are grateful that the children brought them here." As one participant stated "they cannot ask for extra pocket money because they know the children are already struggling with their financial situation. So, they don't want to put more pressures on them."

Arising from their circumstance and cultural norms, Chinese elders felt that they were, in part, responsible for the situation and as a result had to endure the mistreatment and abuse while suffering in silence.

Placing the Blame

Although many of the elders recognized that the elder abuse they experienced was the children's fault, one individual brought up the idea that the elders share some responsibility for the blame. She suggested that, "you also have to understand that the younger generation, they work hard. They have a job to do in the daytime and the elders must understand that." Another offered that "sometimes you can't blame the children for 100 percent of your misfortune because sometimes when you're living with the daughter and the daughter-in-law you treat them differently. Like sometimes you treat the daughter better than you treat the daughter-in-law so of course there would be tensions in between the family."

Enduring the Abuse

Participants expressed strong feelings related to enduring difficult circumstances and abuse. As one woman explained, Chinese elders "are grateful that the children brought them here. Then most of the time, they have to endure whatever they are facing." Another added that "for the first little while, life seems to be alright, but that after a bit things get worse" and older women were expected to bear these hardships.

When asked to elaborate what they undergo, one participant provided the following example:

> It's hard to explain in one word what they have to endure. When the children brought them here, like the husband and wife, it's like I already bring you over here so what else do you want? They can't ask them for money. They always, the feeling is that I already give you a place to live, I feed you, I brought you here but the feeling that whatever they have to endure is almost everything, financial, emotional. It's almost that they lost the dignity or status of whatever they used to hold. So basically the kind of emotion inside, they can't ask them, they can't move out, they aren't eligible for government assistance so what do you do? You have to stay because you have no friends here. You stay, they don't care, they don't care if you're happy; it's very lonely.

Suffering in Silence

Elders acknowledged that they were reluctant to disclosing mistreatment and abuse within the family for cultural reasons. As one woman stated:

> There is a saying in Chinese community that says if bad things happen in family you don't go outside and spread it to other people. So the way they are brought up, that anything that is unpleasant you shouldn't tell people about it so the only thing she can do is try to be patient and try to forgive and hopefully that will reduce the tensions between the family members.

Language Barriers

Language barriers for Chinese elders emerged as a major issue for participants. Many participants suggested it was the largest hurdle to overcome, and the one which caused most of the social isolation. Most participants agreed with the following statement:

> She is saying her biggest problem is because of language barrier. She comes here and she feels totally lost, like a deaf person or a blind person. She can't do anything because of the language barrier. She can't talk or communicate. She's afraid to use any transportation in case she gets lost. It's a very big thing for her and I think it represents others in the community.

Another participant provided an example illustrating the frustration associated with the inability to communicate in English:

> She is totally alone and you know scared and can't speak the language, don't know how to read, don't know where to go . . . she was sitting at the communi-

ty centre for awhile and then people started introducing her to places. And she said one day she wanted to go home after sitting there and the people would tell her if you want to go home, go this way. And she took that direction and then the more she walked the farther she got away from home. And she said at that time she wasn't sure what was going to happen. And she asked another person on the street, and they pointed her back to where she was. At that time she said life is very disappointing.

Participants also discussed the limitations caused by the language barrier in regards to accessing healthcare. As one woman explains "the biggest problem is communication, language barriers. A lot of time they have to go to doctors or appointments, they can't communicate and the families, some of them speak English and some don't." Another participant provided the following example:

She said that getting a family doctor is very difficult because a lot of them don't speak English so they are looking for family doctors who can speak their own language. However, because there is so limited of them, they always have a very high case load so every time they go there they wait for 2 hours and go in for 2 minutes. She said that sometimes they walk in there and not a good 2 minutes and there you go. And she said that with other people she can see the difference that with other English people the doctor seems to give the a little bit more time and they are OK. So it is difficult to go around when you can't speak the language cause you are bounded to see your own kind of doctors, but then because there are not that many of them around the case load is really high.

Suggested Solutions

Participants offered a few suggestions to reduce the challenges that elderly Chinese immigrants experience. One suggested that churches should be used to decrease the loneliness and isolation felt by many of the Chinese elders. Another proposed the creation of Chinese community centres which could have activities for the seniors. She stated that activities should be culturally appropriate, for example, having Tai Chi sessions rather than only having traditional Western activities. Another participant agreed with the creation of church/temple programs and community centres, and also suggested that these activities should be available free of charge as older immigrants often have little money.

Discussion

This study identified three major themes related to abuse of Chinese elders living in Canada including: (i) culturally relevant types of abuse (psychological abuse, disrespect, and the contribution of financial dependency and indebtedness), (ii) cultural factors related to the experience of abuse including placing the blame, enduring the abuse and suffering in silence and finally the (iii) language barriers which heightens the vulnerability of Chinese immigrant seniors.

Empirical evidence on the prevalence of elder abuse among the Chinese population residing in Canada or the United States is rare (Malley-Morrison & Hines, 2004). While members of our study suggested that physical abuse is relatively uncommon among Chinese elders, there is some evidence that suggests this phenomenon is more prevalent, yet often is not detected or underreported due to cultural beliefs or sanctions. Older Chinese Americans are more likely to adhere to traditional beliefs that accept the use of physical force to solve problems than younger Chinese adults (Yick, 2000). A study of the experiences and perceptions of domestic violence among 50 older Chinese American immigrants reported that almost 7 % of the women and 6% of the men had experienced minor physical violence by their spouses during the past 12 months (Shibusawa & Yick, 2007). Among Chinese American elders referred to a health and social services agency the rate of neglect was 60 % followed by 20 % for psychological abuse and abandonment and ten percent each for physical and financial abuse (Fang, 1998, cited in Malley-Morrison & Hines, 2004). In reviewing cases of pf patients with physical elder abuse admitted to a hospital in Singapore, Cham and Seowe (2000) conclude that elder abuse is a significant subset of family violence which may be more widespread than previously thought.

Findings from this study lend support to literature which suggests a relatively high rate of psychological abuse experienced by older Chinese adults and the resultant psychological impact in the form of fear, guilt and lowered self-esteem of the victims (Moon, Tomita & Jung-Kamei, 2001; Tang, 1997; Yan & Tang, 2001). For example, the prevalence rate for a community sample of Chinese elders in Hong Kong (n=355) found that approximately 21 % of respondents reported experiencing verbal abuse compared to 2 percent with physical abuse (Yan & Tang, 2001) and a study of 276 Chinese caregivers in Hong Kong reported a 27 % rate of verbal abuse compared to the 2.5 % rate of physical abuse (Yan & So-Kum Tang, 2004). This concurs with differences in of proclivity to psychological abuse and physical abuse of 20 and 2 %, respectively among Chinese Hong Kong residents (Yan & So-Kum Tang, 2003).

Disrespect was depicted as a common and particularly detrimental occurrence for the elders in this study in agreement with other literature (Carefirst Seniors & Community Services Association, 2002; WHO/INPEA, 2002). Interwoven within older immigrant Chinese women's experiences of abuse and mistreatment was how financial dependency and feelings of indebtedness increased the risk for further abuse and resultant psychological harm. This also means that some seniors feel, in part responsible, for the abuse and mistreatment and as such choose to endure the abuse while suffering in silence.

Disclosure of abuse is prohibited within Chinese culture which emphasizes that a person should not interfere in another's family affairs; individuals should not discuss private matters to outsiders (Manigbas, 2002; Yan & So-Kum Tang, 2001). Abuse against elders by caregivers may induce feelings of guilt and shame on both parties which prohibits seniors from disclosing and caregivers from seeking support or help and thus repeating the cycle (Yan, So-Kum Tang & Yeung, 2002). Disclosure is less likely among Chinese elders as a consequence of language barriers, which further contributes to social isolation and feelings of loneliness exacerbate the risk for abuse (Tam & Neysmith, 2006). Loneliness was found to be a risk factor for mistreatment among older Chinese patients of a major urban health centre in China (Dong, Simon, Gorbien, Percak & Golden, 2007). Lai (2003) indicated that 41% of Chinese elders in Canada do not understand any English while 20% do not speak any English (Lai, 2003). Participants in the present study identified language barriers as the most difficult barrier to overcome. As Manigbas (2002) illustrated, elderly immigrants are dependent and isolated as, "their eyes are blind because they can't read English, their ears are deaf because they do not understand English and their mouths are mute because they do not speak English" (p. 70).

The risk for abuse is also influenced by the decline of traditional values and filial piety observed in Western society (Yan & Tang, 2001). The obligations and rigidity of familial relationships dictated by traditional values and filial piety may serve to protect elders from being abused as older people are to be revered and respected or it may increase the risk for abuse with the strain of care provision in the face of disrupted family networks and increased demands. Further, this risk may be exacerbated with the enhanced demands for care provision arising with increasing life expectancy and dependency of seniors.

In this study participants identified access to free Chinese community-based cultural services and activities may decrease the loneliness and isolation felt by many of Chinese immigrant elders. Language training and social programs tailored specifically for members of the Chinese culture may also be developed. In addition, other culturally sensitive programs dealing with the issues associated with family conflict and violence are important.

Sponsorship requirements results in many Chinese elders being dependent on children or other relatives for financial support, which may aggravate situations of mistreatment or abuse. As with many situations of care-giving for older adults, more supports should be provided to the caregivers as a mechanism to reduce the stress and burden of caregiving and possibly reduce incidences of elder abuse in the Chinese community specifically.

It is imperative to reflect on how social work and human services can be modified to empower disenfranchised communities and provide culturally responsive services appropriate for older adults. Kam (2002) suggests that practitioners should avoid forms of practice with older adults which contribute to older people's sense of powerlessness, incompetence, and low self-esteem including: "negative attitudes toward older people; the use of a medical control model of practice; an unequal relationship with older people; denying older people opportunities to participate in decision making; and limiting older people's choices and alternatives" (p. 161). Tam (2004) advocates that culturally responsive practice with abused Chinese Canadian women requires assurances of confidentiality, recognition of women's ambivalent feelings towards leaving an abusive relationship, and an appreciation of the woman's sense of shame and guilt was requisite to providing services in the women's best interests.

This chapter highlights the need for policies and legislation to be created to protect all elders, echoing recent calls for international convention on the human rights of older people (Tang, 2007).

References

American Geriatrics Society. (2006). *Doorway thoughts: Cross cultural health care for older adults, Volume II*. Sudbury, Massachusetts: Jones and Bartlett.

Brotman, S. (1998). The incidence of poverty among seniors in Canada: Exploring the impact of gender, ethnicity, and race. *Canadian Journal on Aging, 17*(2), 166-185

Brown, J. B. (1999). The use of focus groups in clinical research. In B.F. Crabtree, W.L. Miller (Eds.) *Doing qualitative research, 2nd ed.* (pp. 109-124).Thousand Oaks, CA: Sage,

Buchwald, D., Tomita, S., Hartman, S., Furman, R., Dudden, M. & Manson S.M. (2000). Physical abuse of urban Native Americans. *Journal of General Internal Medicine, 15*(8), 562-564.

Canadian Social Trends. (2005). Chinese Canadians: Enriching the cultural mosaic. (11-008-XIE), Spring

Carefirst Seniors & Community Services Association (2002). *In disguise: Elder abuse and neglect in the Chinese community*. Scarborough, Ontario: Author

Chan, S., & Leong, CW. (1994). Chinese families in transition: Cultural conflicts and adjustment prolems. *Journal of Social Distress and the Homeless, 3*(3), 263-281.

Cham, G.W. & Seow, E. (2000). The pattern of elderly abuse presenting to an emergency department. *Singapore Medical Journal, 41*(12), 571-574.

Citizenship and Immigration Canada. (2002). *Facts and figures – immigration overview.* Ottawa: Policy, Planning and Research, Citizenship and Immigration Canada.

Denzin, N. & Lincoln, Y. (Eds) (2000). *Handbook of Qualitative Research, 2nd edn.,* Thousand Oaks, CA: Sage.

Dong, X., Simon M.A., Gorbien, M., Percak, J. & Golden R. (2007). Loneliness in older Chinese adults: A risk factor for elder mistreatment. *Journal of the American Geriatrics Society, 55* (11), 1831–1835.

Drabenstott, K. M. (1992). Focused group interviews. In J.D. Glazier, R.R. Powell (Eds.) *Qualitative research in information management* (pp. 85-104).Englewood, CO: Libraries Unlimited.

Fulmer, T., Paveza, G., Abraham, I. & Fairchild, S. (2000). Elder neglect assessment in the emergency department. *Journal of Emergency Nursing, 26*(5), 436-443.

Guba, E.G. (1981). Criteria for assessing the trustworthiness of naturalistic inquiries. *Education, Communication and Technology Journal, 29*(2), 75–91.

Health Canada (2002). *Canada's aging population.* Minister of Public Works and Government Services Canada. Cat. H39-608/2002E

Hwang, KK. (2006). Constructive realism and Confucian relationalism: An epistemological strategy for the development of an indigenous psychology. U. Kim, K-S Yang, K-K Hwang (Eds.) *Indigenous and cultural psychology: Understanding people in context* (pp. 73-108). New York: Springer

International Plan of Action on Ageing, 2002. Unanimously adopted at The United Nations Second World Assembly on Ageing (Madrid, 8-12 April 2002).

Kam, P.K. (2002). From disempowering to empowering: Changing the practice of social service professionals with older people. *Hallym International Journal of Aging, 4*(2), 161-183.

Lachs, M.S. & Pillemer, K. (2004). *Elder abuse. Lancet, 364*(9441), 1263-1272.

Lai, D.W. (2005). Prevalence and correlates of depressive symptoms in older Taiwanese immigrants in Canada. *Journal of the Chinese Medical Association, 68*(3), 118-125.

Lai, D.W. & Chau, S.B. (2007a). Effects of service barriers on health status of older Chinese immigrants in Canada. *Social Work, 52*(3), 261-269.

Lai, D.W. & Chau, S.B. (2007b). Predictors of health service barriers for older Chinese immigrants in Canada. *Health & Social Work, 32*(1), 57-65.

Litwin, H. & Zobai, S. (2004). A multivariate examination of explanations for the occurrence of elder abuse. *Social Work Research, 28*(3), 1331-142.

Malley-Morrison, K. & Hines, D. (2004). *Family violence in a cultural perspective: Defining, understanding and combating abuse.* Thousand Oaks, London: Sage Publications,

Manigbas, M. (2002). Multiservice organization combats elder abuse in Chinese community. *Generations, 26*(3), 70-71.

Martin, L.G. (1990). Changing intergenerational family relations in East Asia. *Annals of the American Academy of Political and Social Science, 510*(1), 102-114.

McDonald, L., Colontonio, A., Clarke, D., McCleary, L. George, U. & Marziali, E. (2006). *Health disparities in older visible minorities in Canada.* Presented at the Society for Social Work and Research. Accessed on March 24, 2008 at: http://sswr.confex.com/sswr/2006/techprogram/P4051.HTM

Midlarsky, E., Venkataramani-Kothara, A., & Plante, M. (2006). Domestic violence in the Chinese and South Asian immigrant communities *Annals of the New York Academy of Sciences, 1087,* 279–300.

Moon, A., Tomita, S.K., & Jung-Kamei, S. (2001). Elder mistreatment among four Asian American groups: An exploratory study on tolerance, victim blaming and attitudes toward third-party intervention. *Journal of Gerontological Social Work, 36*(1-2), 153-169

Nurenberg, L. (1998). Culturally specific outreach in elder abuse. In T. Tatara (Ed.) *Understanding elder abuse in minority populations* (pp. 207-220). Brunner/Mazel - Taylor & Francis Group, Philadelphia, PA.

Parra-Cardona, J.R., Meyer, E., Schiamberg, L. & Post, L. (2007). Elder abuse and neglect in Latino families: An ecological and culturally relevant theoretical framework for clinical practice. *Family Process, 46*(4), 451-470.

Patton, M.Q. (1990). *Qualitative Evaluation and Research Methods, 2nd edn.,* Newbury Park, CA: Sage

Potocky-Tripodi, M. (2002). *Best practices for social work with refugees and immigrants.* New York: Columbia University Press.

Rittman, M., Kuzmeskus, L. & Flum, M. (1998). A synthesis of current knowledge on minority elder abuse. In T. Tatara, (Ed.), *Understanding Elder Abuse in Minority Populations* (pp. 221-238). Brunner/Mazel - Taylor & Francis Group: Philadelphia, PA.

Shibusawa, T. & Yick, A. (2007). Experiences and perceptions of intimate partner violence among older Chinese immigrants. *Journal of Elder Abuse & Neglect, 19* (3-4), 1-17.

Simpson, A. (2005). Cultural issues and elder mistreatment. *Clinics in Geriatric Medicine, 21*(2), 355-364.

Statistics Canada (2006). *A portrait of seniors in Canada.* Ottawa: Statistics Canada Social and Aboriginal Statistics Division, Catalogue no. 89-519.

Statistics Canada. (2003). 2001 Census: Analysis Series, Canada's ethnocultural portrait – the changing mosaic. Ottawa: Statistics Canada, Census Operations Division.

Statistics Canada. (2005) *Study: Canada's visible minority population in 2017.* The Daily. Accessed on March 24, 2008 at: http://www.statcan.ca/Daily/English/050322/d050322b.htm

Sung, KT. (2000). Respect for elders: Myths and realities in East Asia. *Journal of Aging and Identity, 5*(4), 197-205.

Tam, D. (2004). Culturally responsive advocacy intervention with abused Chinese-Canadian women. *British Journal of Social Work, 34*(2), 269–277.

Tam, S. & Neysmith, S. (2006). Disrespect and isolation: Elder abuse in Chinese communities. *Canadian Journal of Aging, 25*(2), 141–151.

Tang, C. S.K. (1997). Psychological impact of wife abuse: Experiences of Chinese women and their children. *Journal of Interpersonal Violence, 12*(3), 466-478.

Tang, KL. (2007). Taking older people's rights seriously: The role of international law. *Journal of Aging & Social Policy, 20* (1), 99-117.

Tatara, T. (1998). *Understanding elder abuse in minority populations.* Brunner/Mazel - Taylor & Francis Group, Philadelphia, PA

Walsh, C.A., Ploeg, J., Lohfeld, L., Horne, J., MacMillan, H. & Lai, D. (2007). Violence across the lifespan: Interconnections among forms of abuse as described by marginalized Canadian elders and their caregivers. *British Journal of Social Work Special Issue* - Caring for People: Social Work with Adults in the Next Decade and Beyond, 37(3), 491-514.

Wang, S. & Lo, L. (2005). Chinese immigrants in Canada: Their changing composition and economic performance. *International Migration, 43*(3), 35-71.

Wolf, R.S., Bennett, G. & Daichman, L. (2003). Abuse of older people. In F.L. Green, M.J. Friedman, J.T.V.M. de Jong, S.D. Solomon, T.M. Keane, J.A. Fairbank, et al. (Eds.), *Trauma interventions in war and peace: Prevention, practice, and policy* (pp. 105–128). New York: Kluwer Academic/Plenum Publishers.

World Health Organization, University of Toronto and Ryerson University, *International Network for the Prevention of Elder Abuse. (2002).* The Toronto Declaration on the Global Prevention of Elder Abuse. World Health Organization, Geneva.

WHO/INPEA. (2002). *Missing voices: views of older persons on elder abuse.* Geneva, World Health Organization.

Yan, E. & So-Kum Tang, C. (2003). Proclivity to elder abuse: A community study on Hong Kong Chinese. *Journal of Interpersonal Violence, 18*(9), 999-1017.

Yan, E. So-Kum Tang, C. & Yeung, D. (2002). No safe haven: A review on elder abuse in Chinese families. *Trauma, Violence & Abuse, 3*(3), 167-180.

Yan, E. So-Kum Tang, C. (2001). Prevalence and psychological impact of Chinese elder abuse. *Journal of Interpersonal Violence, 16*(11), 1158-1174.

Yan, E. & So-Kum Tang, C. (2004). Elder abuse by caregivers: A study of prevalence and risk factors in Hong Kong Chinese families. *Journal of Family Violence, 19*(5), 269-277.

Yick, A.G. (2000). Predictors of physical spousal/intimate violence in Chinese American families. *Journal of Family Violence 12,* 249–267.

Zhan, H J. (2005). Joy and sorrow: Explaining Chinese caregivers' reward and stress. *Journal of Aging Studies, 20*(1), 27-38.

Zhang, Y. & Goza, F W. (2006). Who will care for the elderly in China? A review of the problems caused by China's one-child policy and their potential solutions. *Journal of Aging Studies, 20*(2), 151-164.

13

The African Immigrant Experience with Reference to Aging

Douglas Durst and Godknows Kumassah, (University of Regina)

The historical perspective of the immigration of African immigrants and refugees to Canada, research studies on immigrants and refugees, and the conceptual/theoretical perspective of the image of Africans in North America is examined with references to aging and seniors. The history of African immigrants to Canada, which is not a very long one, especially for Black Africans, is the focus of this chapter. It is acknowledged that Canada has its population of Indigenous Black Canadians such as those found in Nova Scotia, south-western Ontario and other regions of Canada. Although these persons are not immigrants, they may experience some of the same issues as African immigrants. There is also a proud population of Caribbean Black Canadians of both French and English heritage. Our current The Right Honorable Governor General, Michaelle Jean, is an immigrant from French-speaking Haiti and is the grandchild of slavery. The Caribbean residents may also relate to some of the experiences of African immigrants but again their backgrounds are unique and it is not correct to make generalizations.

While Blacks of African descent have lived in North America for over three centuries, their history has been characterized by slavery, oppression, and struggles for equality and social justice as have been well documented in literature (McColley, 1988, p. 281). There is evidence of the existence of the slavery of Black people not only in United States of America but also in Canada as early as the seventeenth century (Robinson, 2003). Consequently, over the years, a racist disposition and ideology found its way into the formulation of Canada's immigration policies.

Although Canada's development as a prosperous industrial nation is documented in the literature as being attributed to the efforts of immigrants, it appears that in every period in Canada's history there have been strong sentiments expressed by some members of the general public and those with vested interests against the admission of certain demographic as well as ethnic or racial groups of immigrants, specifically Africans, as undesirable (Dirks, 1995; Knowles, 1997; Kelley & Trebilcock, 1998; Jakubowski, 1997).

Early Canadian Immigration Policies

Dirks (1995), in tracing Canada's immigration tradition, indicates that the first group of immigrants to permanently settle in Canada were Europeans who began to arrive at the beginning of the seventeenth century. He also mentions that, during the next three centuries, Canada's population that comprised mainly of European immigrants grew slowly. In 1763, the European population in the new colony of Canada stood at approximately 60 000. By Confederation in 1867, the number had reached 3 000 000, made up mainly of British and French settlers (Dirks, 1995). At the beginning of the twentieth century, the population had only reached 5 000 000 according to 1901 census. However, by the 1950s, Canada's population had grown to more than 13 000 000, and with marked change in its ethnic composition. Up until then, only Europeans or white Americans were almost exclusively allowed into Canada (Dirks, 1995). The only exception in terms of other ethnic groups was the free and fugitive Black slaves from the United States, and Chinese laborers who were used in building the Canadian Pacific Railway in the late 1880s (Knowles, 1997). Persons of African heritage were some of the first non-European immigrants to arrive on Canada's soil.

Knowles (1997), and Kelley and Trebilcock (1998), in describing the first large influx of refugees to Canada in 1783, mention that 3 000 free Blacks were among the British loyalists from the American Revolution to settle in Nova Scotia. The free Blacks, who expected that they would be dealt with on the same terms as white Loyalists in their new home, were faced with a scourge of racism and a host of other obstacles with regard to land grants and provisions. "Bitterly disappointed in their hopes of finding equality and a good life in Nova Scotia, nearly 1 200 of them sailed in 1792 for Sierra Leone to start afresh on the west coast of Africa" (Knowles, 1997, p. 24 -25).

Effects of Canadian Immigration Policies on African Applicants

As observed through the immigration tradition of Canada, before the 1960s as a policy, people other than those of European descent were mainly excluded from immigrating to Canada. Whenever any other racial or ethnic group had been admitted into Canada over the years, it had always been in a refugee situation and public and international pressure had been involved. While the earlier immigration policies were racially discriminative and restrictive, a careful examination of the later policies when overt racism was no longer an issue still contained restrictive provisions, especially with regard to third world applicants. These restrictive provisions could be identified in the features and criteria for determining eligibility of immigrant applicants; namely, within the family, independent, and business classes (Dirks, 1995; Kelley & Trebilcock, 1998; Knowles, 1997).

First, while the family class provision in the immigration policy provided for family members to be reunited in Canada, the high priority attached to the criteria for family reunification placed most third world applicants, particularly Africans, at a disadvantage. Since Africans (except South African whites) had traditionally been excluded, it was obvious that none of them ever had relatives living in Canada to become their sponsors unless through the generosity of a white Canadian humanitarian or philanthropist (Kelley & Trebilcock, 1998, p. 320).

Second, although the immigration policy's criteria for independent class eligibility attempted to provide an objective and fair system that would give equal opportunity to all applicants regardless of race or nationality, it still ignored other forms of discrimination contained within the nine categories of the points system. People from poor third world countries with all their disadvantages find it a major obstacle when factors like their education, job opportunity in Canada, age, personal characteristics, degree of fluency in English or French, and degree of kinship with people already living in Canada are taken into consideration in determining their eligibility to immigrate to Canada. The reasons for most of these people's desire to immigrate include the opportunity to acquire these very qualities, abilities, and skills that are being required of them. Ironically, many refugees are allowed into Canada without possessing many of these requirements.

Finally, the business class, with its three categories, is the most restrictive and discriminative to African immigrants in particular. This aspect of the immigration policy reflects the ideological perspective of the government toward neo-liberalism. It reinforces the belief in free-market capitalist system and private enterprises' ability to meet the economic and social needs of the nation (O'Connor, Orloff & Shaver, 1999). It is, therefore, very difficult, if not impossible, for a poor African immigrant to qualify for any of the three business-class categories, and, thereby, giving the rich and wealthy self-employed, entrepreneur, or investor the opportunity to buy their way into Canada by virtue (or vice) of their money.

Knowles (1997) compares the immigration statistics of 1962 when the white-only immigration policy was abolished to that of 1963 when the Canadian economy began to recover from the recession. In one year, most immigration from non-European countries more than doubled. From Africa (not including South Africa), the numbers jumped from 104 in 1962 to 264 in 1963 (Knowles, 1997, p. 154) but compared to the total immigration, African immigrants remained few in number.

Although no specific reasons are given in the literature for the low number of immigrants from Africa admitted into Canada prior to 1963, it is possible that the restrictive factors played a part in who was admitted. Besides, the fact that racial discrimination had been eliminated from the letter of the immigration policy does not mean that it did not exist in the minds and attitudes of the immigration officials and did not persist (Jakubowski, 1997). The literature gives examples of incidents where, with the discretionary powers at their disposal, officials could refuse admission to an immigrant with a passing mark and allow admission to one without it, or refuse an immigrant admission for a frivolous reason like un-adaptability to the Canadian climate (Kelley & Trebilcock, 1998; Knowles, 1997).

The African Immigrants in Canada

Before 1961, when Canada's restrictive immigration policy was still in force, the total immigrant population in Canada was 894 465 out of which 4 635 were African immigrants and refugees (Statistic Canada, 2001). When this population is divided according to regions of Africa, Western African region accounted for only 75 people out of 4 635. There were only 535 immigrants from the Eastern African region and 2 595 people from the Northern. It is quite obvious that, before 1961, the Western, Eastern, and Central regions of African had the fewest number of immigrants which are regions predominantly populated by Black Africans. The Northern and Southern regions of Africa represented the population of white settlers in Africa, especially the Republic of South Africa which was still oppressing the Blacks under the Apartheid policy (Statistic Canada, 2001).

After 1961, when Canada's restrictive immigration policy was changed, the African immigrant and refugee population in Canada increased considerably from 4 636 to 23 825 out of a total immigrant population of 745 565 between 1961 and 1970. From 1971 to 1980, the African immigrant population was 54 650 out of a total immigrant population of 936 275. Between 1981 and 1990, it was 59 715 out of 1 041 495, and 139 770 out of 1 830 680 for the period 1991 to 2001. However, in the past five years, the numbers have more than doubled to 374 565. Correspondingly, all the five regions of Africa represented in Canada also experienced increases in their immigrant populations. However, there still existed the disparity in terms of fewer numbers of immigrants coming from the Western, Eastern, and Central regions of Africa which are predominantly Black as compared to white dominated Northern and Southern regions of Africa.

Table 1 presents data on senior African immigrants in the year of 2006 from all five regions. It is important to recognize that not all of the immigrants are Black Africans. Of the total immigrants living in Canada (6 186 950), only 374 565 (6.1%) immigrants were from Africa and from the predominantly Black regions only 0.8% from the Western region, 2.1% from the Eastern region and 0.4% from the Central region. As a percentage of African immigrants, 13.0% are from the Western region, 34.7% from the Eastern region and 6.0% form the Central region.

Table 1
Senior African Immigrants in Canada (2006)

Place of Birth	Total	% of Total	African	Total 65+	%of 65+	+% of Region
Total Immigrants	6 186 950					
Africa	374 565	6.1%		32 500		8.7%
Western Africa	48 645	0.8%	13.0%	980	3.0%	2.0%
Eastern Africa	129 920	2.1%	34.7%	12 005	36.8%	9.2%
Northern Africa	134 505	2.2%	35.9%	13 645	41.9%	10.1%
Central Africa	22 405	0.4%	6.0%	360	1.1%	1.6%
Southern Africa	39 090	0.6%	10.4%	5 595	17.2%	14.3%
		6.1%	100.0%		100%	8.7%
Canada Census, 2006						

When examining the senior African population, some interesting trends emerge. Overall the senior population is quite low and the African population in Canada is one of the youngest of the immigrant groups. Of all of the African seniors, Northern Africa has the highest percentage of residents 65 or more years of age at 41.9% of all African seniors and includes countries such as Egypt, Libya, and Morocco. The Eastern Africa, which is heavily populated with Black Africans, has the second largest percentage of the African seniors at 36.8%. The Southern African region holds 17.2% of the seniors and includes many white South Africans who left Africa after the fall of Apartheid and the following years of economic and social instability. Not surprisingly, the Western and Central areas of Africa have the lowest of the African senior population at 3.0% and 1.1% respectively. Western regions include countries such as Ghana, Nigeria, Togo and the Central region includes such countries as Angola, Cameroon, Chad, and the Congo.

When examining the percentage of seniors from the African regions, the total African seniors represent only 8.7% of all Africans which is well below the national average of seniors in Canada at 13.7%. However, the Southern region has 14.3% of its population as 65 years or more. Its composition reflects and is slightly greater than the percentage of the senior population in the Canadian population (13.7%). In start contrast, in the regions of high percentage of Black Africans, the senior population is low at 2.0% for the Western region and only 1.6% for Central Africa. The Black Africans are a young population.

Historically, Africans represent the most recent arrivals of immigrants to Canada with the majority of them immigrating to Canada after 1961. Prior to 1961, the Canadian immigration policies were formulated to exclude nonwhites. Africans, specifically Black Africans, were not deemed desirable candidates for immigration to Canada. They were not considered part of the preferred ethnicity. However, as a result of strong criticism and condemnation of the discriminatory nature of Canada's immigration policy from the Canadian public, significant change was made in 1962 (Kelley & Trebilcock, 1998, p. 345). The change abolished the "White Canada immigration policy" and incorporated a points system that made it possible for any independent immigrant, regardless of ethnicity, skin color, or nationality to be considered a suitable candidate for admission into Canada.

This change gave Black Africans equal opportunity, in theory, to be admitted into Canada as immigrants. As a result, there has been a slow but steady increase of the African immigrant population from 4 635 before 1961 to 139 770 in 2001 and more than double to 374 565 in 2006. Since 1961, the numbers have multiplied by 80 making Africa an accelerating immigration source!

Spiritual Well-being and Immigration Adjustment

In his study of African immigrants to the USA, Kamya (1997) employed quantitative exploratory cross-sectional design in his research. He examined the integration of African immigrants into the social environment of their host country. His report reinforces the fact that African immigrants encounter social and cultural integration difficulties in their host countries. His examination of African immigrants' experiences with stress, self-esteem, spiritual well-being, and coping resources found a high and positive correlations between spiritual well-being and hardiness as well as between self-esteem and coping resources. He also found a negative but strong relationship between stress and self-esteem. Consequently, he concludes that immigrants with strong support and spiritual well-being are able to cope better. The importance of the African's belief in a Supreme Being who controls the natural order of things is noted by Kamya (1997) as necessary for understanding the immigrant experience of African immigrants. Although Kamya generalizes, this point is summarized in the following quote:

> Spiritual well-being is defined as satisfaction with one's religious well-being
> reflected in one's relationship with a Supreme Being, one's existential well-being,

and one's sense of meaning and purpose in life. For Africans, the spiritual has a personal and a communal aspect. It also implies the community's preparedness and acknowledgment of something outside itself and the community's experience and involvement of this "other-ness." Self-esteem and spiritual well-being are intimately tied into the individual's coping resources, defined as characteristics or ongoing behaviors that enable individuals and communities to handle stressors more effectively, to experience fewer symptoms on exposure to stressors, or to recover faster from exposure. For Africans, therefore, coping, be it cognitive or social, emotional or physical, is derived from the personal and collective understanding of the spiritual in people's lives. (Kamya, 1997, p. 156)

While Christianity and Islam have become the predominant religions and sources of spirituality for most Africans, traditional religions and beliefs also play a major role in the spiritual lives of many Africans (Golding, 1997). The belief of communicating with the creator through the spirits of the ancestors is one of the major components of the traditional religions. Worshippers of the ancestral spirits seek to obtain power, protection and provision through animal sacrifices and offerings (Matthews, 1998; Mezzana, 2002). The ancestors are honored as spirits who preserve the moral standards and are regarded as intermediaries between the living and the divine powers (Matthews, 1998).

Although 91.7 percent of the African immigrants in Godknow's study (2008) indicated Christianity as their religion, more than half of them also admit that ancestral spirits play roles in their spirituality. However, they experienced conflicts in terms of performing certain common rituals they grew up with here in Canada for fear of being ridiculed and stigmatized. This aspect of the spiritual dimension is important in understanding how many Africans integrate or adjust to immigration and their perspectives on aging.

Conceptual/Theoretical Analysis

A look at the past and present Western perception of the image of the continent of Africa and its people is necessary in understanding the feelings and expectations of Africans who immigrate to North America. While, like other visible minority groups, the experiences of immigrants and refugees from Africa have been characterized by issues of race, class and gender, African immigrants and refugees experience further prejudice and discrimination as a result of their ethnic origin particularly as Black Africans (Royster, 2003).

The theoretical perspective identified by Deirdre A. Royster (2003) as "Racial Deficit Theory" in which wealthier and ethnically homogenous white North Americans view, particularly, African immigrants as less intelligent, less capable of controlling their emotions, less capable of governing themselves, and so forth, shall form the basis for understanding the African immigrant experience in this study. This deficit theory manifests itself in several ways including how the Western news media perpetuates this theoretical perspective.

Impacts of Racism and Discrimination

Since the mid 1700s, when Europeans conceived and implemented the idea of using Black Africans as slaves in the New World, the concept of racism and discrimination based on people's skin color was intensified (Bay, 2000). The rise of ideological racism during the slavery era and long after perpetuated the perception and treatment of Black Africans as inferior. Although no scientific or philosophic case could be made for the perceived moral and intellectual inferiority of African Americans, the words of notable early American politicians such as Thomas Jefferson strongly influenced the racial thought of Americans. One of the less-celebrated distinctions attributed to Thomas Jefferson was the thought "that the Blacks, whether originally a distinct race, or made distinct by time and circumstances, are inferior to the whites in the endowments both of body and mind" (Jefferson, *Notes on Virginia*. 1780s, in Bay, 2000, p. 15). The intellectuals among the Black community were not silent but held little influence in stemming the tide of ideological racism (Bay, 2000).

Over the years, white Americans came to embrace a number of religious, historical, and biological theories that were postulating the natural inferiority Blacks as historical truths of scientific knowledge (Royster, 2003; Bay 2000). These theories provided the rationalization for the enslavement of Africans in the Americas and the marginalization of the Black people in North America. Today, these theories continue to govern the social and economic relations between white and Black people (Royster, 2003). Royster (2003) explains the discrimination Black people encounter in their relationship with white people from the "racial deficit" theoretical perspective.

The racial deficit theory attempts to explain the differences between the Black and white races as well as identify the characteristics that, supposedly, make white people superior to Black people (Bay 2000; Royster, 2003). The whites that embrace this theory view Black Africans as less civilized than their counterparts in North America (Bay 2000). This unique view of Africans stems from the perception that the Western world has of the continent of Africa and its people. This image of Africa is further reinforced and perpetuated by the North American media (Belleh, 2003; Chavis, 1998; Hawk, 1992; Kunihira, 2007; Makunike, 1993).

Media Portrayal of Africans

Most North Americans have never visited Africa and will never visit Africa, yet there is an image of Africa and Africans embedded in the minds of North Americans

(Hawk, 1992). The knowledge of Africa that North Americans have is derived from sources such as school textbooks, the news media, church missionaries, and the entertainment industry. Of all these sources, the news media's role as the one that gives meaning to current events in the world for North Americans is considered the most important. This is because the media is responsible for the interpretation of the events they report which, in turn, define the understanding of the events by their readers and viewers (Hawk, 1992). The news media give meaning to current events and identify for the reader those events that are important (Bellah, 2003).

Due to commercial and financial considerations and priorities of editors among many others, news about Africa is mainly limited to events that are of a violent nature like tribal wars and coups, and catastrophes such as famine, hunger and disease (Bellah, 2003; Chavis, 1998; Ebo, 1992). Very little is portrayed about the people of Africa in terms of their culture, history, and values except in relation to violence and catastrophic events. Ebo (1992) observes that "much of what the American people know about Africa is derived from the negative and misguided images of Africa portrayed in the American media" (p. 15). He further indicates that this negative portrayal of Africa by the Western media is a deliberate and systematic process as a way of perpetuating and reinforcing the "racial deficits theory" as far as Africans' ability to govern and manage themselves as sovereign nations are concerned. Bellah states that "this pattern of news coverage is a carefully choreographed mechanism designed to give the Western viewer a sense of comfort and superiority over other peoples and nations" (Ebo, 2003, p. 3). The three images of Africans that feature prominently in North American media can be described as primitive, impoverished, and diseased images (Chavis, 1998).

Primitive African Image

Africa, as the least-known continent, has had the stigma of being the place of savages and portrayed in Western media as a crocodile-infested dark continent "where jungle life has perpetually eluded civilization" (Hacker, 1995; Ebo, 1992, p. 15). Hollywood and western television programs about Africa always feature Africans as half naked, living in mud houses with thatch roofs and the men wielding locally made spears and shields. Even political leaders who should know better make ignorant and insensitive gaffes about Blacks. Recently, the former Alberta premier made a public comment about visiting Africa and ending up in a pot of boiling water. Andrew Hacker (1995) in his book, *Two Nations,* confirms the persistence of the belief that Blacks represent an inferior strain of the human species. As such, he observed that Africans are seen as languishing at the lower level than members of other races. While this belief is not expressed publicly or overtly, the fact remains that most white people believe that, compared with other races, persons of African ancestry are most likely to carry primitive traits in their genes (Hacker, 1995, p. 24).

Given this prejudice, the presumption is that most individuals of African heritage lack the intellectual and organizational capacities required in the industrial and civilized world. Hence, Africans are considered only fit for physical work or jobs that require very little or no intellectual activities (Hacker, 1995). This also explains the difficulties African immigrants encounter in having their academic qualifications recognized, particularly, in Canada because education received in Africa is neither trusted nor respected as of an equivalent value. It also accounts for the over-representation of African immigrants, especially women, in low level jobs and occupations (Omene, 2000). In reference to Africa as the "dark continent" by the West, Hawk (1992) indicates that this has not only the allusion to the skin color of the inhabitants of Africa but to their ignorance of the Western ways.

Impoverished African Image

Africa is not only regarded as the primal continent and the most backward but also the least developed by almost every measure. The media reporting of Africa perpetuate this image by couching it in terms of economic degradation and describing the cure as economic intervention (Kunihira, 2007). The following quote from Hawk (1992) illustrates this point:

> Like anthropologists and explorers of the colonial era, journalists are empowered to paint an image of Africa by listing its deficiencies with respect to Western norms. Coverage of Africa which emphasizes poverty, disease, and famine corresponds to the existing view of Africans as have-nots. By comparing them to Western economic and technological standards, an image of Africa is created in the American mind that is a chronicle of Africa's deficiencies to the Western standard. (Hawk, 1992, p. 9)

Church missionaries, non-governmental organizations and other relief groups working in Africa, supposedly, to assist the impoverished and less fortunate Africans also contribute to further perpetuate this image in the minds of North Americans (van der Heyden, 1998). In their fundraising efforts, most of these organizations portray images of malnourished and orphaned African children in the most deplorable conditions to their sponsors in North America and Europe in order to generate support for higher donations. Bob Geldof, Bono and Oprah Winfrey are examples of celebrities who, although are genuine and passionate, perpetuate the impoverished image (Bellah, 2003).

While the condition of poverty is an undeniable reality for most African nations and the need for resolution very critical, there are many individual Africans who can be classified as belonging to the middle and upper classes in terms of their economic status. In other words, not everybody in Africa is poor. There exist affluent Africans by Western standards who have succeeded in providing the necessities for their families as well as making it possible for their children to attain the highest level of education and employable skills possible. There can also be found communities and neighborhoods in African cities and towns that have beautiful and well-built houses, streets, businesses, and industries comparable to those in most Western cities and towns. The omission of these details from the media reporting on Africa has created in the Western mind the impression that Africans who immigrate need intervention or rescuing from their economic problems (Hacker, 1995).

Diseased African Image

Another image of Africa that many Westerners have is the impression that most of the deadliest diseases in the world today originate from the jungles of Africa. Included in the list are malaria, the "ebola" fever and the west Nile virus (Close, 2001; Kunihira, 2007). Human Immunodeficiency Virus/Acquired Immune Deficiency Syndrome (HIV/AIDS) is the deadliest of such diseases whose origin is traced to the continent of Africa by the news media (Kanabus & Allen, 2004). As a result, the news media is often biased in reporting the cases of the disease in Africa as one of an unprecedented epidemic. While poverty and lack of access to modern medical treatments and resources may account for the visibility of and exposure given to the cases of the disease among the afflicted in Africa, it does not isolate Africa as the only continent most suffering in terms of the epidemic numbers of infected people in the world (UNAIDS, 2001).

In respect to the origin of AIDS and HIV, Annabel Kanabus and Sarah Allen (2004), in their research, point to the interesting and controversial debate this issue has generated since the beginning of the AIDS epidemic. They indicate that the first cases of AIDS occurred in the United States in 1981 with very little information provided about the source of the disease. While there is clear evidence that the virus HIV causes the AIDS disease and that the virus has been found to be part of a family of viruses known as simian immunodeficiency virus (SIV) found in the sooty mangabey (green) monkey which is indigenous to western Africa, Kanabus and Allen (2004) also mention that there are several controversial theories circulating as to how the HIV crossed over from animal (monkey) to humans. One such theory, proposed by the journalist Edward Hooper (1999), has suggested that HIV could be traced to an oral polio vaccine developed from chimpanzee kidney cells which was tested on about a million people in the Belgian Congo, Rwanda and Burundi in the late 1950s (Kanabus & Allen, 2004).

The presumption of the diseased image of Africans is that African immigrants are viewed with suspicion, particularly, as to their healthiness to live and function within their new communities. While mandatory medical examination is a requirement for admission into most Western countries as an immigrant (Knowles, 1997), African immigrants often encounter certain discriminating attitudes in Canada that could be attributed to the diseased image perception held by certain people about the continent of Africa and its people. Notably, in respect to the theory of HIV being transmitted through polio vaccine which was administered to unsuspecting Africans, though refuted, this theory supports the racial deficit theory which considered Africans as less than humans (Hooper, 1999, p. 86-87).

The racial deficit theory, as identified by Royster (2003) in which she explains that wealthier and ethnically homogenous white North Americans view people of African descent, particularly Black Africans, as less intelligent, less capable of controlling their emotions, less capable of governing themselves and so forth, conceptualizes the theoretical perspective of the thesis topic and forms the basis for understanding the African immigrant experience in this study. The outcome of this unique perspective of racism and discrimination provided the rationalization for the enslavement of Africans in the Americas and the marginalization of the Black people in North America.

In comparison to indigenous Blacks of North America, Bay (2000) reported that Black Africans are viewed by mainstream society as less civilized. This view is maintained and perpetuated by the Western media in terms of how the image of the continent of Africa and its inhabitants are portrayed to the American public. The primitive, impoverished, and diseased images of Africans are the ones that are featured prominently in North American media. Consequently, these images inform as well as form the basis of how many Canadians react to and interact with African immigrants socially (Royster, 2003).

Conclusion

A qualitative study with 12 African immigrants and refugees who settled in a prairie city has implications for adult Africans who age in their new country (Kumassah, 2008). The study found that coming from a third world situation, the transition into a western industrialized society had been difficult. During their maturing years, they had developed lifestyles that appropriately fitted into the cultural norms of the various African societies from which they came. Being forced by their circumstances as immigrants and refugees in a foreign land to adopt new lifestyles or alter certain aspects of their normal ways of life was both difficult and challenging for most of them. For instance, the absence of the extended family support network they depended on in Africa meant they needed to rebuild a new support system in a society that they felt was more individualistic than communal. They soon realized that building such support network in a different cultural context was quite overwhelming.

The participants migrated from a society where they were the majority, as with most African immigrants. Therefore, to be in a society where they were suddenly the minority was not only unfamiliar and strange to them but also created self-consciousness with regard to how they were perceived by the majority in their new country. Consequently, this self-consciousness also led to the whole issue of value conflicts as well as the perceptions of racism and discrimination discussed above (Kumassah, 2008).

Three themes that impacted the African adult immigrant that included (1) the effects of the absence of the extended family network and support, (2) the clash of cultures, and (3) perceived racism and discrimination among others on their immigrant experiences (Kumassah, 2008).

The participants noted that each of them had felt lonely and socially isolated at one point or another in their immigrant experience. This feeling of loneliness was attributed to the lack of strong social support network of family and friends in their host country. Although most of the participants appreciate the opportunity to make a better life for themselves in Canada, they also constantly miss the relationships and support of the extended family and friends they have grown to depend on socially, emotionally and sometimes financially in their countries of origin. While they understood that it would be difficult to bring over all the members of their support network from Africa, they felt that the government could make the family reunification section of the immigration policy less stringent in terms of eligibility and requirements, less expensive and with a shorter processing time. Hence, they encountered difficulty in applying for reunification of their aging parents.

Secondly, the issue of raising and disciplining their children in an African traditional way was one of the concerns of the participants. They emphasized the need to be able to instil in their children the sense of community and a lifelong respect for people especially loyalty to their parents and the members of the extended family as is done in Africa. While some agree that there are several good values worth emulating within the Canadian culture, others felt that their children are losing their identity as Africans within the individualistic and competitive nature of the Canadian culture. They wished that immigrant parents, particularly those from the third world, could be allowed to raise and discipline their children without government interference as long as the children's physical and emotional well-beings were not jeopardized.

Thirdly, the participants also suggested the need to provide easy access to essential services that would help make the transition into the Canadian culture easier for new African immigrants and refugees. They sought assistance with settlement and integration programs such as initial English language, job seeking and resume writing skills training.

For elderly African immigrants, the local African cultural association can assist in connecting and assisting in finding meaningful relationships. One cannot overemphasize the importance of African immigrants and refugees helping their fellow African immigrants. Africans already in Canada are familiar with the culture of the newcomers and can identify with their settlement, adaptation and integration issues, conflicts and needs. Many of the participants recommended the need for government to allocate specific funding to the African cultural association with the mandate to hire its own members, and train them to assist African newcomers from the time they first arrive in Canada. The funding should also cover the provision of a resource centre where new African immigrants and refugees could go for information on available services and assistance with other adjustment and integration needs in a culturally sensitive environment.

Lastly, with regard to racism and discrimination as they pertain to the negative portrayal of the image of Africans in the western media, some of the participants suggested that the responsibility for creating a positive public image of Africans should rest mostly on the African immigrant community themselves. To change the perception of North Americans about Africa and its people, the participants recommended that the African immigrant community should use the same media to make their voice heard.

With the demographic changes in the population of Canada, the African immigrants are making Canada their new home. As with the Canadian population as a whole, they will age in Canada and have new needs for service. Policy makers and service providers need to include knowledge about immigrants, especially those from the developing countries like African immigrants and refugees in order to provide relevant, sensitive and effective services to these culturally unique segments of the immigrant population. Meeting these emerging needs represents a challenge to social researchers to examine the complexity of issues facing immigrants from Africa as they age in their new homeland.

References

Bay, Mia. (2000). *The White image in the Black mind: African-American Ideas about White people, 1830 - 1925.* New York: Oxford University Press.

Belleh, Raymond Tarek. (2003). *Western media and Africa: The western media and Iits exploitation of Africa.* Retrieved September 23, 2007. (http://www.africanevents.com/Essay-RaymondTB-WesternMedia.htm

Canada. (2001). *2001 census Canada.* Ottawa: Statistics Canada.

Canada. (2006). *2006 census Canada.* Ottawa: Statistics Canada.

Chavis, Rod. (1998). Africa in the western media. University of Pennsylvania-African Studies Center. Retrieved on 8/29/2007. http://www.africa.upenn.edu/Workshop/chavis/98.html

Close, W.T. (2001). *Ebola: Through the eyes of the people.* Big Piney: Meadowlark Springs Productions.

Dirks, G.E. (1995). *Controversy and complexity: Canadian immigration policy during the 1980s.* Montréal: McGill-Queen University Press.

Hacker, A. (1995). *Two nations: Black and White, separate, hostile, unequal.* New York: Ballantine Books.

Hawk, Beverly. G. (Ed.). (1992). *Africa's media image.* New York: Praeger

Hooper, E. (1999). *The river: A journey to the source of HIV and AIDS.* Boston, MA: Little, Brown and Company

Golding, V. (1999). *Traditions from Africa.* Austin, TX: Raintree Steck-Vaughn Publishers.

Kamya, H.A. (1997). African immigrants in the U.S.: The challenge for research and practice. *Social Work, 42*(2), 154-165.

Kanabus, Annabel & Allen, Sarah. (2004). *The origin of HIV and the first cases of AIDS.* West Sussex: AVERT. http://www.avert.org/origins.htm

Kelley, N. & Trebilcock, M.J. (1998). *The making of the mosaic: A history of Canadian immigration policy.* Toronto: University of Toronto Press.

Knowles, V. (1997). *Strangers at our gates: Canadian immigration and immigration policy, 1540-1997.* Toronto: Dundurn Press.

Kumassah, Godknows, (2008). Giving voice: The lived experiences of African immigrants and refugees in the City of Regina. M.S.W. Thesis. Faculty of Social Work. Regina: University of Regina.

Kunihira, Stella M. (2007). Africa in American media: A content analysis of Newsweek Magazine's portrayal of Africa, 1988-2006. Unpublished research. Saint Mary's College. Notre Dame, IN. www.saintmarys.edu/~socio/SeniorSem%20F2007/Stella%20Maris%20Pap.doc

Jakubowski, Lisa M. (1997). *Immigration and the legalization of racism.* Halifax, NS: Fernwood Publishing.

Matthews, D.H. (1998). *Honoring the ancestors: An African cultural interpretation of Black religion and literature.* Oxford: Oxford University Press.

McColley, R. (1988). *Slavery. Dictionary of Afro-American slavery,* Edited by Randall M. Miller and John David Smith. Westport: Greenwood Press.

Mezzana, D. (2002). African traditional religions and modernity. *Online Journal, African Societies.* http://www.africansocieties.org/n3/eng_dic2002/religionitrad.htm

O'Connor, J., Orloff, A. & Shaver, S. (1999). *States, markets, families: Gender, liberalism and social policy in Australia, Canada, Great Britian and the United States.* Cambridge, UK: Cambridge University Press.

Omene, M. (2000). *A study of the experiences of black Caribbean women in the Saskatchewan labour force.* Regina: University of Regina.

Robinson, B.A. (2003). *A brief history of slavery in North America.* New York: CRT Press.

Royster, D A. (2003). *Race and the invisible hand: How White networks exclude Black men from blue-collar jobs.* Berkeley & Los Angeles, CA: University of California Press.

UNAIDS. (2001). *Sub-Saharan Africa: AIDS epidemic Update. 2001 report on the global AIDS epidemic.* http://www.who.int/hiv/pub/epidemiology

van der Heyden, Tina. (1998). *Africa in international media.* Seminar paper. African Media Debates. www.journ.ru.ac.ca/amd/int.htm

14

Socio-Cultural Determinants of Mental Health Among Elderly Iranian Immigrants

Siavash Jafari, Richard Mathias, (University of British Columbia), and Souzan Baharlou, (Association of Medical Doctors of British Columbia)

Historically, the immigration of people is a universal phenomenon and over time has occurred in all nations. Individuals may immigrate to seek better employment, to improve their future, to avoid political and religious persecution, or to seek religious freedom. According to Statistics Canada's 2006 census (Statistics Canada, 2006), there were some 121 510 Iranian immigrants (96% first generation) living in Canada, with the highest number living in Toronto (47%), Vancouver (22%), and Montreal (9%). Massive numbers of Iranian immigrants came to Canada mainly after the Iranian Revolution in 1979. Initiation of war by Iraq soon after the revolution was another factor that caused social and religious turmoil and added to the hardships brought on by political pressures. These events caused Iranians to experience changes in social structure, economic status, security, and other areas, resulting in high levels of stress (Bagheri, 1992; Hassen & Sardashti, 2000; Khavarpour & Rissel, 1997; Pliskin, 1992; Zangeneh, Sadeghi & Sharp, 2002). As a result, this group of Iranian immigrants was identified to be prone to developing psychosocial stress and mental disorders (Bagheri, 1992; Jalali, 1996; Zangeneh et al., 2002). These factors are assumed to have interfered with their integration into Canadian society by separating them from their normal surroundings.

According to the 2001 report of the World Health Organization, mental disorders are growing health problems worldwide and are expected to affect more than 25% of all people at some time in their lives (WHO, 2001). According to the same report, 450 million people worldwide suffer from some form of mental disorder including alcohol and substance abuse disorders. Of the ten leading causes of disability worldwide, five are mental disorders: major depression, schizophrenia, bipolar disorder, alcohol use disorder, and obsessive-compulsive disorder (Goldner, Snider & Mozel, 2001). It is also expected that the burden of mental disorders will continue to increase due to the changes in the age of the population and also due to social and economic factors. It is expected that within the next two decades, depressive illnesses will become the second leading cause of disease burden worldwide and the principal cause in developed countries such as Canada (Murray & Lopez, 1996).

Like many other industrialized countries, Canada is facing an increasingly aging population. The presence of an aging immigrant population raises important concerns about the well-being of this population. Estimates suggest that by 2016 there will be six million seniors, comprising 16 percent of the population (Statistics Canada, 2004). As Canada's population continues to age, mental health care for seniors is becoming a greater priority. For seniors with mental disorders, the challenges of aging can be even more overwhelming and complex as they deal with a multitude of issues. For instance, among Canadian elderly living in the community, approximately 10 to 15 percent exhibit depressive symptom;, whereas, for elderly living in long-term care institutions, the estimates are as high as 50 percent (Conn, Lee, Steingart & Silberfeld, 1992).

Although much is known about the overall immigrant populations of Canada, the scale and diversity of research on elderly Iranians is extremely limited. It was felt such research was needed in order to develop a systematic approach to review the important but often subtle roles of immigration, ethnicity, and culture in the clinical care of elderly Iranian immigrants in British Columbia (BC), Canada. For this purpose, a qualitative approach was used to investigate the factors that might affect the mental health of Iranian immigrants. While the main focus of this chapter is the mental health of Iranian elderly immigrants living in BC, every effort was made to identify published articles on Iranian immigrants from other provinces and from other countries and have included them in our discussion.

Methods

An ethnographic approach was adopted combining observation, informal interviews and triangulated case studies (Hammersley & Atkinson, 1995) to investigate the perceived definition of mental health among participants, and factors that might affect their mental health. Sample recruitment started after obtaining approval from the University of British Columbia (UBC) Ethics Committee. Both focus group (FG) discussions and in-depth interviews were conducted with 24 elderly and ten key informants. These methods are well established in social science studies (Gibbs, 1997) and they are particularly suitable for identifying, exploring and explaining complex attitudes, perceptions and beliefs (Kitzinger, 1995), and explaining the level of consensus around a given subject (Morgan & Kreuger, 1993).

After obtaining permission from the proposed participants, the two investigators contacted them and described the project and its purposes. The sample ages of the elderly participants and key informants ranged from 59 to 75 years and 46 to 58 years respectively. The length of residency in Canada was revealed to be between 3 and 10 years. The number of men and women were evenly distributed and the focus groups were relatively homogenous (Morgan & Kreuger, 1993). Fieldwork included diverse data sources to help build a detailed picture of the context in which mental health was imagined. Participants were selected through snowball sampling. After identifying the most knowledgeable elderly who were interested in participating in this study, we asked them to introduce some friends and family members that were older than 55 and were interested in our discussions. Key informants were selected from among the family counsellors, immigrant settlers, interpreters, and community-based professionals. Themes arising from these interviews were used along with themes from the literature review and community-based fieldwork to develop a topic guide for use in the focus group discussions and in-depth interviews.

Overall, six focus groups, each consisting of five to seven participants, lasted between one and half to two hours and ten in-depth interviews were conducted. Focus group discussions and in-depth interviews elicited data on demographics, mental health knowledge of participants, and their experience with immigration and subsequent life experiences in Canada. The interviewers read the consent form to the subjects and gave each one a copy to sign. The form assured confidentiality. Each group discussion was recorded with a digital recorder for later analysis. Following each interview, the facilitators met to discuss and record field notes containing data on the researchers' impressions, insights, interpretations and observations on the process of the study. The learning gained through this process was used to improve future sessions. Sources of data in this study included transcripts from the group discussions and in-depth interviews, field notes and findings of our observations from participation in Iranian community events and two elderly day cares in Vancouver. Informal contact with people in the community was also an important source of data for this study.

Findings

Definition of Mental Health

There were rich sets of descriptions to define mental health among our participants. *"Gam o gosseh"* (sadness), *"narahati"* (being uncomfortable), *"deltangi"* (heart distress), *"afsordegi"* (depression), *"beihoselegei"* (lack of patience), *"narahati e aasab"* (neural illness), and *"beimari e rohei"* (spiritual sickness) were among the most common terms being used. Indeed, among these definitions the last two were less likely to be used than the other five definitions because of their associated stigma. Some participants referred to both emotional and psychosocial aspects of mental health simultaneously. One participant, for instance, said:

> To me, mental health means a good co-ordination between the person's mind, emotions and his behavior in the community.

Some participants identified an aspect of mental health as "not having a psychological illness." Depression, anxiety, and sadness were some of the essential terms used to describe poor mental health. The majority of participants perceived mental health in relation to concepts such as good relationships, proper manners, effective communication with people, and being honest and trustworthy. Also, mental health was defined as a balance between internal feelings and external expressions by some participants. A 66-year-old female participant stated:

> Good mental health means having a stable personality and behaving properly . . . It means that we act according to our internal feeling.

The Iranian concept of health derives from the central concept of balance between the mind, body, and society. Mental illnesses are believed to be created as reflections of one's own behaviors. In Iranian culture, it is strongly believed that whatever you do to others will be paid back to you. Interestingly, Iranians believe that what adults do may even affect their children's health and future. It is also believed that if you are good to others, God will be good to you and your family. Two main concepts can be inferred from this notion. First, it is believed that illness and health are reflections of our own actions. Second, illness and health, disease and its cure, and poor and good mental health are all provided by God as a punishment or reward for one's actions and beliefs. Many participants in our interviews believed that mental illnesses arise from a lack of morals, sinful activities, and interpersonal conflicts. Elderly Iranians are also more likely to attribute the development and cure of mental illness to spiritual causes. They tend to attribute illness recovery and effectiveness of treatment to God's will. This notion is obvious on their recurrent use of the term "*en-sha-allah*" which means "if God wills." In Iranian culture, it is believed that nothing, good or bad, can happen unless God wishes.

Effects of Immigration on Mental Health

Our participants believed that it is not simple to cope with leaving one's families, assets, homeland, friends, and sometimes even one's memories and culture. Differences in language and culture were among the most important concerns mentioned by participants in the focus groups and the in-depth interview groups. Most informants (men and women alike) described the initial years of resettlement as filled with shock and distress. A female participant who had been in Canada for only three years, said:

> The problems start even before arrival to a new community, when you are leaving your assets, toys, books, friends and family in particular.

Participants agreed on five major concerns that the elderly immigrants encounter: English proficiency, employment, cultural ties, social isolation, and lack of social supports.

English Insufficiency

Our participants believed that the lack of English mastery was the first and main factor affecting the mental health of elderly Iranian Immigrants. One participant, who was a 64-year-old elderly male and had been in Canada for five years, said:

> If English is not your first language, even if you are highly educated and successful in your own country, you cannot make progress in your new home . . . It's not just the issue of speaking a language, it is communication with the host society.

Some of the participants stated that learning the new language is the best way of enhancing communication. One respondent, who had been in Canada for seven years, stated:

> I believe that those immigrants who want to make progress in the host society must learn the [English] language . . . It helps you to enhance your communication skills.

Participants believed that an inability to speak English may create isolation, marginalization, anxiety, and mental health problems. In fact, participants believed that proper communication was an essential part of their integration into the mainstream culture but there were problems communicating because of poor English skills. Fluency in the language of the recipient society should facilitate the process of culture adjustment (Westermeyer & Her, 1996). Several studies have demonstrated that not knowing the local language can influence adjustment and cause distress. Akiyama (1996) in Japan and Hussain, Creed and Tamenson (1977) in the United Kingdom (UK) have demonstrated that not knowing the local language results in distress. Participants in our study regarded language as an important skill or tool for proper communication and social interactions. The identification of immigrants lacking English proficiency can provide a basis for designing more effective public policies regarding immigration, language training, the labor market, and immigrants' social and integration (Charette & Meng, 1998).

Employment and Financial Resources

Unemployment, underemployment, and financial hardship were other factors mentioned as determinants of mental health among our participants. Participants stated that employment was one of the main concerns among their families and friends. Our interviews with elderly participants and key informants revealed that few economic resources were available for elderly Iranian immigrants. Only three participants were currently employed, of them two were running their pre-immigration business in Iran and one participant was working in a department store in Vancouver. One participant, for instance, said:

> I am a civil engineer. I immigrated to Canada to make a better life for my fami-ly. In the immigration process you get a high score as a civil engineer. It means that there is a demand for your profession. But, when you come here everything is different . . . I have more than 27 years of job experience, but I am not eligi-ble to work in Canada. I have no other choice except working in Iran while my family is living in Canada. Isn't it a big stress?

Some participants reported having difficulty finding employment that matched their skills and education. Most of them were not qualified to work in their profession. One of the participants whose husband was a flight engineer, best described these issues as:

> My husband could not find a job in his field, so he went back to Iran to work at his previous job and I am here with my two children, 24 and 27 years old . . . They [employers] do not accept his credentials in Canada . . . He must work four more years before he retires and then come back here.

The main source of income for the majority of elderly immigrants in our study (25 people) was revealed to be from their retirement benefits in Iran. The maximum amount of earnings for this group was $430 Canadian dollars per month. Indeed, 16 participants were financially dependent on their children or their husbands. Interestingly, even those participants who had enough financial support from Iran and had immigrated to Canada as investors stated they had employment problems. Lack of Canadian business knowledge and experience, along with poor understanding of the Western business culture were some of the areas of concern among these respon-dents. Results of a study conducted by Garousi (2005) of Iranian immigrants in Canada showed that 35% of Iranian immigrants in Canada were unemployed and among those who were employed only 28% had a full-time job. Results of the same study revealed that the incidence of low income was substantially higher among Iranian families (34%) compared to all Canadians (11%). Those elderly who try to keep their job and source of income in Iran need to live away from their families. With the increase in this separation a high proportion of the elderly live alone without the support of their spouse. For Iranian elderly women who have been economically dependent on their spouse, the problems of being unattached are even greater. These women, left alone in Canada, may feel more deprived of emotional, physical, as well as financial support.

As a consequence of barriers to successful integration into the Canadian labor force, immigrants may experience a decline in their present status in Canada compared to their country of origin (Greenberger & Chen, 1996; Rick & Forward, 1992). Parallel to the findings of Kiray (1985) in Turkish culture, status is very much determined by one's occupation and income in Iranian culture. One of the main concerns of Iranian immigrants in our study was repeated questioning by friends and families in Iran about their status in Canada. Given these cultural characteristics, employment-related difficulties and accompanying loss of status are expected to have significant adverse effects on mental health of this ethnic group.

Basran & Zong (1998) studied 404 foreign-trained professionals living in Vancouver who had immigrated from India, Taiwan, Hong Kong, and China. Their results showed that professional immigrants had experienced considerable downward mobility after immigrating to Canada and were currently living on a relatively low income (70% under $30 000 CDN per year). Interestingly, although 88% of them had worked in their profession of choice in their home country, only 18.8% had done so in Canada. Another study conducted by Grant and Nadin (2005) in Saskatchewan revealed that although most respondents were highly skilled in their country of origin, on average, they had worked only nine months at a job that used their skills and 31% indicated that they had never had a job that used their credentials and work experience.

The effect of employment status on mental health is well documented. The results of a large scale meta-analysis of almost 500 studies (Faragher, Cass & Cooper, 2005) provided a clear indication of the immensely strong relationship between job satisfaction and both mental and physical health. According to the same study, the relationships were particularly impressive for aspects of mental health, specifically burnout, lowered self-esteem, anxiety, and depression (Faragher, Cass & Cooper, 2005).

Interest Regarding Culture of Origin

Iranian immigrants come from a culture that originated in the Middle East, where cultural norms are far different than Western norms. It was revealed that our participants do not like to accept the mainstream culture, nor do they want their children to absorb the new culture. For instance, a 64-year-old male, who had been in Canada for 6 years, said:

> I love my culture and I will follow it as long as I am alive . . . I ask my children
> to take care of this heritage.

Elderly Iranians prefer their children to keep their culture of origin and avoid Westernization. This was most obvious in the statement of one participant who said:

> I prefer that my daughter practices our religious and cultural norms in Canada. I
> am not a fanatic, but I am concerned about my kids . . . Our culture is rich and
> emphasizes family values, morality, humanity, charity, and so on.

Importantly, the maintenance of an Iranian cultural identity was fundamental to most participants' sense of self and many people retained strong emotional ties to Iran and Iranian culture. Most elderly Iranian immigrants are strongly embedded in the Iranian communities in Vancouver. They participate in weekly events, workshops and meetings in their area, socialize with their friends, and discuss the most recent events related to Iran's political issues. Those elderly, who move back and forth between Iran and Canada, are usually the centre of discussions. They carry the most recent news about the social, political, and economical situation of Iran and share their findings with their friends in Canada. Findings of our observational phase revealed that discussions on issues related to Iran's current national and international policies are an area of particular interest among elderly Iranians.

One of the most salient social situations that framed the discourse on poor mental health for participants in our study was the post-immigration cut-off from their homeland culture. For many Iranians, the move to Canada has entailed major changes in family structure and lifestyle. This perhaps is even more applicable to elderly immigrants, because compared to younger immigrants they live more on memories than on thoughts of the future. Elderly Iranians believe they belong to Iran and most of them wish to be buried in Iran. Death in "Gorbat" – a strange country – is viewed as a failure and it is commonplace in Iranian culture to hear that: "wherever you live, you must die in your own land." In his study of Iranian immigrants of Canada, Garousi (2005) found that the majority of Iranian immigrants who participated in their study were most interested in the Iranian languages, literature, and foods. He also found that the first generation Iranians had stronger feelings of connection to Iranian culture than the second generation Iranians. In her study of Iranian immigrants in the United States, Ghaffarian (1998) found that elderly participants had higher levels of cultural resistance and poorer mental health compared to younger participants.

Other studies have supported the line of thinking that integration into the host culture to some extent produces more favorable mental health outcomes. For example, among Southeast Asian refugees, Pacific Islander immigrants, and British immigrants who had lived in New Zealand, time spent with one's own ethnic group predicted higher reported levels of anxiety (Pernice & Brooks, 1996). In their study of first-generation Chinese immigrants in Britain Furnham and Li, (1993) found that the more traditional orientations were associated with poorer mental health outcomes. Specifically, the belief that Chinese values are important and should be sustained was found to be associated with poor mental health.

Social Isolation

Involvement in the social mainstream culture is limited for many elderly Iranian immigrants. Barriers such as small family and friendship networks, economic restrictions, physical health issues, and difficulty getting around because of inability to drive can prevent appropriate and effective communication of elderly immigrants with mainstream culture (Ferguson & Browne 1991). Elderly Iranian immigrants in our study felt socially isolated and dissatisfied with their social relationships. One participant, for example, stated:

> What can we do except go to shopping centres and wander around for a couple of hours? We are happier at home . . . We watch Iranian satellite channels. At least we understand them.

Another 66-year-old man, stated:

> Sometimes I go to the pool that is located in our neighborhood. A couple of Iranian friends come there and we have some quality time . . . The rest of the day I have nowhere to go . . . Going out means you have to spend money [laughter].

Several studies have shown social connections to be crucial in influencing both mental and physical health. People who volunteer and are involved in social activities are more likely to report better overall health than people who are not involved in regular social activities (Grzywacz & Keyes, 2004). In her study of South Asian women in Canada, Naidoo (1992) found that traditional, conservatism, and isolation were correlated with greater feelings of disturbance. Likewise, membership in South Asian organizations and unwillingness to adapt to the Canadian way of life were positively correlated with greater feelings of stress (Nidoo, 1992).

Social and Family Support

Another related factor introduced by elderly Iranian immigrants as a determinant of mental health was lack of social and family support. Some participants reported they did not have friends from the mainstream culture to socialize with and often relied primarily on their spouse for social and spiritual support. Participants believe this issue may be influenced by cultural differences. A 71-year-old male participant, stated:

> Back in Iran, I knew my neighbors and they knew me as well. I used to greet people and socialize with them. It was very pleasant and I felt fresh and alive.

The importance of social and family support was pointed out repeatedly by our participants. A 70 year-old female who has been in Canada for five years, said:

> Friends are very important in Iranian life. We always try to have good relationships with our friends . . . As an immigrant there are so many barriers, such as language and cultural differences that might prevent you from making friends . . . the outcome will be loneliness and isolation.

Some elderly immigrants were forced by their children to leave Iran and join them in Canada. One participant stated her concerns as:

> Back there you have the feeling that there is always somebody that you can count on . . . Whenever I had an illness or any concern there were so many people to help me but, here nobody . . . They forced me to come here, and now I cannot see them for days.

Poor social support and loss of connection with families and friends in Iran along with the hardships of immigration have negative impacts on the mental health and well-being of elderly Iranian immigrants. Our findings suggest that elderly immigrants face a lack of family and friend support. This finding is similar to the findings of Coehlo and Ahmad (1980) on Iranian immigrants of the United States. Their study revealed that loss of family and friends, changes in lifestyle, and serious post-immigration pressures were the most important reasons for depression among their participants.

Empirical works have demonstrated that greater social support among the elderly is associated with better health (Auslander & Litwin, 1991) including mental health (Aquino, Russell, Cutrona & Altmaier, 1996; Dean, Kolody & Wood, 1990; Kogan, Van Hasselt, Hersen & Kabacoff, 1995; Lynch et al., 1999; Russell & Cutrona, 1991). Indeed, common life events may jeopardize the support networks of this age group. The elderly immigrants who leave their home country to a new one may lose their social and family support systems (Kahn, Hessling & Russell, 2003). Furthermore, physical impairments, chronic diseases, and later-life related illnesses can limit their ability to interact with others (Newsom & Schulz, 1996; Penninx, van Tilburg, Boeke, Deeg, Kriegsman & van Eijk, 1998).

The process by which social support produces these benefits is complex, and this has been studied in immigrants in general. These studies showed that well-being is uniquely predicted by factors such as the access to support networks and the characteristics of the host society (Rhodes & Lakey, 1999). Indeed, health and well-being are most strongly predicted by the availability of support rather than the actual use of this support (Auslander & Litwin, 1991; Newsom & Schulz, 1996). In other words, the highest levels of well-being are found among people who believe that they have a high level of social support regardless of how much support they receive (Kahn, Hessling & Russell, 2003).

Previous studies have documented that the most common sources of support for elderly are their spouse and children, followed by their close friends (Campbell, Connidis & Davies, 1999; Lynch, 1998). The prevalence of each type of support can also vary according to the socioeconomic status of the elderly person, as well as his/her gender, age, and ethnicity (Barrett, 1999; Chipperfield, 1994; Choi, 1996; Connidis & McMullin, 1994; Shye, Mullooly, Freeborn & Pope, 1995; Wu & Pollard,

1998). Several researchers (Connidis & McMullin, 1994; Litwak, 1985; Lynch, 1998) found that both the availability and receipt of support for the elderly increased when their children were available. Because children are valued as an investment and one of the primary sources of support during old age, the presence of children and measures of support for Iranian elderly are interrelated.

Discussion

This chapter examined the definition of mental health among elderly Iranian immigrants of British Columbia and factors that might influence their mental health. Iranian immigrants who participated in this study experienced a number of immigration-related stressors including: lack of English language knowledge, employment problems, financial dependency, loss of status, lack of social support, differences in values and norms, and concerns about their families in Iran. Lack of English proficiency can affect immigrants of any age, gender, and cultural background. The elderly, in particular, need special attention, as well as interventions to help them to improve their English and communication skills. In elderly immigrants mental illnesses usually occur in the context of physical illnesses, disability, culture, and psychosocial impoverishment. High crossover of these physical and psychosocial factors makes the assessment of elderly immigrants very complex.

Our participants viewed unemployment and underemployment as status deprivation. In the Iranian community, like most other Asian societies, education, occupation, income, and wealth are usually thought of as the main determinants of the achieved status. Social mobility that comes with immigration forces immigrants to move to a different status. It was common to hear from participants that immigrants lost three main types of capital that they had gained over their life: social capital (family, friends, connections, prestige, and employment), cultural capital (e.g., respect for the elderly, cultural norms) and economical capital (housing, assets, properties, and income). Some studies show that the immigration experience and disadvantaged socioeconomic status often cause elderly immigrants to be vulnerable to depression and other mental health illnesses (Gelfand & Yee, 1991; Yu Esh, 1986). The negative impact of financial dependency on depression, as shown in several studies (Raguram, Weiss, Mitchell, Keval & Channabasavanna, 2001; Lai, 2004) adds further support to this argument. Income can have an impact on mental health because it influences a person's ability to meet basic needs, make choices in life and deal with unexpected problems (Frey, Stutzer 2002; Kasser, 2002). According to data from the Government of Canada, 30% of immigrant families live below the poverty level during their first ten years in Canada. Mental illnesses such as depression can arise when immigrants are unable to find meaningful and economically sustaining employment (Government of Canada, 2006).

Family and friends were viewed by the elderly Iranians as their most important source of emotional and physical support. Among the resources available for the elderly Iranian immigrants, family support was revealed to be the most important factor for mental health maintenance. The emotional care provided by family members and friends was deemed to be more important than financial and physical care. When the immigrant elderly access mental health services, they relay on their community, particularly families, friends and neighbors. In Canada, it has been estimated that family members and friends provide between 75% and 85% of all care for elderly people in the community (National Advisory Council on Aging, 1993). But, as elderly immigrants get older, their need for personal care services increases greatly while their children, families, and friends are not available or cannot be expected to assume sole responsibility.

The findings in the present study have several limitations. First, the findings are based on only 44 participants. Qualitative research typically involves a small number of participants and the question is whether the results are can be generalized to the elderly Iranian population of Canada. Hence, the findings in the present study should be further examined using a larger sample size, and mixed methods. Second, in this study the focus was on elderly immigrants in British Columbia who might be different than their counterparts in other provinces. Lastly, using a convenience sample makes it impossible to suggest that the sample was a fair representation of the elderly Iranian immigrant population.

Despite these limitations, the findings have implications for health care professionals who work with elderly Iranian immigrants. The results of this study underline that personal characteristics such as employment status, knowledge of English language, social and family support, and cultural ties can influence the mental health of elderly Iranian immigrants. A better understanding of these barriers would help planners in designing more realistic and effective programs for adequate mental health services for ethnic minorities. Special attention is needed to enhance the language skills of elderly immigrants to help them get involved in the host society. It is also crucial to create employment opportunities that utilize the knowledge and expertise of elderly immigrants. Employment not only provides a reliable source of income for this age group, but also facilitates their communication with the mainstream culture.

References

Akiyama T. (1996). Onset study of English speaking temporary residents in Japan. *Social Psychiatry and Psychiatric Epidemiology, 31,* 194–198.

Aquino, J.A., Russell, D.W., Cutrona, C.E. & Altmaier, E.M. (1996). Employment status, social support, and life satisfaction among the elderly. *Journal of Counseling Psychology, 43,* 480–489.

Auslander, G.K. & Litwin, G.K. (1991). Social networks, social support, and self-ratings of health among the elderly. *Journal of Aging and Health, 3,* 493–510.

Bagheri, A. (1992). Psychiatric problems among Iranian Immigrants in Canada. *Canadian Journal of Psychiatry, 37*(1), 7-11.

Barrett, A.E. (1999). Social support and life satisfaction among the never married: Examining the effects of age. *Research on Aging, 21,* 46-72.

Basran, G.S. & Zong, L. (1998). Devaluation of foreign credentials as perceived by visible minority professional immigrants. *Canadian Ethnic Studies, 30,* (3) 6-23.

Bowen, J.M. & Nelson, J.M. (2002). Caring for elderly immigrants. Challenges and opportunities. *Minn Med, 85,* 25-7.

Campbell, L.D., Connidis, I.A. & Davies, L. (1999). Sibling ties in later life: A social network analysis. *Journal of Family Issues, 20,* 114-148.

Charette M.F & Meng R. (1998). The Determinants of literacy and numeracy, and the effect of literacy and numeracy on labour market outcomes *The Canadian Journal of Economics / Revue canadienne d'Economique, 31,* 3, 495-517.

Chipperfield, J.G. (1994). The support source mix: A comparison of elderly men and women from two decades. *Canadian Journal on Aging, 13,* 435-453.

Choi, N.G. (1996). The never married and divorced elderly: Comparison of economic and health status, social support, and living arrangement. *Journal of Gerontological Social Work, 26,* 3-25.

Conn, D.K., Lee, V., Steingart, A. & Silberfeld, M. (1992). Psychiatric services: A survey of nursing homes and homes for the aged in Ontario. *Canadian Journal of Psychiatry, 37,* 525-530.

Connidis, I.A. & McMullin, J.A. (1994). Social support in older age: Assessing the impact of marital and parent status. *Canadian Journal on Aging, 13,* 510-527.

Dean, A., Kolody, B, & Wood, P. (1990). Effects of social support from various sources on depression in elderly persons. *Journal of Health & Social Behavior, 31,* 148–161.

Faragher, E.B., Cass, M. & Cooper, C. (2005). The relationship between job satisfaction and health: a meta-analysis. *Occupational and Environmental Medicine, 62,* 105-112.

Frey, B. & Stutzer, A. (2002). *Happiness and economics.* Princeton, New Jersey: Princeton University Press.

Furnham, A. & Li, Y.H. (1993). The psychological adjustment of the Chinese community in Britain: A study of two generations. *British Journal of Psychiatry, 162,* 109-113.

Gelfand, D. & Yee, B. W.K. (1991). Influence of immigration, migration, and acculturation on the fabric of aging in America. *Generations, 15,* 7-10.

Ghaffarian, S. (1998). The Acculturation of Iranian Immigrants in the United States and the implications for mental health. *Journal of Social Psychology, 138,* 645-654.

Gibbs, A. (1997). *Focus groups. Social research update 19.* University of Surrey. Department of Sociology.

Goldner, E.M., Snider, B. & Mozel, M. (2001). *Defining the challenge: epidemiology of mental disorders in British Columbia. 1. Estimating the prevalence of mental disorders in adults.* Vancouver (BC): Department of Psychiatry, University of British Columbia.

Government of Canada. *The Human face of mental health and mental illness in Canada.* (2006). Retrieved July 28, 2007 from: http://www.mooddisorderscanada.ca/docs/Human_Face_of_-Mental_Illness_in_Canada_October_2006.pdf.

Grant, P.R. & Nadin, S. (2005). The difficulties faced by immigrants with ongoing credentialing problems: A social psychological analysis. A paper presented at the Tenth International Metropolis Conference, Toronto, Ontario.

Greenberger, E. & Chen, C. (1996). Perceived family relationships and depressed mood in early and late adolescence: A comparison of European and Asian Americans. *Developmental Psychology, 32,* 707-716.

Grzywacz, J.G. & Keyes, C.L. (2004). Toward health promotion: physical and social behaviors in complete health. *AM J Health Behavior; 28,* 2, 99-111.

Hassen, C. & Sardashti, H. (2000). Relationship between depression and psychosocial stress among Iranian immigrants. *Psychiatry Prax (Germany), 27,* 2, 74-76.

Husain, N., Creed, F. & Tamenson, B. (1971). Adverse social circumstances and depression in people of Pakistani origin in the U.K. *British Journal of Psychiatry, 171,* 434–438.

Jalali, B. (1996). Iranian families. In McGoldrick, M., Giordano, J. and Pearce, J. (Eds.), *Ethnicity and family therapy.* New York, NY:Guilford Publications, Inc.

Kahn, J.H., Hessling, R.M. & Russell, D.W. (2003). Social support, health, and well-being among the elderly: What is the role of negative affectivity? *Personality and Individual Differences, 35,* 5–17.

Kasser, T. (2002). *The high price of materialism.* Cambridge, Mass.: The MIT Press.

Kazemi, M.S. (1986). *Iranians in Ontario,* Mihan Publishing Inc., Toronto, Canada.

Khavarpour, F. & Rissel, C. (1997). Mental health status of Iranian migrants in Sydney. Australian and New Zealand. *Journal of Psychiatry (Australia), 31,* 6, 828-34.

Kiray, M.B. (1985). Metropolitan city and changing family. In T. Erder (Ed.). *Family in Turkish society* (pp. 79-93), Turkey: Turkish Social Science Association.

Kitzinger, J. (1995). Introducing focus groups. *British Medical Journal, 311,* 299-302.

Kogan, E.S., Van Hasselt, V.B., Hersen, M. & Kabacoff, R.I. (1995). Relationship of depression, assertiveness, and social support in community-dwelling older adults. *Journal of Clinical Geropsychology, 1,* 157–163.

Lai, D.W.L. (2004). Impact of culture on depressive symptoms of elderly Chinese immigrants. *Canadian Journal of Psychiatry, 49,* 820-827.

Litwak, E. (1985). *Helping the elderly: The complementary roles of informal networks and formal systems.* New York: The Guilford Press.

Lynch, S.A. (1998). Who supports whom? How age and gender affect the perceived quality of support from family and friends. *The Gerontologist, 38,* 231-238.

Lynch, T.R., Mendelson, T., Robins, C.J., Krishman, K.R.R., George, L.K., Johnson, C.S. & Blazer, D.G. (1999). Perceived social support among depressed elderly, middle-aged, and young-adult samples: cross-sectional and longitudinal analyses. *Journal of Affective Disorders, 55,* 159–170.

Morgan, D.L. & Kreuger, R.A. (1993). When to use focus groups and why. In Morgan D. L. (ed). *Successful focus groups.* London: Sage.

Murray, C.J. & Lopez, A.D. (1996). Evidence-based health policy – lessons from the Global Burden of Disease Study. *Science, 6,* 274, 5293, 1593-4

National Advisory Council on Aging (1993), A quick portrait of Canadian seniors: needing support for daily living? From whom? *Aging Vignette, 11.*

Newsom, J.T. & Schulz, R. (1996). Social support as a mediator in the relation between functional status and quality of life in older adults. *Psychology and Aging, 11,* 34–44.

Nidoo, J.C. (1992). The mental health of visible ethnic minorities in Canada. *Psychology and Developing Societies, 4,* 165-187.

Penninx, B.W.J.H., van Tilburg, T., Boeke, A.J.P., Deeg, D.J.H., Kriegsman, D.M.W. & van Eijk, J.T.M. (1998). Effects of social support and personal coping resources on depressive symptoms: different for various chronic diseases? *Health Psychology, 17,* 551–558.

Pernice, R. & Brooks, J. (1996). Refugees' and immigrants' mental health: Association of demographic and post-immigration factors. *The Journal of Social Psychology, 136,* 511-519.

Plawecki, H.M. (2000). The elderly immigrant. An isolated experience. *Journal of Gerontological Nursing, 26,* 2: 6-7.

Pliskin, K.L. (1992). Dysphoria and somatization in Iranian culture. *Western Journal of Medicine, 65,* 225-37.

Raguram, R., Weiss, M.G., Harshad, K. & Channabasavanna, S.M. (2001). Cultural dimensions of clinical depression in Bangalore, India. *Anthropology & Medicine, 8,* 31–46.

Rhodes, G.L. & Lakey, B. (1999). Social support and psychological disorder: Insights from social psychology. In R.M. Kowalski, & M.R. Leary (Eds.), *The social psychology of emotional and behavioral problems.* (pp. 281–309). Washington, DC: American Psychological Association.

Rick, K. & Forward, J. (1992). Acculturation and perceived intergenerational differences among youth. *Journal of Cross-Cultural Psychology, 23,* 85-94.

Russell, D.W. & Cutrona, C.E. (1991). Social support, stress, and depressive symptoms among the elderly: Test of a process model. *Psychology and Aging, 6,* 190–201.

Shye, D., Mullooly, J.P., Freeborn, D.K. & Pope, C.R. (1995). Gender differences in the relationship between social network support and mortality: A longitudinal study of an elderly cohort. *Social Science and Medicine, 41,* 935-947.

Statistics Canada, (2000). *Aging and health practices.* (2001). Retrieved November 13, 2007 from: http://www.hc-sc.gc.ca/seniors-aines/pubs/workshop_healthyaging/pdf/workshop1_e.pdf

Statistics Canada. (2004). Retrieved December 2004 from:www12.statcan.ca/English/sensus01/-Producets/Standard/Index.cfm

Statistics Canada. (2001). *Stress and well-being. Health reports (Statistics Canada. Catalogue 82-003)* 2001; 12, 21-32.

Statistics Canada. (2006). Census 2006. http://www12.statcan.ca/census-recensement/2006.

Vahid Garousi. (2005) *Iranians in Canada: A Statistical Analysis.* Retrieved March 12, 2007 from: http://www.iranian.com/News/2005/June/IraniansCanada.pdf

Westermeyer, J. & Her, C. (1996). English fluency and social adjustment among Hmong refugees in Minnesota. *Journal of Nervous and Mental Disease, 184,* 130-132.

World Health Organization. *The world health report 2001. Mental health: New understanding,* New Hope. Geneva: World Health Organization, 2001.

Wu, Z. & Pollard, M.S. (1998). Social support among unmarried childless elderly persons. *Journal of Gerontology: Social Sciences, 53,* S324-S335.

Yu Esh. (1986). Health of the Chinese elderly in America. *Research on Aging, 8,* 84-109.

Zangeneh, M., Sadeghi, N. & Sharp, N. (2002). Iranians living in Toronto: Attitudes and practices of gambling and help-seeking behavior, a preliminary study about Iranian refugees and immigrants in Toronto. *Shiraz E-Medical Journal. 3* (6). http://semj.sums.ac.ir.

Acknowledgements

The authors would like to extend their gratitude to everyone who contributed in one way or another to the success of this study. They are most grateful to the "Iranian Elderly Daycare" facilities located in Vancouver for their support of this study. Furthermore, they thank all those who made the data collection exercise a success. The authors extend special thanks to the participants and key informants for their participation.

WE extend special thanks and appreciation to Dr. Patricia Spittal (Anthropologist and Assistant Professor of the Department of Health Care and Epidemiology, at the University of British Columbia, Vancouver) for her support, guidance and assistance in this study. Her timely readings, corrections and encouragement made the writing of this chapter a learning process and a gratifying exercise.

15

South Asian Immigrant Seniors Living in Edmonton: Diverse Experiences

Cheuk Fan Ng, (Athabasca University) and Herbert C. Northcott, (University of Alberta)

Introduction

The elderly population in Canada is becoming more diverse. In 2001, most of the 28 per cent of Canadian seniors who were immigrants had come from Europe when relatively young (Statistics Canada, 2003). In contrast, of the seniors who immigrated to Canada when they were elderly, about half were from Asia (McDonald, George, Daciuk, Yan & Rowan, 2001). While gerontological research has been concerned about the "minority elderly" (e.g., Kamo & Zhou, 1994), research about the *migrant* elder is just emerging (Longino, Jr., & Bradley, 2006).

South Asians are the second largest visible minority group in Canada (Tran, Kaddatz & Allard, 2005). A growing body of research focuses on South Asian immigrants, for example, their life satisfaction (Vohra & Adair, 2000) and the health of immigrant women (Grewal, Bottorff & Hilton, 2005) and elderly men (Oliffe, Grewal, Bottorff, Luke & Toor, 2007), and the challenges elderly women face as aging immigrants (Choudhry, 2001). Nevertheless, there is a lack of research on elderly South Asian immigrants (Burr, 1992).

A growing body of research suggests that age at immigration is a significant factor in successful resettlement (Angel & Angel, 2006). For older migrants, immigration involves not only the disruptive severing of ties with their country of origin but the challenge of building new relationships and learning new skills in the host country later in life (Angel & Angel, 2006; Choudhry, 2001). Thus, there is a need to examine the experiences of South Asian immigrant seniors who have come to Canada in different stages of life.

Gender roles are likely to have a significant impact on the experiences of immigrants (Chappell, Gee, McDonald & Stones, 2003), particularly those coming from traditional, non-Westernized societies such as South Asia (Choudhry, 2001; Dhruvarajan, 1993; Grewal et al., 2005; Ollife et al., 2007). For persons who immigrated at an older

301

age, traditional gender roles may be an even more significant factor in their experiences in Canada.

Theories Relevant to Successful Aging of Immigrants

Humans of all ages have needs. According to Abraham Maslow, these needs are, in ascending order: physiological needs, safety needs, belongingness and love needs, esteem needs, self-actualization (Maslow, 1943, 1954), and self-transcendence (Maslow, 1969). (Note: There are debates about whether Maslow (1969) added a top level called "self-transcendence," as discussed in Koltko-Rivera, 2006). These needs may be met in somewhat different ways as a person ages and "successful aging" (Baltes, 1997; Baltes & Baltes, 1990; Kahn, 2002; Riley & Riley, 1990; Rowe & Kahn, 1998) may be particularly challenging for the person who immigrates at an older age. Another set of models (e.g., Carp, 1976; Kahana, Lovegreen, Kahana & Kahana, 2003; Lawton, 1982) emphasizes the fit between the person and the physical and social environment and older immigrants may have more difficulty attaining a desirable "fit."

As Scheidt and Windley (2006) state, "The complex question of *whether, where, and how* culture affects residential adaptations and healthy aging over time remains largely unaddressed" (p. 121). Nevertheless, theories of acculturation (Ward, Bochner & Furnham, 2001) stipulate that any cross-cultural transition leads to stress and skills deficits, and that personal characteristics (e.g., language fluency), group characteristics (e.g., culture gap), and situational factors (e.g., length of cultural contact) may mediate the process of acculturation. Thus, those immigrant seniors who aged in their homeland are likely to be less acculturated than those who immigrated earlier in life.

How the needs of aging immigrants are met shapes their experience in Canada. The objective of this study is to examine how age at immigration, length of time in Canada, and gender contribute to the diversity of South Asian immigrants' experiences in older age in Canada. This question is explored focusing on the following groups:

1. Immigrant seniors who arrived in Canada before the end of mid-life (age 54 or younger) and have ten or more years residency ("established-when-younger" immigrants);

2. Immigrant seniors who arrived in Canada after mid-life (age 55 or older) and have ten or more years residency ("established-when-older" immigrants); and

3. Immigrant seniors who arrived in Canada after mid-life and have less than ten years residency ("recent" immigrants).

Ten years of residency is used because family-class immigrants in Alberta are not eligible for government benefits until after ten years (Chappell et al., 2003). Fifty-five years old is used because it is touted as a common age for early retirement in Canada and has been used in previous research as a definition of "elderly" immigrant (Basavarajappa, 1998; Burr, 1992).

In this chapter, Maslow's hierarchy of human needs described before is used as the organizational framework. The basic needs include physical shelter and safety (e.g., housing, neighborhood safety), financial security, and mobility (i.e., transportation). The next level focuses on social relationships (e.g., living arrangements, family relations, inter-generational relationships, social contacts with friends and community, and loneliness). The highest level includes identity (e.g., ethnic/cultural and Canadian identity, cultural customs and practices), religion, meaning and values of life, and life satisfaction. We end with immigrant seniors' reflections on the advantages and disadvantages of immigrating to Canada.

Physical and Financial Security

Financial resources are crucial in providing the basic necessities of life (i.e., food, clothing, and shelter). Low personal incomes characterize those elderly women who immigrated after age 65 or from Third World regions (Boyd, 1989). "Migrant elders" are admitted into Canada primarily under the family reunification class, often sponsored by their children or other family members who are obliged to provide financial support. Recent migrant elders, then, tend to be financially dependent on their family members and lack an independent source of income (Choudhry, 2001).

Living with family or relatives minimizes the effects of low personal incomes and it may represent a deliberate strategy used by the elderly and their families (Christenson & Slesinger, 1985, as cited in Boyd, 1989). But do such living arrangements offer optimal economic and social benefits for the elderly immigrant? Little research has examined the extent to which economic resources are extended to the elderly in family settings (Boyd, 1989).

Previous studies on housing have focused on either immigrants in general (e.g., Canada Mortgage and Housing Corporation (CMHC), 2005a) or Canadian seniors in general (e.g., CMHC, 2005b), but rarely on immigrant seniors. Besides housing, neighborhood safety is an important factor in residential satisfaction for older people (Kahana et al., 2003). For some immigrant seniors, unfamiliarity with the new environment, language and culture may reduce their sense of safety (e.g., Chan, 1983). Feeling socially accepted in the neighborhood may also be an important issue (Novac, Darden, Hulchanski, & Seguin, 2002).

Regarding transportation, access to automobiles declines with age (Rittner & Kirk, 1995) and access to public transportation may increase residential satisfaction (Kahana et al., 2003). A recent study of non-seniors showed that recent immigrants were much more likely than the Canadian-born to use public transit to commute to work, and women were heavier users of public transportation than men (Heisz & Schellenberg, 2004). It is not clear whether these findings apply to immigrant seniors. Lack of proficiency in English is likely to reduce elderly immigrants' ability to use public transportation (Choudhry, 2001).

Social Relationships: Family and Social Networks

The social connections of older people can be conceptualized to include several layers including living arrangements, family, and organizations such as the church and voluntary associations. These interlocking relationships serve a social integration function, with poor social integration resulting in loneliness (Knipscheer, Dykstra, de Jong, Gierveld & de Tilburg, 1995). Furthermore, living arrangements strongly influence the needs and opportunities for social interaction (Knipscheer et al., 1995). Older immigrants and especially those with Asian background, rarely live alone and are more likely to live with extended families than non-immigrants (e.g., Basavarajappa, 1998; Kritz, Gurak & Chen, 2000). In 2002, South Asian seniors in Canada lived in predominately family-oriented households: 66% with their spouse, 25% with other family members and just eight percent lived alone (Tran, Kaddatz & Allard, 2005). These studies, however, do not tell us what older immigrants' preferences are or whether they are satisfied with their living arrangements.

The inter- and intra-generational families play a key role in integrating older people in society (Knipscheer, 1995). In South Asia, the family is the centre of social organization. The core familial value is respect for elders and filial piety. Family solidarity and mutual dependence are encouraged. Furthermore, the community is seen as an extended family (Ibrahim, Ohnishi & Sandhu, 1997, as cited in Choudhry, 2001).

In Canada, the 2002 Ethnic Diversity Survey showed that 93% of South Asian respondents reported a strong sense of belonging to their family. Most still have close ties with their country of origin or their parents' country of birth (Tran et al., 2005). Family members offered emotional support, instrumental support (e.g., transportation), and advice (Grewal et al., 2005). However, elderly immigrant women may find that their traditional roles (e.g., retention and transmission of culture and religion) are not as valued as they were in South Asia (Choudhry, 2001; Grewal et al., 2005). Further, family members in Canada are not always available to meet the elderly women's social needs. Finally, the language barrier can add to these women's isolation or create distance between them and their grandchildren (Choudhry, 2001).

Social networks outside the family are also important (Knipscheer et al., 1995). The 2002 Ethnic Diversity Survey showed that South Asians attach a great deal of importance to and maintain their social networks within their ethno-cultural community in Canada. The survey also showed that 39% of South Asians were involved in sport teams, hobby clubs, community organizations and other such activities (Tran et al., 2005). However, it is not clear what the participation of elderly immigrants is in these activities.

Identity, Meaning, and Life Satisfaction

Research suggests that South Asian immigrants to North America have brought with them a strong sense of their native culture and customs (Dhruvarajan, 1993; Inman, Howard, Beaumont & Walker, 2007). They hold onto core values (e.g., family and religion) and a behavioral style (e.g., language and eating habits) at home (Dhruvarajan, 1993) but adapt to interactions and dress etiquette in their professional life (Inman, Howard, Beaumont & Walker, 2007). The 2002 Ethnic Diversity Survey showed that 69% of South Asians in Canada felt a strong or very strong sense of belonging to their ethnic or cultural group (Tran et al., 2005).

The core value of family is retained through respecting elders and family, and maintaining family ties and connections (via letters, phone calls, visits) with people in their native country and with family in the host country (Dhruvarajan, 1993; Inman et al., 2007; Tran et al., 2005). Religion is moderately related to ethnic/cultural identity (Walters, Kelli & Paul, 2007). The majority (83%) of South Asian respondents in the 2002 Ethnic Diversity Survey said that their religion was important or very important to them and that they had participated in religious activities in the previous 12 months (Tran et al., 2005). Similarly, the Asian Indian immigrants in the Dhruvarajan (1993) study visited the temple frequently.

The retention of native language and the maintenance of certain behavioral styles are important aspects of ethnic identity for South Asians in Canada. Over half (58%) of South Asian parents in the 2002 Ethnic Diversity Survey believed that it was important for their children to learn their own first language. More than eight in ten considered maintaining their ethnic customs and traditions such as holidays and celebrations, food, clothing and art are important or very important (Tran et al., 2005). Social support (e.g., having friends from their own ethnic group, and belonging to cultural/ethnic or religious organizations) (Dhruvarajan, 1993; Inman et al., 2007) and approval of the ethnic group also play a significant role in preserving their cultural identity (Inman, Constantine & Ladany, 1999, as cited in Inman et al., 2007).

Traditionally, parents and elders in Indian families socialize young children into culturally expected behaviors through modelling, maintaining religious practices, and imparting cultural knowledge (Inman et al., 2007). When in the host country, the majority of Asian Indian immigrants encourage their children to practice customs and rituals at least to some extent. Those immigrants who are religious and have been in Canada for a shorter period of time are more likely to retain and transmit behavioral aspects of ethnic culture (Dhruvarajan, 1993).

Identification with the host society is important for national unity (Walters, Kelli & Paul, 2007). The 2002 Ethnic Diversity Survey showed that the majority of South Asians reported a strong or very strong sense of belonging to Canada, their province, and town, city or municipality and, if eligible, voted in at least one of the last elections (Tran et al., 2005). In a further analysis of the Survey data, Walters et al., (2007) reported that South Asian immigrants were most likely to choose "Canadian" as their only response to the ethnicity question and are the least likely to report belonging to at least one other ethnic group, in addition to being Canadian. Time since migration has the strongest relationship with identity formation.

Method

This study was conducted in Edmonton, Alberta. Potential respondents (i.e., 60 years of age or older, born in South Asia, and a permanent resident or citizen of Canada) were recruited through a local ethnic association and an immigrant settlement agency. A face-to-face, structured interview in the senior's language of choice (English, Hindi, or Punjabi) and lasting about two hours was conducted at the senior's home or other place of the senior's choice. The senior was given $20 for participation in the study. Although the respondents constitute a convenience sample, attempts were made to obtain as representative a sample as possible. For the purposes of this study, the emphasis is on comparisons internal to the sample, that is, between interviewees who are female and male, and who came to Canada earlier and later in life.

The questionnaire obtained demographic and immigration information and included questions about housing, neighborhood safety, transportation, financial security, feelings of isolation and loneliness, living arrangements, family and intergenerational relations, social connections with friends and community in Canada and country of origin, cultural retention and practices, religious practices, Canadian and ethnic/cultural identity, perception of discrimination, voting participation, life satisfaction, and perceived advantages and disadvantages of immigrating to Canada. The questionnaire was translated into Hindi and Punjabi, and then translated back into English to ensure accuracy of translation (Brislin, 1986). The final questionnaire incorporated feedback from community representatives on earlier drafts of the questionnaire and from pretests of each language version.

A total of 161 interviews were conducted (99 in English, 31 in Hindi, and 31 in Punjabi). Chi-square tests and one-way ANOVAs were used to assess significant differences among recent immigrants (n = 57), established-when-older immigrants (n = 36), and established-when-younger immigrants (n = 68), and between men (n = 80) and women (n = 81).

Results

Most of our respondents were born in India (82%), Punjabi was the predominant mother tongue (61%); most were either Sikh (52%) or Hindu (33%), and the average age was 68.5 years (range 60-92 years). Over half rated their health as excellent (25%) or good (30%), and 33% reported some activity limitations. The majority (83%) was sponsored as immigrants, with 67 per cent immigrating to Canada to be with their families. Differences among the three immigrant groups and between men and women on several demographic and immigration variables are shown in Table 1.

Financial Security

If they were married, most of our respondents and their spouses were either retired (66% and 46%, respectively) or keeping house (15% and 27%). Twenty-eight percent of our respondents received at least one government benefit and 18% received a non-government pension. Table 2 shows that recent immigrants were significantly less likely than established immigrants to be receiving the old age security, guaranteed income supplement, Canada Pension Plan, spousal allowance, or a personal pension. Established-when-older immigrants were the most likely to receive Alberta Senior Benefits.

Awareness of the most common government benefits was generally high (62-87%). Recent immigrants were less likely than established immigrants to be aware of old age security, guaranteed income supplement, and spousal allowance benefits (see Table 2). Men were significantly more aware of Canada Pension plan than were women (94% vs. 80%; p = .011). To increase awareness, respondents suggested distributing information through the mass media, government departments and agencies, and seminars and workshops.

Recent immigrants were more likely than established immigrants to have received money from someone in their family and were less likely to have given money to a family member in the past year. Most respondents (84%) said that they had control over their own money, with recent immigrants less likely to say they had control over their own money. (see Table 2).

Overall, 66 per cent of our respondents currently living with a spouse and 52 per cent of our respondents not living with a spouse indicated that their income as a couple or their personal income was adequate for their needs. Recent immigrants were less likely than established immigrants to indicate that their income was adequate (see Table 2).

Table 1
Sample Characteristics: Significant Differences for Immigrant Groups and by Gender

Sample Characteristics	Recent Immigrants %	Established-When-Older Immigrants %	Established-When-Younger Immigrants %	X^2	Males %	Females %	X^2	Total %
Widowed	35	44	16	16.65*	16	42	12.89**	29
Secondary School or Lower	63	80	18	22.57***	49	64	9.49*	57
Sponsored by Children	98	100	62	37.86***	93	82		87
Reason for Immigration: Family	83	81	47	21.41***	58	72	6.61**	67
	Mean	Mean	Mean	F	Mean	Mean	F	Mean
Rating of English Ability[a]	2.36	2.47	3.39	18.99***	3.05	2.59	7.25**	2.82
Age	66.56	74.47	67.06	27.05***	69.58	69.51		68.54
Age at Immigration	61.30	59.11	40.94	145.97***	52.19	52.23		52.21
Years in Canada	5.18	15.36	26.10	162.71***	16.36	16.23		16.30
n	57	36	68		80	81		161

Note: ***p<.001; **p<.01; *<.05
[a]A four-point scale ranging from 1 (understand/speak/read/write not at all) to 4 (very well).

Table 2

Percentage Distributions of Financial Security Variables by Immigrant Group

	Recent Immigrants		Established-When-Older Immigrants		Established-When-Younger Immigrants		p		Total	
	%		%		%				%	
Received Money from Family	49		22		13		***		28	
Given Money to Family	36		72		67		***		57	
Control Over Own Money	67		94		93		***		84	
Income Adequate – Couple[a]	34		61		90		***		66	
Income Adequate – Single Person[b]	19		88		56		***		52	
Income Adequate (Couple or Single)	29		74		81		***		61	
Benefits: Receive (R), Aware of (A)	R	A	R	A	R	A	R	A	R	A
Old Age Security	5	74	86	97	63	93	***	**	48	87
Guaranteed Income Supplement	5	57	67	86	27	72	***	*	28	70
Spousal Allowance	—	46	11	77	9	67	*	**	6	62
Widowed Persons Allowance	6	59	6	79	6	76			6	71
Canada Pension Plan	5	83	53	86	59	91	***		39	87
Alberta Seniors Program	39	81	61	83	31	74	*		40	78
Home Repair/Modification Program	2	35	6	40	2	42			3	39
Seniors Apartment & Lodges	4	60	—	77	—	65			1	66
Other Financial Benefits	11	39	14	63	10	44	***		11	46
Personal Pension	2	18	18	36	31	68			18	
n	57	57	36	36	68	68			161	161

Notes: *** p<.001; ** p<.01; * p<.05   [a] n=102; [b] n=56

Housing

Most of the respondents (74%) lived in single-detached houses, 12 per cent lived in townhouses and duplexes and eight per cent lived in apartments. The majority rated the condition of their dwelling as either good (45%) or excellent (40%). Recent immigrants and established-when-older immigrants lived in significantly higher-density dwellings (1.44 and 1.37 persons per room, respectively) than established-when-younger immigrants (0.91 persons per room) (p< .001). However, the mean dwelling densities that seniors perceived to be "just right" were higher for recent immigrants (1.39) and established-when-older immigrants (1.36), than for established-when-younger immigrants (0.95) (p<.001), suggesting that acculturation to Canadian standards has occurred among the latter.

Nine per cent indicated that they or their families had experienced discrimination when looking for housing. For established-when-younger immigrants only, a significantly higher percentage of men (21%) than women (0%) reported such incidents, experienced mostly when they were younger. Most incidents involved landlords lying about the non-availability of vacant accommodation and landlords refusing to show their houses (7 of the 11 responses).

The majority of seniors (90%) felt very safe at home alone. Most of the respondents were either very satisfied (54%) or satisfied (38%) with their housing. Most (83%) did not want to move from their current residence. For those who wanted to move, the most frequently cited barrier to living in the accommodation of their choice was cost (21 of 34 responses given by 26 respondents).

Neighborhood

Most of the respondents (82%) said that they went out alone in their neighborhood, more often in summer (79% daily; 12% several times a week) than in winter (37% daily; 25% several times a week; 22% weekly). For women, recent immigrants and established-when-older immigrants were significantly less likely to go out alone in the neighborhood and went out less frequently in both summer and winter than established-when-younger immigrants. Women were also less likely to go out alone than men. The majority (91%) of the 132 seniors who went out alone reported that they felt very safe walking alone in the neighborhood. While ten per cent of men (but none of the women) in our sample indicated that they or their families had experienced discrimination while living in the neighborhood (p = .004) nevertheless, in general, our respondents were either very satisfied (72%) or satisfied (27%) with their neighbourhood.

Transportation

Most of the respondents did not have a valid driver's license (65%) or the use of a vehicle (64%). Men were more likely to drive than women (39% versus 14%) and established-when-younger immigrants (49%) were more likely to drive than recent immigrants (9%) or established-when-older immigrants (11%). None of the recent immigrant women drove.

Forty-two per cent said they used public transportation. Men (63%), recent immigrants (51%), or established-when-older immigrants (50%) were more likely to use public transportation than women (22%) or established-when-younger immigrants (31%). A common means of transportation was a ride provided by someone in their household (61%), especially for women (82%), recent immigrants (67%), or established-when-older immigrants (72%). Getting a ride from someone outside the household was also quite common (29%).

Despite reliance on public transportation and rides provided by others, the majority of seniors reported that it was very easy (57%) or somewhat easy (13%) to get to places they needed to go. However, needing a ride was the most frequently cited reason for difficulty getting to places they needed to go (16 of 34 responses).

Family Relationships and Social Connections

Intra- and Inter-generational Families

Only a small percentage of our respondents reported having no living sons or daughters (14%), or no grandchildren (11%); however, with respect to proximity to children and grandchildren 37% reported having no sons, 36% no daughters, and 9% no grandchildren living in the Edmonton area. Recent immigrants and established-when-older immigrants were significantly less likely than established-when-younger immigrants to have no sons living in Edmonton (35%, 28% vs. 43%, respectively; p < .05) or no grandchildren living in Edmonton (6%, 0%, versus 19%; p =.013). The majority (66%) said that they did not have any family members living in the Edmonton area beside their children and grandchildren.

Respondents with grandchildren living in the Edmonton area indicated that they helped their grandchildren in multiple ways (34%), providing childcare and helping with household chores (33%), providing emotional and cultural support (25%), and financial support (9%). In return, their grandchildren helped the respondents in several ways and by giving love, respect and emotional support. However, 32% of respondents said that their grandchildren did not help them or were too young to help.

Living Arrangements

Living alone was very rare (5%) and living in extended families was the most common living arrangement for our respondents (56%). Among the married, the established-when-younger immigrants were the least likely to live in multi-generational families (19%) and most likely to live with their spouse only (54%), suggesting that acculturation to Canadian norms tends to occur over time. Among the unmarried, even the established-when-younger immigrants tended to live in multi-generational families than to live alone (16% versus 6%). For those respondents living without a spouse, men were more likely than women to live alone (9% versus 1%), while women were much more likely than men to live in an extended family (40% versus 13%).

Recent immigrant seniors (74%) and established-when-older immigrants (64%) were more likely to live in dwellings headed (owned or rented) by their children while established-when-younger immigrants (71%) were more likely to own or rent themselves. Further, those respondents who lived in extended families were more likely to live in dwellings owned or rented by their children.

The majority of our respondents (87%) contributed to their households in various ways: 23% provided childcare, 14% contributed to household expenses, 10% prepared meals, and 30% contributed in multiple ways. Men were more likely than women to say they were providing childcare and contributing to household expenses; whereas, women were more likely than men to say they were preparing meals and doing household work. Recent immigrants were most likely to contribute by providing childcare and preparing meals.

Most of our respondents (88%) did not prefer a different living arrangement than the one they had. Of the few who preferred a different living arrangement, the most frequently cited barrier was cost (11 of 24 responses given by 19 respondents).

Family Contacts and Relationships

Table 3 shows that most respondents had at least weekly contact by phone, letter or email with family, friends or relatives or had at least weekly visits with family, friends or relatives in Edmonton. About one in five would prefer more frequent contact or visits. Recent immigrants and established-when-older immigrants reported significantly less frequent visits than established-when-younger immigrants and were significantly more likely to prefer additional contact than were established-when-younger immigrants.

Almost all respondents (92%-99%) said that they have someone to confide in, help out in a crisis, get advice from, or to make them feel loved. Respondents indicated that family was most likely to make them feel loved. Sons, daughters and family generally were most likely to help out in a crisis. Established-when-younger immi-

Table 3

Percentage Distribution of Family and Social Relationships Variables by Immigrant Groups and by Gender

Variable	Recent Immigrants %	Established-When-Older Immigrants %	Established-When-Younger Immigrants %	p	Men %	Women %	p	Total %
Family Members[a]								
Ask for seniors' opinion (advice/guidance)	72	72	65		69	69		69
Respect seniors' decisions	61	72	71		65	70		68
Share seniors' values	73	89	74	*	68	85	*	77
Make it easy for seniors to eat the kind of food they like	91	97	96		90	99	*	94
Make it easy for seniors to practice their customs and traditions	95	97	91		87	100	**	94
Ensure seniors get enough rest and are not overworked	89	97	88		89	93	*	91
Take care of seniors when sick	98	95	94		94	98		96
Ensure seniors get a good diet and any needed medication	96	97	94		95	96		96
Ensure seniors get enough exercise	66	82	78		76	73		75
Social Contact								
At least weekly contact with family, relative, or friends	65	65	93	*	76	78		77
Prefer more contact with family, relatives, and friends	27	17	10	*	21	15		18
At least weekly visits with family, relatives, or friends in Edmonton	44	58	75	*	63	58		60
Prefer more visits in Edmonton	33	8	19		22	20		21
n	36	68			80	81		161

*** p<.001; ** p<.01; * p<.05. [a]Percentage respondents indicating 4 on a 4-point scale ranging from 1 (never) to 4 (all the time)

grants also relied on friends to help out. Advisors and confidants were typically a spouse, son or daughter, friend or other family member. Women were more likely than men to confide in a son or daughter and men were more likely than women to confide in a friend and in family members in general.

Table 3 shows that the majority of our respondents (69%-96%) indicated that their family showed respect and caring in several ways by doing the following frequently or all the time: ask for their advice or guidance, respect their decisions, share their values, make it easy for them to eat the food they like or practice their customs and traditions, ensure they get enough rest or exercise, a good diet and any needed medication, or take care of them when they are sick. Men were less likely than women to report that their family share their values, make it easy for them to eat the food they like, practice their customs and traditions, or ensure that they get enough rest.

Social Contact With Community

One in five (20%) of the respondents were doing volunteer work. Men were more likely than women to be doing volunteer work (30% versus 10%) (p = .003). The most popular involvement for those doing volunteer work was in community or cultural activities (41%), followed by temple activities (28%).

Most of our respondents (75%) participated in social group activities in the past 12 months, with 69% participating weekly or more often. These activities allowed them to meet people and socialize (45%), or gave them peace of mind (32%). Age or health problems (29%), transportation problems or distance (26%), and lack of time (24%) were the common reasons given for not participating.

Close to half (45%) of the respondents, especially men and established immigrants said that they used community and recreational services. Library use was the most popular (men: 41%; women 7%), followed by physical exercise programs (established-when-younger immigrants: 25%; recent or established-when-older immigrants: 3%). Most respondents learned about these services either from friends or relatives (31%), cultural, community, or religious organizations (26%), or family (23%). Men were more likely to learn of these services from cultural, community, or religious organizations than women (39% versus 15%): whereas, women were more likely than men to learn of these services from family (36% versus 10%) (p = .001). Those who used these services found it easier to access these services in summer (very easy 74%; somewhat easy 19%) than in winter (very easy 39%; somewhat easy 22%). Weather conditions and lack of transportation were the primary obstacles to access.

Isolation and Loneliness

Most respondents (58%) spent some time alone at home each day. One in eight (13%) indicated that they would prefer to spend less time alone, although 4% would like more time alone. Sixty-three per cent of respondents indicated that they never feel lonely themselves. Men were more likely than women to say that they were lonely "frequently" (15% versus 4%). In addition, 3% of women (but none of the men) said that they were lonely "all of the time." (p = .016)

Identity, Religion, and Life Satisfaction

Connections to Homeland

Table 4 shows that over half of the respondents (56%) had occasional or frequent contact by telephone and visits with family and friends in their homeland (38%). Most (74%) have visited their homeland in the past five years at least once. Recent immigrants were least likely to have made a return visit in the past five years and established immigrants were more likely to have made several return visits (p = .042). About half of those (52%) who made a return visit or visits in the past five years stayed longer than two months. Family and friends from their homeland visited respondents in Edmonton less often than respondents visited family and friends in their homeland. Established immigrants were significantly more likely than recent immigrants to have visits in Edmonton with family and friends from their homeland and to visit family and friends in their homeland.

Cultural Customs and Practices

Table 4 shows that the respondents incorporated various cultural practices and South Asian traditions into their daily lives in Canada, including practicing their religion, speaking native language, wearing South Asian clothing, eating South Asian food, and celebrating South Asian holidays. Recent immigrants were most likely to report wearing South Asian clothing outside. Men were much more likely to read South Asian newspapers than were women.

Identity in Canada

Our respondents saw themselves as more South Asian than Canadian (59%), as equally South Asian and Canadian (32%), and more Canadian than South Asian (7%). Interestingly, established-when-older immigrants were most likely (86%) to report see ing themselves as more South Asian than Canadian, followed by recent immigrants (67%), while established-when-younger immigrants were most likely to see themselves

Table 4

Percentage Distribution of Cultural Practices and Identity Variables by Immigrant Groups and by Gender

Variable	Recent Immigrants %	Established-When-Younger Immigrants %	Established When-Younger Immigrants %	x^2	Men	Women	x^2	Total %
Connection with Homeland[a]								
Phone contact with family/friends	54	64	53		60	52		56
E-mail/fax contact with family/friends	12	8	31	**	19	20		19
Letter contact with family/friends	18	17	18		23	12		18
Have family/friends visit in Edmonton	7	11	18	*	9	16		13
Visit family/friends in homeland	29	39	46	**	44	33		38
Never back in homeland in last 5 yrs	42	22	13	*	23	28		26
Up to 2 months average stay during homeland visit	42	25	63	*	45	52		48
Cultural Practices[b]								
Wear South Asian clothing	68	47	40	**	52	52		52
Eat South Asian food	56	61	53	*	53	60		56
Celebrate South Asian holidays	77	64	66		65	74		69
Watch South Asian videos/movies	39	36	46		34	48		41
Listen to South Asia radio	42	36	34		41	35		38
Watch South Asian television	32	31	40		28	42		35
Read local South Asian newspapers	28	28	29		39	19	**	28
Visit South Asian internet sites	4	3	6	*	5	4		4
Listen to, view, or participate in South Asian music/dance or art	16	9	33	*	20	22		21
Speak native language/dialect	88	97	75		82	86		84
Practice religion	91	94	81		84	91		88
Read Canadian newspapers	19	25	47	**	43	22	**	32

National Identity									
Self more South Asian than Canadian	67	86	38	***	53	65		59	**
Children more South Asian than Canadian	27	8	8	***	11	18		15	*
Grand-children more south Asian than Canadian	11	—	6		3	8		6	*
Life in Canada[c]									
Family and relatives close by	79	89	74		74	84		79	
Friends from the same cultural background	72	75	63		63	75		69	
Feeling welcome in Canada	67	78	78		65	83		74	*
Knowing English	73	72	90	*	86	74		80	
Canadian citizenship	66	75	87		85	69		77	
A source of income	88	92	92		91	90		91	
Employed or self-employed	50	38	58		61	40		51	*
Canadian-born friends	14	17	25	**	24	15		19	
Member of a political party	9	11	10	**	13	7		10	**
Feelings about Canadian Society[a]									
Like the way of life in Canadian Society	69	83	75		78	71		75	
Understand Canadian culture	59	81	86		76	75		76	*
Feel accepted by most Canadians	77	73	88		74	90		81	
Canadians appreciate the contributions of immigrants	76	82	79		79	79		79	
Acceptance by Canadians depends on international political events	46	40	34		49	26		39	
n	57	36	68		80	81		161	

Notes for Table 4
*** p < .001, ** p < .01, * p< .05 aPercentage of respondents indicating 3 and 4 on a four-point scale ranging from 1 (never) to 4 (all the time). bPercentage of respondents indicating 4 on a four-point scale ranging from 1 (never) to 4 (all the time). cPercentage of respondents indicating 5 on a five-point scale ranging from 1 (not at all important) to 5 (very important). dPercentage of respondents indicating 4 and 5 on a five-point scale ranging from 1 (strongly disagree) to 5 (strongly agree).

as equally South Asian and Canadian (53%) (p = .000). Men were more likely than women to see themselves as more Canadian than South Asian (13% versus 1%; p = .006). However, men were significantly more likely than women (26% versus 12%; p = .031) to cite barriers to developing their identities as Canadians. The most commonly cited barriers included language (43%), cultural differences (39%), or skin color/ethnicity (18%).

Most of the respondents saw the identity of their children and grandchildren becoming more and more Canadian. Established-when-younger immigrants (60%) were more likely to describe their children as seeing themselves as more Canadian than South Asian than either recent immigrants (32%) or established-when-older immigrants (25%). Men were more likely than women to feel that their own children (53% versus 31%, p = .026) or grandchildren (84% versus 61%, p = .014) saw themselves as more Canadian than South Asian.

Life in Canada

Table 4 shows that the majority of the respondents indicated that the following were "important" or "very important" for living in Canada: having family and relatives close by, having friends from the same cultural background, feeling welcome in Canada, knowing English, having Canadian citizenship, and having a source of income. Established-when-younger immigrants were more likely to say knowing English is important or very important than were recent or established-when-older immigrants. Women were more likely than men to say feeling welcome in Canada is important or very important. Being employed or self-employed was considered important or very important by 51% of our respondents, with men more likely than women to indicate so.

In contrast, relatively few rated having Canadian-born friends as important or very important, with established-when-younger immigrants the most likely to say it is important (Table 4). Women (57%), recent immigrants (53%), or established-when-older immigrants (56%) were more likely to say that they do not know people from other cultural or ethnic groups. Few thought that being a member of a political party was important or very important, with men, recent or established-when-younger immigrants more likely to say it is important (Table 4). Among those recent immigrants who were eligible, only 28%-33% voted all the time and 56%-68% never voted in city, provincial, or federal elections. In contrast, among established-when-younger immigrants, 84-86% voted "all of the time" (p = .000). Reading Canadian newspapers such as the *Edmonton Journal* or the *Globe and Mail* regularly is most common among established-when-younger immigrants (48%) (p < .001). Men were more likely than women to read Canadian newspapers regularly (43% versus 22%) (p < .01).

About 60% of respondents said that they were "concerned" or "very concerned" about certain issues: money (60%), being part of Canadian society (58%), quality of family life in Canada (61%), moral standards in Canada (68%), and friends, family or relatives outside of Canada (62%). Almost half of our respondents (42%) were concerned about prejudice and discrimination in Canada, with men significantly more likely to say so than women (50% vs. 35%). Of the 140 respondents who answered the question: "In the past three years, have you experienced racism in Canada?" "Never" was said by 79% and 1% said "all of the time." Men were less likely than women (66% versus 92%) to say that they have never experienced racism in Canada in the past three years (p = .001). Experiences of racism included references to religion, traditional dress and attire, and skin color. On the other hand, some commented positively about the friendliness, generosity, acceptance, and fairness of people in Canada.

The majority of respondents either agreed or strongly agreed with the following statements: "I like the way of life in Canadian society" (75%), "I understand Canadian culture" (76%), "I feel accepted by most Canadians" (81%), and "Canadians appreciate the contributions of immigrants" (79%). Thirty-nine per cent agreed or strongly agreed that their acceptance by Canadians depended on international political events.

Satisfaction with Life as an Immigrant Living in Canada
The great majority of respondents (91%) were satisfied or very satisfied with their life as a whole. Had they lived in South Asia today, respondents indicated that their life would be good to excellent (50%) or poor to very poor (18%). In contrast, 89% said that life in Canada for them was good or excellent (89%) and none said life in Canada was poor or very poor.

The perceived advantages of immigrating to Canada included being with family (26%), better health care (20%), and financial benefits (14%). Men were more likely than women to say good government, safety, or freedom, good quality of life, and better educational or job opportunities; whereas, women were more likely than men to say being with family. The main advantages of immigrating to Canada reported by recent immigrants and established-when-older immigrants were being with family and better health care. For established-when-younger immigrants, the advantages were more varied: opportunity for children and grandchildren, better educational or job opportunities, good quality of life, financial benefits, and good government, security, or freedom, better health care, and family.

One in three of our respondents (32%) could not cite any disadvantages of immigrating to Canada. One-third (31%) cited missing family, friends, or relatives as the main disadvantage, 10% said missing homeland, and 9% said missing or losing culture or identity. Women were more likely than men to say missing family, friends, or relatives as the main disadvantage. Men's responses were more varied. Finally, additional information offered by our respondents about their experiences as immigrants to Canada suggests that established immigrants were more likely to emphasize that they had a good life in Canada or that Canada was a good country; whereas, recent immigrants were more likely to emphasize the need for more financial assistance.

Discussion

Overall, the South Asian immigrant seniors in this study were satisfied with many aspects of their life in Canada: housing and neighborhood; living arrangement, contact with and emotional support from their family and friends, and social contact through community, cultural, and religious organizations. The majority of our respondents indicated that having family and relatives close by was very important to them and there is evidence of mutual help within the family, with the senior helping with childcare and household maintenance, and adult children and grandchildren helping the senior with daily living and providing emotional support. Most of our respondents indicated that the advantages of immigrating to Canada have outweighed the disadvantages.

However, some respondents have experienced difficulties in their lives. The common difficulty was with financial security, a concern expressed by Boyd (1989). About two in five of the respondents reported not having adequate income for their needs. Another difficulty was isolation and loneliness. About one in ten said they felt lonely frequently or all the time; a similar observation was expressed by Choudhry (2001). Some seniors had difficulty getting to places because of the lack of a ride and poor public transportation. To some, language and cultural differences were the main barriers to developing their identity as Canadians.

Maintaining ties to their homeland and their South Asian identity was important for our respondents, findings that are consistent with Dhruvarajan (1993) and Tran et al. (2005). Most of our respondents still had connections with family and friends in their homeland, maintained some cultural practices and traditions in their daily life, and considered having friends from the same cultural background very important to them (as in Inman et al., 2007). Most saw themselves as more South Asian than Canadian, but noted that the next generations tended to become more Canadian.

Participating in the Canadian mainstream society is very important to the respondents in some respects (feeling welcome in Canada, knowing English, having Canadian citizenship, being financially secure). Other aspects of Canadian life (being a member of a political party or having Canadian-born friends) were less important.

Age at Immigration and Length of Residency

The most significant finding of this study is that those immigrants who came to Canada at older and younger ages have different experiences with different consequences. Those immigrant seniors who came to Canada at a younger age are the most acculturated to independent living (e.g., live alone or with their spouse only, drive a car), as is the norm in the aging Canadian population generally. They participate in Canadian society actively (e.g., voting, meeting people from other cultural or ethnic groups). On the other hand, those who came at an older age are more likely to lack skills essential to independent living in Canada (e.g., English language skills, driving), be more dependent on their children (e.g., for transportation, living in the homes of their children), maintain the lifestyle of their homeland (e.g., living arrangement, language spoken), and have a stronger South Asian identity. Those who came to Canada when they were older and have resided in Canada for more than 10 years, apart from better financial circumstances (primarily as a result of becoming eligible for government benefits such as old age security), are not any more acculturated to independent living than those who came recently in their old age. Recent immigrants are less likely to say that their income was adequate, a finding consistent with Boyd (1989). It is possible that immigration policy and the immigrant screening process may predispose a dependence on adult children (Turcotte & Schellenberg, 2007). Note that dependence on children in old age is not considered undesirable in South Asian culture (Choudhry, 2001).

Gender

In this study of older immigrants, women were more likely than men to lack the skills essential for independent living; for example, they tended to have poorer English-language skills, were more likely to live in three-generation families, and were less likely to drive and more likely to rely on family and friends for transportation. Women were less likely than men to participate in the mainstream society (e.g., voting, using community and recreational facilities, knowing people from other cultural or ethnic groups).

Women were also less likely than men to see themselves, their children, or their grandchildren as more Canadian than South Asian.

Marital and family status may play a role in these gender differences. For example, whereas currently unmarried men were more likely than unmarried women to live alone, unmarried women were more likely to live in an extended family with their adult children, as they responded to subtle pressure from family and community (Choudhry, 2001). Devotion to the family and children by women is an important value to the South Asian community, especially first-generation immigrants (Naidoo, 2003). While self-reports of discrimination were infrequent, discrimination was reported more by older men than women. In their relative isolation from the larger society, the women were less likely to experience directly the discrimination that occurs when looking for housing or participating in the labor market.

Conclusion

Our findings are consistent with "successful aging" models (e.g., Baltes and Baltes, 1990) and models that focus on person-environment fit (e.g., Lawton, 1982). Most South Asian immigrant seniors who have immigrated to Canada later in life are able to use familial resources (e.g., extended family living arrangement, social network within the ethnic-cultural community) to compensate for their lower level of skills in independent living. One result of living with their extended family is that these seniors can live in reasonably good-quality dwellings in safe neighborhoods and have their transportation needs met reasonably well. Contrary to common belief, these findings suggest that aging immigrant seniors are quite satisfied with their housing and neighborhood, living arrangements, family and social relationships, and life in general.

Like many other studies about immigrant seniors, the sample is small and selective so the findings need be interpreted with some caution. Also, in any study of a relatively cohesive community where data are obtained through interview, there is the possibility of a social desirability effect. First, respondents may present themselves and their community in the best possible light. Second, using interviewers from within the community may increase discomfort with disclosure.

In summary, this study has provided insights into the diversity of experiences of older immigrants as influenced by their age at immigration, length of time in Canada, and gender. Older immigrants and especially older recent immigrants are more dependent on their family than immigrants who came to Canada at a younger age and have grown old in Canada. At the same time, these aging immigrants often enjoy family contact and support, have a strong traditional identity, and can be satisfied with life in Canada even if they acquire relatively few of the cultural values and customs of Canadian mainstream society. It may be that the older immigrant who is most

"Canadian" and by extrapolation older Canadians in general can be the most vulnerable given that Canadians and "Canadianized" immigrants are most likely to live alone in old age, less likely to have family contacts and supports, and more likely to have their identity undermined by an agist society which de-values and stigmatizes the old. Traditional cultural values can function as a "moral medicine" that is protective against depression, despair, anomie, and alienation (Acharya, 2004). In a multi-cultural society, there is room for one to learn from another.

This study has policy implications for housing, income support programs, family assistance, and community integration of seniors. The challenge for policy makers and program providers is to develop policies and services that are inclusive, that meet the needs of older immigrants with increasingly diverse backgrounds as well as Canadian-born seniors.

References

Acharya, Manju (2004). *Constructing the meaning of mental distress: Coping strategies of elderly East Indian immigrant women in Alberta.* Doctoral Dissertation. Edmonton: University of Alberta.

Angel, R.J. & Angel, J.L. (2006). Diversity and aging in the United States. In R.H. Binstock & L.K. George (Eds.), *Handbook of aging and the social sciences* (6th ed.), (pp. 94-110). New York: Academic Press.

Baltes, P.B. (1997). On the incomplete architecture of human ontogeny: Selection, optimization, and compensation as foundation of developmental theory. *American Psychologist, 52,* 366-380.

Baltes, P.B. & Baltes, M.M. (1990). Psychological perspectives on successful aging: The model of selective optimization with compensation. In P.B. Baltes, & M.M. Baltes (Ed.), *Successful aging: Perspectives from the behavioral sciences* (pp. 1-34). Cambridge, England: Cambridge University Press.

Basavarajappa, K.G. (1998). Living arrangements and residential overcrowding among older immigrants in Canada. *Asian and Pacific Migration Journal, 7*(4), 409-432.

Boyd, M. (1989). Immigration and income security policies in Canada: Implications for elderly immigrant women. *Population Research and Policy Review, 8,* 5-24.

Brislin, R.W. (1986). The wording and translation of research instruments. In W.S. Lonnor & J.W. Berry (Eds.), *Field methods in cross-cultural research* (pp. 137-164). Beverly Hills, CA: Sage.

Burr, J.A. (1992). Household status and headship among unmarried Asian Indian women in later life: Availability, feasibility, and desirability factors. *Research on Aging, 14,* 199-225.

Canada Mortgage and Housing Corporation (CMHC) (2005a). *2001 Census housing series issue 7 revised: Immigrant households* (Research Highlights, Social-Economic Series, Issue 04-042). Ottawa: CMHC.

Canada Mortgage and Housing Corporation (CMHC) (2005b). *2001 Census housing series issue 9 revised: The housing conditions of Canada's seniors.* (Research Highlights, Social-Economic Series, Issue 05-006). Ottawa: CMHC.

Carp, F.M. (1976). Housing and living arrangements: A transactional perspective. In R.H. Binstock & E. Shanas (Eds.), *Handbook of aging and the social sciences.* (pp. 426-443). New York: Van Nostrand.

Chan, K.B. (1983). Coping with aging and managing self-identity: The social world of elderly Chinese women. *Canadian Ethnic Studies, 15,* 36-50.

Chappell, N., Gee, E., McDonald, L. & Stones, M. (2003). *Aging in contemporary Canada.* Toronto, ON: Prentice Hall.

Choudhry, U.K. (2001). Uprooting and resettlement experiences of South Asian immigrant women. *Western Journal of Nursing Research, 23*(4), 376-393.

Dhruvarajan, V. (1993). Ethnic cultural retention and transmission among first generation Hindu Asian Indians in a Canadian prairie city. *Journal of Comparative Family Studies, 24*(1), 63-79.

Grewal, S., Bottorff, J.L. & Hilton, B.A. (2005). The influence of family on immigrant South Asian women's health. *Journal of Family Nursing, 11*(3), 242-263.

Heisz, A. & Schellenberg, G. (2004). *Public transit use among immigrants.* (A report by Statistics Canada, Business and Labour Market Analysis Division, Catalogue no.: 11F0019MIE – No. 224). Ottawa: Minister of Industry.

Inman, A.G., Howard, E.E., Beaumont, R.L. & Walker, J.A. (2007). Cultural transmission: Influence of contextual factors in Asian Indian immigrant parents' experiences. *Journal of Counseling Psychology, 54*(1), 93-100.

Kahana, E., Lovegreen, L., Kahana, B. & Kahana. M. (2003). Person, environment, and person-environment fit as influences on residential satisfaction of elders. *Environment and Behavior, 35,* 434-453.

Kahn, R.L. (2002). On "successful aging and well-being: Self-rated compared with Rowe and Kahn." The Gerontologist, 42, 725-726.

Kamo, Y., & Zhou, M. (1994). Living arrangements of elderly Chinese and Japanese in the United States. *Journal of Marriage and the Family, 56,* 544-558.

Knipscheer, K., Dykstra, P., de Jong Gierveld, J. & de Tilburg, T. (1995). Living arrangements and social networks as interlocking mediating structures. In C.P.M. Knipscheer, J., de Jong Gierveld, T. G. van Tilburg & P.A. Dykstra, (Eds.). *Living arrangements and social networks of older adults.* Amsterdam: VU University Press.

Koltko-Rivera, M.E. (2006). Rediscovering the later version of Maslow's hierarchy of needs: Self-transcendence and opportunities for theory, research, and unification. *Review of General Psychology, 10,* 302-317.

Kritz, M.M., Gurak, D.T. & Chen, L. (2000). Elderly immigrants: their composition and living arrangements. *Journal of Sociology and Social Welfare, 27*(1), 85-114.

Lawton, M.P. (1982). Competence, environment press and the adaptation of older people. In M. P. Lawton, P.G. Windley & T.O. Byerts (Eds.), *Aging and the environment: Theoretical approaches* (pp. 33-59). New York: Springer.

Longino, C.F., Jr. & Bradley, D.E. (2006). Internal and international migration. In R.H. Binstock & L.K. George (Eds.), *Handbook of aging and the social sciences* (6th ed., Chapter 5). New York: Academic Press.

Maslow, A.H. (1943). A theory of human motivation. *Psychological Review, 50,* 370-319.

Maslow, A.H. (1954). *Motivation and personality.* New York: Harper.

Maslow, A.H. (1969). The farther reaches of human nature. *Journal of Transpersonal Psychology,* 1, 1-9.

McDonald, L., George, U., Daciuk, J., Yan, M.C. & Rowan, H. (2001). *A study on the settlement related needs of newly arrived immigrant seniors in Ontario.* Toronto: Centre for Applied Research, Faculty of Social Work, University of Toronto. Retrieved July 18, 2006, from http://www.socialwork.utoronto.ca/fsw/fswsupport/casr/report.html

Naidoo, J.C. (2003). South Asian Canadian women: A contemporary portrait. *Psychology and Developing Societies, 15*(1), 51-67.

Novac, S., Darden, J., Hulchanski, D. & Seguin, AM. (2002). *Housing discrimination in Canada: The state of knowledge.* Ottawa, ON: Canada Mortgage and Housing Corporation.

Oliffe, J.L., Grewal, S., Bottorff, J.L., Luke, H. & Toor, H. (2007). Elderly South Asian Canadian immigrant men: Confirming and disrupting dominant discourses about masculinity and men's health. *Community Health, 30*(3), 224-236.

Riley, M.W. & Riley, J.W. (1990). Structural lag: Past and future. In M.W. Riley, R.L. Kahn, & A. Foner (Eds.), *Aging and structural lag.* (pp. 15-36). New York: Wiley.

Rittner, B. & Kirk, A.B. (1995). Health care and public transportation use by poor and frail elderly people. *Social Work, 40*, 365-373.

Rowe, J.W. & Kahn, R.L. (1998). *Successful aging.* New York: Random House (Panthcon).

Scheidt, R.J. & Windley, P.G. (2006). Environmental gerontology: Progress in the post-Lawton era. In J.E. Birren & K.W. Schaie (Eds.), *Handbook of the psychology of aging* (6th ed.). (pp. 105-125) New York: Academic Press.

Statistics Canada (2003). Immigration status and place of birth, sex, and age groups for population, for Canada, provinces, territories, Census Metropolitan areas and census agglomerations, 2001 Census, 20% sample data. Tabulation 95F0357XCB01004. Retrieved March 18, 2004, from http://www12statcan.ca/english/census01

Tran, K., Kaddatz, J. & Allard, P. (2005). South Asians in Canada: Unity through diversity. *Canadian Social Trends, 78,* 20-25. Ottawa: Statistics Canada.

Turcotte, M. & Schellenberg, G. (2007). *A Portrait of seniors in Canada 2006* (Catalogue No.: 89-519-XIE). Ottawa: Minister of Industry.

Walters, D., Kelli, P. & Paul, A. (2007). The acculturation of Canadian immigrants: Determinants of ethnic identification with the host society. *Canadian Review of Sociology and Anthropology, 44*(1), 37-64.

Ward, C., Bochner, S. & Furnham, A. (2001). *The psychology of culture shock* (2nd ed). East Sussex, UK: Routledge.

Acknowledgements

This study was initiated by Dr. Gita Das, the Indo-Canadian Women's Association in Edmonton, and Dr. Baha Abu-Laban, Director of the Prairie Centre of Excellence for Research on Immigration and Integration (PCERII) at the University of Alberta. The PCERII provided funding and the Population Research Laboratory at the University of Alberta conducted the interviews. We acknowledge the assistance of many individuals in the immigrant settlement field and the South Asian community, in particular, Dr. Nayanika Kumar and Dr. Gita Das of the Indo-Canadian Women's Association of Edmonton. We thank Liz White for the management of this project.

16

Gentrification, Displacement, and Resistance: A Case Study of Portuguese Seniors In Toronto's "Little Portugal"

Carlos Teixeira, (University of British Columbia)

Introduction

Toronto, the largest and most multicultural city of Canada, has been for the last five decades the major "port of entry" for Portuguese immigrants arriving in Canada. Portuguese immigration to Toronto began in the early 1950s, and attained its peak in the late 1960s and early 1970s. In 2001, according to the Canadian Census, 357 690 Portuguese were living in Canada. Of this total, the Toronto Census Metropolitan Area is home to the largest concentration of Portuguese, 171 545, in the country (Statistics Canada, 2001). The majority of this group is first generation immigrants (born in Portugal) and live in the downtown core of the community: "Little Portugal."

Toronto's "Little Portugal" is located in the St. Christopher House catchment area of west central Toronto (see Figure 1). In this neighborhood, Portuguese immigrants have created an institutionally complete community that is also one of the most visible ethnic neighborhoods in Toronto (Teixeira, 2000; Qadeer, 2003). Today, this neighborhood contains most of the community's social, cultural, commercial and religious institutions. In addition, as this concentration might suggest, the Portuguese have also been among the most segregated groups in Toronto (Murdie and Teixeira, 2006).

Evidence from census data reveals that the Portuguese community in Toronto has expanded in two areas of new settlement in recent years. The first of these is northwest of "Little Portugal" along the traditional "immigrant corridor" where the Portuguese are replacing the Italians. The second is in the western suburbs and, in particular, in the cities of Mississauga and Brampton. These cities have become primary suburban destinations for the Portuguese families who have left the Toronto core. However, although many Portuguese have moved to other parts of the Greater Toronto Area, most of this immigrant community's social, cultural, commercial and religious institutions remain in "Little Portugal."

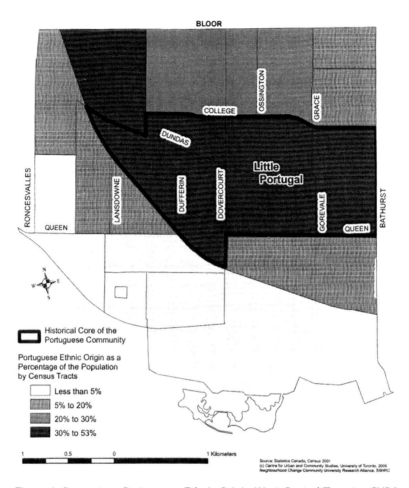

Figure 1. Percentage Portuguese Ethnic Origin West Central Toronto, CURA
Study Area, 2001

This being said, "Little Portugal" is today a neighborhood in transition. This transition has resulted from three major changes:

1. the movement of a large number of Portuguese to the suburbs;

2. an in-movement of immigrants and refugees from the Portuguese diaspora (Brazil and Portugal's former African colonies); and

3. an in-movement of an increasing number of the urban professional class who see an opportunity to obtain relatively low cost housing with potential for renovation in close proximity to the city's downtown core.

These characteristics serve to explain why "Little Portugal" has today become an area of emerging gentrification.

This residential and commercial gentrification, and the "invasion/succession" of different populations (Portuguese and non-Portuguese speaking immigrants, African refugees and white middle-class Canadians), has implications for the "life-cycle" of "Little Portugal." These processes, together with the out-movement of economically mobile Portuguese residents and the continued presence of an aging first generation, may significantly impact continued social cohesion in the neighborhood and the viability of an existing Portuguese commercial and institutional infrastructure.

This chapter explores issues related to neighborhood change in Toronto's "Little Portugal" with a particular focus on Portuguese seniors; the aging first generation immigrant population who built the community but who are today facing pressures for displacement. It addresses the following research questions: What are the main positive and negative impacts of gentrification on "Little Portugal"? Does gentrification mean the displacement of lower income households, including the aging first generation Portuguese, or are there viable strategies of resistance?

Gentrification

The process of "gentrification" plays a critical role in this migratory process, as the Portuguese (and other immigrant groups) are displaced from their older settlement areas in our Canadian inner cities (Meligrana & Skaburskis, 2005; Slater, 2004; Ley 1996; Caulfield, 1994). Gentrification has been defined as "the loss of affordable older inner-city housing through their renovation and upgrade by middle and upper-income households" (Meligrana & Skaburskis, 2005, p. 1571). In the Canadian context, most of the opportunities for gentrification and its greatest potential to displace low-income households are found within low-income inner city neighborhoods (often ethnic/immigrant neighborhoods) with a high proportion of older dwellings (Meligrana & Skaburskis, 2005, p. 1571).

While this view of gentrification, associating the process with the displacement of populations, has negative connotations, it should be noted that there has been protracted debate on gentrification's causes, consequences, and relative significance in various cities and national contexts. For example, David Ley (1993, p. 232) defines gentrification more simply as "an upward movement in the social status of a census tract." As well, in the United Kingdom the process has been often defined in notably positive terms as "the rehabilitation of working-class and derelict housing and the consequent transformation of an area into a middle-class neighborhood" (Atkinson, 2004). This being said, in the Canadian context very little is known about the costs of gentrification upon ethnic neighborhoods, and much less regarding its impact upon one segment of these neighborhoods' populations – immigrant seniors.

Methodology

In order to accurately represent the "voices" of Portuguese seniors and other residents of "Little Portugal" regarding the phenomenon of gentrification, the author:

a. spent 2 months (July and August, 2006) conducting informal interviews with "key" informants – Portuguese (20) and non-Portuguese (20); and

b. conducted 6 focus groups with three Portuguese-speaking immigrants and three non-Portuguese people who are especially familiar with the study area.

With reference to Portuguese seniors, this chapter draws in particular upon the responses of thirty-three first and second generation participants who have roots in Portugal (twenty informal interviews and thirteen participants from the focus groups). Most respondents were women (54.6%), homeowners (81.8%) and over fifty years of age (60.6%).

The Portuguese ethnic background of the researcher and experience of participant observation within "Little Portugal," as well as extensive contacts with local residents, helped develop a list of potential key informants to participate in both the informal interviews and focus groups. Various community organizations and institutions (e.g., ABRIGO, BIA-Dundas St. West, St. Christopher House) also assisted in the recruitment of key informants. The author of this research conducted the informal interviews and moderated the focus groups. Both key informant interviews and focus group discussions were taped and transcribed and, after a careful reading, themes were selected around which to summarize the material.

"Little Portugal" in Transition

All of the Portuguese informants in this study agreed that "Little Portugal" is a neighborhood in transition. However, there was no agreement among respondents on the degree of change and/or on the main "forces" at play in the neighborhood. As is evident from the comments of respondents, the "forces" currently shaping the neighborhood are diverse and complex. The major trends are summarized in the following sections.

Seniors on the Move: Why are First Generation Portuguese Moving Out?

With regard to the question, "Who moves out of "Little Portugal?" respondents identified three main groups leaving the area for reasons both voluntary and forced. The first group moving out is Portuguese in their 40s or 50s, who are currently homeowners in "Little Portugal." This is a group with some assets and financial stability, which aspires to move to the suburbs in order to improve their housing conditions. The second group moving out of "Little Portugal" is well-off Portuguese seniors, with their house mortgages paid, who move in order to join their children already established in the suburbs. The third group that is moving out of "Little Portugal" is also Portuguese seniors, but these are retired on fixed incomes. This group faces a "constrained" housing market because they do not own a dwelling and cannot afford high rents, or else own their own home but cannot keep up with the high maintenance costs of their dwellings, including increasing property taxes. For this group, the solution is an involuntary move out of "Little Portugal."

Opinions in the Portuguese community are quite divided vis-à-vis the pros and cons of Portuguese seniors moving from "Little Portugal" to the suburbs. Some argue that the move to the suburbs only leads to isolation for these seniors:

> This old generation spent a lot of years in Little Portugal and they were used to do almost everything in Portuguese [businesses, services . . .] In the suburbs is different . . . they will be more isolated. Some return back after a few years in the suburbs.

In other cases, they maintain a close contact with the Portuguese neighborhood of "Little Portugal" via frequent visits to shop in the Portuguese businesses and/or participating in the social, cultural and/or religious life of the Portuguese community. A Portuguese bank manager who deals frequently with Portuguese retired seniors now living in the suburbs also noted:

> I have seen a lot of my clients living far away from "Little Portugal" . . . in the suburbs. However, they return to do their shopping in "Little Portugal." My Bank [Portuguese owned] decided to open on Saturdays because we have clients that come from Mississauga, Brampton Kitchener, Cambridge . . . to do their banking with us . . . coming/visiting on weekends our "Little Portugal" is like going home.

Clearly, many Portuguese seniors are wary of the move to the suburbs, and prefer the security of their traditional home in "Little Portugal." However, the steady increases in housing property taxes and the problems of housing maintenance have become sources of preoccupation for Portuguese seniors. Now on fixed incomes, and many with their children already living in the suburbs, they find themselves becoming increasingly dependent on others. Thus, many of this group feel they must move, but not by choice! One respondent explained:

> Some Portuguese seniors have problems maintaining their houses . . . some houses are already in bad conditions . . . I would say in some cases unsafe to live . . . if they are on a fixed income – a pension of $1 000 . . . it's not going very far. How can they put [pay] the repairs? The bills still have to be paid . . . and we know how most Portuguese don't like to be owing anybody money . . . no debts . . . but they have no choice – sell the house.

It should be noted that some respondents see a lot of financial advantages in this move, which represents an excellent opportunity for Portuguese seniors to profit from Toronto's real estate market. However, it is clear that even in the best cases Portuguese seniors approach this prospect with mixed feelings.

The Gentrifiers: Why is "Little Portugal" Attractive?

Portuguese respondents agree that "Little Portugal" has, in the last two decades or so, been "invaded" by different groups of people interested in buying housing in Toronto's downtown. One of the most important of these groups is urban profession-al Canadians ("white collar" workers). The prime location of "Little Portugal" vis-à-vis the Central Business District is likely an important "pull" force on urban professionals' decisions to move into "Little Portugal" as it eliminates a long commute to the sub-urbs. The other major "pull" factor, and probably one of the most important ones, attracting them to the neighborhood is the nature of the existing housing stock – old Victorian-era/early twentieth century housing – with historical value and often large and well preserved.

Gentrification was highlighted by the respondents as one of the major causes of the noticeable changes in the neighborhood's housing market and, in particular, of the escalating housing prices and high rents which are affecting both Portuguese and non-Portuguese residents of "Little Portugal." As one respondent noted:

> Presently the housing prices are increasing almost every day and a lot of Portuguese who own houses in "Little Portugal" are selling the ones they own here and are moving to areas where they can buy brand new homes.

However, urban professionals are not the only new residents of "Little Portugal." New immigrants to Canada are also settling in the neighborhood. These immigrants from Asia, particularly from China and Vietnam, tend to be working class ("blue col-lar") and are in search of large, comparatively inexpensive houses in "Little Portugal" to accommodate their large families. As well, there are new Brazilian immigrants and Portuguese-speaking immigrants from the former Portuguese colonies in Africa (e.g., Angola, Mozambique or Cape Verde Islands) who have settled in Toronto's "Little Portugal." Respondents are aware of how gentrification and the resources of urban professionals are also displacing these new residents:

> I have also seen the arrival of other ethnic groups, the Asiatics [sic], the Chinese . . . but if "Little Portugal" is going through gentrification this area will stop being a hub/reception area for new immigrants . . . they cannot afford the rents . . . Like Chinatown [Dundas/Spadina], Queen St. West [Bathurst to Dufferin] . . . which are in transition . . . "Little Portugal" too will follow.

The Seniors Who Stay: Why Do They Remain?

Most of the Portuguese who decided to stay in "Little Portugal" are first generation, born in Portugal, "blue collar" workers with low levels of education and little
knowledge of the English language. This group is the least assimilated of all
Portuguese, and is also a population that is aging fast with an important number of
them already retired. When Portuguese started buying homes in the 1950s and 1960s,
housing was inexpensive and, with a small down payment, they could become homeowners in Toronto. Partly as a result, the Portuguese have today one of the highest levels of homeownership of all immigrant groups living in Toronto.

For some of these established homeowners, nothing would make them want to
leave their houses, the homes they renovated and where their children were born. In
fact, this group seems to be resisting gentrification. Regarding those Portuguese who
resist gentrification to stay in "Little Portugal," two respondents noted:

> The majority of those that stay here are first generation Portuguese . . . the ones
> who arrived in the 1950s, 1960s, and 1970s . . . the ones that were able to ren-
> ovate their houses to accommodate their housing needs . . . and some due to
> lack of mobility, both social and physical, decided to stay.

> A lot of senior Portuguese are managing a house at the expense of their health
> . . . what a price! But this shows to me how important that is for them.

Key to this resistance to gentrification is the importance of proximity to "Little
Portugal," mainly to Portuguese services, businesses, cultural and religious institutions,
as a source of security for this particular group of Portuguese.

The Seniors' Perspective: Benefits of Gentrification

For almost two thirds (64.5%) of the Portuguese respondents, the "increased
property values" as well as the "increased social mix" of peoples (58.1%) into "Little
Portugal" represent by far the two most positive impacts of gentrification in the neighborhood.

Given the escalating housing prices that define Toronto's housing market today,
it is not surprising that many respondents see the "increase of property values" as the
most positive impact of gentrification upon "Little Portugal." On this issue, most respondents agreed that the Portuguese homeowners benefited from gentrification.
Respondents also noted that the housing renovations undertaken by urban professionals had improved the quality of the existing housing stock and the overall housing
prices in "Little Portugal." In their words:

> The Portuguese are the winners with this "invasion" of urban professionals to the
> city and to "Little Portugal." Their houses are worth today a fortune . . . and if it
> was not this invasion of these urban professionals . . . speculators the housing

prices would have been much lower. So I don't see anything negative here with their arrival.

The Portuguese that own housing in "Little Portugal" . . . have "richness under their feet' ["riqueza debaixo dos pez"]. Those who sell tend to buy smaller residences so they make money on the transaction . . . it's a natural process. That happens in all major cities in the world.

However, the increased property values in the neighborhood represent a "mixed blessing" for with increased property prices in "Little Portugal" also comes increases in property taxes. This aspect of the gentrification phenomenon particularly affects Portuguese seniors, who are often retired and living on fixed incomes.

The "increased social mix" of peoples coming to "Little Portugal" in the last few years was highly valued by some Portuguese respondents as a positive impact of gentrification. As they observed:

It is positive to the City of Toronto and to "Little Portugal" as well because it's wonderful thing to see all these different peoples enjoying the area, restaurants, cafes . . . and Portuguese enjoy them here too. Some Portuguese interact with them.

Respondents agree that the increase in social mix in "Little Portugal" has been beneficial to the Portuguese community, and particularly to older, first generation seniors, in that it has assisted their integrating into Canadian society; an integration that was postponed by the institutionally complete nature of the "Little Portugal" community where immigrants could find all businesses and services in their own language and cultural practices. As one respondent observed on this issue of "integration":

It's positive . . . the arrival of gentrifiers into "Little Portugal" . . . it destroys the "ghetto" that we had for decades. We are here highly concentrated and Portuguese didn't need to learn English because their lives were done in Portuguese within the Portuguese community . . . now our "ghetto" is diluting/disintegrating and we are integrating ourselves more into the Canadian society.

From this perspective, it is clear that Portuguese respondents recognize positive aspects in the gentrification of "Little Portugal" in terms of economics and culture. However, while the Portuguese, and particularly Portuguese seniors, appreciate some of the positive things the gentrifiers have brought with them to the neighborhood, they are not blind to the more negative aspects of this phenomenon on their community.

The Seniors' Perspective: The Downside of Gentrification

For Portuguese respondents the "loss of affordable housing" (77.4%) in "Little Portugal" is the most important negative impact of gentrification in the area, followed by "displacement through rent/price increases" (58.6%) and "unsustainable speculative property price increases" (48.4%).

By far, the "loss of affordable housing" was the most important negative impact of gentrification noted by respondents in regard to "Little Portugal." As a consequence of this relatively new phenomenon in the area, two related negative impacts of gentrification are already visible in the area – high rents and high housing prices – which are making this area more and more unaffordable for low income people, including both Portuguese seniors retired on fixed incomes and new immigrants arriving in Toronto. There is agreement among the Portuguese respondents that "Little Portugal" is still an affordable neighborhood of Toronto in which to buy housing and/or to rent. The key question is, however: For how much longer will this be the case?

Most respondents were concerned about the future with regard to this issue. Respondents pointed out that the majority of urban professionals, the potential gentrifiers in "Little Portugal," are still living mostly on the "periphery" of "Little Portugal." Thus, for most of our respondents, the (re)discovery and "invasion" in mass by urban gentrifiers into "Little Portugal" is just a question of time. After the gentrification of "Little Italy" (to the north) and Queen St West (to the south), both processes almost completed, it seems "Little Portugal" (sandwiched between the two areas) will be next. As respondents noted:

> I live [West of Bathurst] . . . the value of the houses has skyrocketed . . . My parents bought our house for $30 000 [in the 1960s] . . . now it's half a million. My neighbor's house is small and was listed for $630 000 and who bought it? Professionals!

In the face of this new trend of high resale housing costs, there is the question of whether the Portuguese homeowner will actually benefit from it. Some respondents say "yes" if the Portuguese family sells the house for good money and buys another one in a less expensive area of the city of Toronto or in the suburbs. For others, and particularly for established Portuguese seniors, selling their house in "Little Portugal" is not an option at all since they do not want to leave. Regarding this dilemma, one respondent noted:

> Houses are selling for a very good price . . . but what is the point . . . most of the first generation Portuguese [50 years of age and on] don't want to move . . . they want to die where they spent most of their lives . . . here in "Little Portugal." What's the point to sell for good bucks, cash some money and go to the suburbs

. . . far away from the Portuguese community? That's not what they want. So
. . . what's the point of having this huge housing prices here . . . who benefits?

According to the Portuguese key informants, Portuguese seniors are perhaps the segment of the Portuguese population most impacted by gentrification, followed by low income renters. The steadily rising housing property taxes in the past few years, and the high housing maintenance costs, are major preoccupations and may "force" some seniors to sell their property because of lack of financial means.

As some respondents noted, the Portuguese have been known for being a resourceful community where through the help of internal "informal" ethnic networks of contacts (friends and relatives) they have been able to improve considerably their housing conditions/quality through renovations. However, some noted that things have changed for Portuguese seniors:

> A few years ago, few were those Portuguese in the age bracket 60-65 who talked about selling their houses and/or renting part of it to help pay the bills . . . the majority thought they would die in their own house . . . the house they lived for four/five decades . . . but times changed and they cannot afford it anymore.

Similarly, a Portuguese aide to a provincial member of parliament who is also a community activist describes his experience in assisting Portuguese seniors in search of help from the government. As he states, the challenges are numerous:

> Everyday, my number one job is dealing with people complaining to me because they are seniors and they can't afford . . . hydro. They can't afford to pay for the water; they cannot afford to pay their property taxes. They are all Portuguese. That's why they come to my office, because I speak Portuguese, and that's the number one issue that we are dealing with now . . . There's no way, except to sell the house but many of these people don't want to do that . . . the way to deal with this issue is to change the evaluation system to make sure it isn't dependent on your neighbor's property, so that if one person is stupid to pay a million for a $500 000 house, it's not automatically going (to) increase the prices of the other houses. I mean, that's one way of doing it.

Portuguese Seniors Resisting Gentrification

Some respondents (the most optimistic ones) also argued that the Portuguese, particularly the homeowners, are to a certain degree resisting the "forces" of gentrification in "Little Portugal." This argument is based on the fact that most first generation Portuguese in the area own their own homes and/or some of them get an extra income from their housing by renting part of it.

Respondents noted, however, that every time a Portuguese sells a house in the area the same house is not bought by a Portuguese family, but instead by gentrifiers; speculators and/or by members of other immigrant groups. Thus the number of Portuguese homeowners in the area will tend to decrease with time and with it some of the existing affordable rental units such as flats and basement apartments. Also, it is expected that the "informal renting" that characterized the Portuguese homeowners will also decrease. On this issue of "resistance" to the forces of gentrification by some of the Portuguese living in "Little Portugal," some respondents observed:

> So far, Portuguese are resisting gentrification because they own their own prop-
> erties/houses . . . The first generation is aging. But a lot of houses are subdivid-
> ed in flats, and this means an extra income for them. In fact "Little Portugal" still
> is a very economically viable neighborhood.

Portuguese Seniors - Renting Part of the House as a "Survival Strategy"

Some Portuguese senior homeowners are already facing serious challenges to keep their houses. In the face of drastic increases in property taxes and maintenance/utilities costs as a consequence of gentrification, they are coping by rent-ing parts of their houses. This strategy seems to work for most of the Portuguese sen-iors, particularly the ones more in need of cash, who will rent part of their dwellings in a very "informal" (verbal) way where receipts are not necessary (avoiding taxes). It should be noted that this has been a traditional strategy in Toronto's Portuguese com-munity, beginning in the 1950s, and continuing through to the 1960s and 1970s, when renting was used as a means for new Portuguese homeowners to pay their mortgages. Now, however, this has become a "survival" strategy for Portuguese seniors. Most of their renters are Portuguese speaking immigrants, with the Portuguese language serv-ing as a major bridge/facilitator in this "informal" process of renting housing in Little Portugal.

Accommodating the Housing Needs and Preferences of Portuguese Seniors: Housing Policy Implications

A major source of concern in "Little Portugal" are the issues of an aging of the community. There is agreement among our respondents that more needs to be done in order to accommodate the housing needs/preferences of our Portuguese seniors:

> The solution for an aging population is more incentives for them to take care of
> their own homes . . . Aging in place is a good way to go. Also there is an urgent
> need in our community for more housing for seniors . . . Some of them do not
> need any type of assistance so far, neither physically or financially . . . The only

problem they have is that they can not take care of their homes anymore and the expenses to keep up a house today are very high. What they need is a place where they can spent the rest of their lives in peace . . . feeling at home ["ambiente Portugues"] . . . It's a group of citizens that is growing in a scary kind of way.

There is a great need for seniors' housing like Terra Nova in here. Lots of people want to go there. People come from Orangeville to come and live here . . . now that they are seniors they want to have what they are used to around them . . . I find the Portuguese speaking community wants more buildings like that where there's high concentration, not necessarily all of them, but where it's close to "Little Portugal" . . . because to most of the Portuguese going to the nursing home is the last resort.

Criticism of the Portuguese community regarding its failure to support building affordable housing for seniors is evident in the following quotation:

I am a social worker . . . I see the problems they face. "Aging in place" is the first choice for the majority of Portuguese seniors and they will do their best to stay in their homes. We should also follow the lead of other immigrant groups like the Italians, the Chinese . . . in Toronto that built specific seniors housing that caters to their cultural needs and preferences, linguistic, food . . . I mean ethnic-oriented senior homes. After 50 years in this country, we could have done better . . . the Portuguese community need to put their mouth where the money is . . . building and catering specifically to the needs of the Portuguese community seniors . . . From a business point of view they would make a lot of money. At my knowledge the demand is there but the need has not been filled.

Respondents also note that much more needs to be done by the Portuguese community to accommodate the housing needs/preferences of its increasingly aging population, and to take a more active role by building (with or without support of the government) affordable senior housing that caters to the cultural needs and preferences of an aging Portuguese population.

Conclusion

In general, all of the Portuguese respondents in this study agreed that "Little Portugal" is a neighborhood in transition. There was also a general consensus that the population most impacted by the forces of gentrification that are now re-shaping the residential areas of downtown Toronto such as "Little Portugal" are the aging first generation Portuguese immigrants, now seniors, who originally bought and renovated their homes decades earlier in a less expensive housing market.

As the responses indicate, there is widespread recognition in Toronto's Portuguese community today that many Portuguese seniors are confronted by the dilemma of being "land rich and cash poor." Gentrifiers, mostly urban professionals, are seeking to move into downtown areas such as "Little Portugal" and this demand is having a significant impact upon housing prices in the area. While respondents generally regard this as a good thing, they also note that for Portuguese seniors this increase in property values is a mixed blessing, for it is accompanied by increasing property taxes and maintenance costs which they, often retired and living on fixed incomes, are not able to support.

Although in other contexts this would merely be an economic dilemma that is readily solved through the homeowner selling his/her home and buying a cheaper dwelling in another area, making a substantial profit in the process, for Portuguese seniors the process of gentrification is not simply a matter of dollars and cents. Members of this group concentrated together in "Little Portugal" where they built an institutionally complete community with businesses and services providing them with everything that they need to live in the Portuguese language and in a Portuguese cultural "way." These seniors have lived most of their lives in this community, where they raised their children, and are understandably resistant to the idea of dispersing to the suburbs where housing costs are cheaper, but where they would be missing the language, culture and friendships that they enjoyed in "Little Portugal."

There are no easy solutions, at either the policymaking level or the community level, for the housing challenges facing Portuguese seniors who wish to keep their community alive, but who are confronted by the economic realities of gentrification, including higher property taxes. Some respondents have suggested the government provide more information and supports to members of this group on the possibility of entering the formal housing rental market. Many members of this group subdivided parts of their homes decades earlier, after they initially purchased the houses, in order to take in renters so as to quickly pay off their mortgages. If Portuguese seniors were to resort to this strategy again, with their properties now in a highly desirable location in the city of Toronto, they would go a long way towards not only easing the cost dilemmas of this group but also to providing much needed affordable housing for Toronto's constrained rental market.

However, while this might resolve the dilemmas facing Portuguese seniors from gentrification in the short term, in the long term this group are confronted by the realities of an aging population. Some of the respondents cited this as an issue of grave concern, and one requiring state and community intervention:

> We are aging as a community . . . we will have more and more Portuguese seniors here. We will see a bipolarization . . . and we have not worked hard enough with the other Portuguese speaking communities living in and around "Little

Portugal." We have a lot to do to break down the isolation that separates us . . .
It's urgent . . . We need more seniors' housing in our community . . . I am pes-
simistic . . . I get the feeling that we missed the "boat" already. We are one of
the few communities among the largest communities in Toronto that didn't
invest enough or at all in seniors' housing . . . a disaster. The major challenge
now is how to accommodate our seniors in terms of housing in a cultural space
where they feel at home.

From this perspective, while Portuguese seniors and "Little Portugal" may survive
the forces of gentrification, in time this group and the community will be confronted
by serious housing challenges of an aging population that may, in conjunction with
gentrification, ultimately mean the end of "Little Portugal" as it is known today. Thus,
while the question of the impact of gentrification upon immigrant groups, and particularly seniors, has received little attention from scholars and policymakers to date, it
is clear from this case study that this issue will demand more detailed attention in
future as Canada's "baby boom" and first generation immigrant populations age and,
in the process, transform Canada's residential urban and suburban housing markets.

References

Atkinson, R. (2004). The evidence on the impact of gentrification: New lessons for the urban ren-
aissance. *European Journal of Housing Policy, 4*: 107-131.

Caulfield, J. (1994). *City form and everyday life: Toronto's gentrification and critical social practice.* Toronto: University of Toronto Press.

Ley, D. (1996). *The new middle class and the remaking of the central city.* Oxford:: Oxford
University Press.

Meligrana, J. and Skaburskis, A. (2005). Extent, location and profiles of continuing gentrification
in Canadian metropolitan areas, 1981-2001. *Urban Studies, 42:* 1569-1592.

Murdie, R.A. & Teixeira, C. (2006). *Urban social space. In Canadian Cities in Transition: Local
Through Global Perspectives,* In T. Bunting and P. Filion, ed. (154-170). Toronto: Oxford
University Press.

Qadeer, M. (2003). *Ethnic segregation in a multicultural city: The case of Toronto, Canada.* CERIS
Working Paper Series, no. 28, Joint Centre of Excellence for Research on Immigration and
Settlement, Toronto.

Teixeira, C. (2006). Residential segregation and ethnic economies in a multicultural city: The little
Portugal of Toronto. In *Landscapes of the Ethnic Economy,* In. D.H. Kaplan and W. Li, (Ed.).
(pp. 49-65). New York: Rowman & Littlefield.

Slater, T. (2004). North American gentrification? Revanchist and emancipatory perspectives
explored. *Environment and Planning A, 36:* 1191-1213.

17

Caring for Older Haitian Parents: The Impact of Immigration on Family Dynamics and Caring Activities on Family Caregivers

Louise Racine, (University of Saskatchewan)

Introduction

Caring for aging parents at home represents a challenge for first generation Haitian immigrants in Canada. Haitian traditional values pertaining to men's and women's traditional roles, gendered division of domestic work, immigration, and the constraints of a free market economy, has an impact on the gendering of caring among Haitian Canadian family caregivers. These contextual factors also influence the family patterns of negotiation used by Haitian Canadian women to involve husbands or spouses in the sharing of domestic tasks, and to facilitate caring activities. Covan (1997) conceptualizes the gendering of caring in elder's care as an outcome of the sexual division of labor that imparts to women the sphere of caring and nurturing. This position can be seen as being limited to gender since it overlooks the influence of the broader social context within which caring unfolds. On the other hand, Hooyman and Gonyea (1999) argue that gender cannot be studied in isolation from structural factors like race, social class, ethnicity, and economy.

In this chapter, the everyday struggle of Haitian Canadian women caregivers to reconcile paid work with caring activities is described. More specifically, the extent to which both men and women caregivers are torn between Haitian cultural traditions and the need to adapt to the Canadian market economy are examined. Traditionalism and patriarchy represent the cultural premises upon which conflicts on the sexual division of household labor arise between Haitian Canadian men and women. Second, the influence of immigration in redefining family dynamics of Haitian Canadian traditional roles is examined. The patterns of negotiation used by Haitian Canadian women caregivers to achieve this reconfiguration are described. The influence of caring on caregivers' familial and social life is scrutinized. Finally, the impact of caring on paid work is examined and the blurring boundaries between private and public spheres in women's lives delineated.

Research Methods

Theoretical Perspective

A postcolonial feminist framework guided data collection and analysis in this ethnographic study. Postcolonial feminism is a paradigm of inquiry from which the hegemonic practices of Western science in marginalizing other forms of knowledge can be counteracted. It aims at disrupting the relations of ruling that silence the voices of culturally different "others," at integrating subjugated knowledge, at unveiling asymmetrical power relations, and at developing transformative knowledge directed at achieving social justice by correcting inequities arising from social discrepancies affecting non-Western immigrants (Racine 2003). Postcolonial feminist epistemology focuses on patriarchy as a source of oppression for it allows us to locate social inequalities within a political, historical, cultural and economic context, and to examine how they are constructed (Quayson, 2000). Such a perspective enables researchers to integrate the knowledge of immigrants and refugees and to "give a voice to racialized women who have been silenced. It provides the analytic lens to examine how politics and history have variously positioned us and shaped our lives, knowledge, opportunities, and choices" (Anderson, 2000a). The onus of presenting subjugated racialized voices is on the postcolonial feminist researcher. Anderson (2000b), Meleis and Im (1999), Quayson (2000), Schutte (2000), and Smith (1987) define postcolonial feminism as a critical perspective aimed at addressing health problems stemming from social inequities that affect the well-being of non-Western people (Racine, 2003; Racine, 2004). In this critical ethnography, the use of a postcolonial feminist perspective addresses issues in the context of caring to uncover the social, political, economic, and cultural determinants that construct experiences of caring for aging relatives at home.

Description of the Participants

In this study, 12 out of 16 participants were women (mostly daughters, but also one daughter-in-law) caring for aging mothers or mother-in-law. Six women were married; five were divorced, and one was single. One participant worked in paid employment for 20 hours a week while another was retired. The ten other women caregivers were working full-time in the paid labor force. Most of them were parenting young children, adolescents, or grandchildren, while caring for their aging parents at home. On the other hand, the four men caregivers were married (two of them were retired). The fact that women outnumbered men as caregivers and care-receivers can be partly explained by women's longer life expectancy at birth, but demographic data alone cannot explain the gendering of caring among Haitian Canadian caregivers. Structural factors that model caring activities as well as the roles of men and women must be examined.

The Impact of Haitian Traditional Values in Shaping Haitian Men and Women Immigrants Roles in Canada

During fieldwork, it was noticed that Haitian Canadian women, like other Canadian women, juggle the triple-task issue, which consists of working in the labor force, parenting young children or adolescents, and caring for aging parents at home. Meanwhile, women remain totally accountable for performing almost all domestic duties. Haitian traditional and patriarchal values, like patriarchal values in other societies, have an impact on the gendering of caring activities. In this section, how traditionalism and patriarchy influence the roles of men and women in the household are explored, in their patterns of negotiation to share housekeeping tasks, and in the approaches to problem-solving that are used within the family to support or not support women caregivers' commitment.

The traditional authority of Haitian Canadian men, embedded in a culture of machismo, was reported in a prior study aimed at exploring the construction of Haitian ethnicity in the Montreal area (Massé, 1983). In fact, Massé (1983) documented the occurrence of asymmetrical relations of power in structuring men's and women's social relations. Attention is made before asserting that asymmetrical power relations and machismo are observed only among Haitian Canadian men since this would be inscribing their identities in an essentialist cultural discourse. The point is that machismo is a social and cultural construction of colonialism. Hall (1997) emphasizes that colonialism and slavery have had an impact on Black men's masculinity. As well, Hall (1997) defines machismo as a means of resistance to oppose the hegemony of White men in separating Black men's roles. Therefore, when examining some Haitian Canadian men's machismo, one must be aware that it has been aimed at resisting and counteracting the effects of negative stereotypes that have affected Black men's identities, an effect created by colonialism and by the derived ideology of Whiteness. To avoid generalizing machismo to all Haitian Canadian men, its historical, cultural, and social constructs must be examined. These attitudes and behaviors arise from colonial hegemony and were inscribed as normative practice aimed at disenfranchising Black men of their human rights. Machismo is deeply rooted in hegemonic discourses on race. As Hall (1997b) states:

> During slavery, the white slave master often exercised his authority over the black male slave, by depriving him of *all* [italics added] the attributes of responsibility, paternal and familial authority, treating him as a child. This "infantilization" of difference is a common representational strategy for both men and women . . . Infantilization can also be understood as a way of symbolically "castrating" the black man (i.e., depriving him of his "masculinity") . . . Treated as "childish," some blacks in reaction, adopted a "macho," aggressive-masculine style. (p. 262-263)

As a product of colonialism and imperialism, machismo must be questioned, and therefore, not used uncritically to label the decisions or behaviors of Haitian Canadian men in pertaining to marital and familial roles. Keeping in mind that machismo is a colonial construct, one may understand the nuances of participants about Haitian Canadian men. In this participant observation excerpt, Margaret* described Haitian traditional family roles:

> In Haiti, children were the safety net, to care for their parents when they grew older. It was not uncommon to see large families of six or eight children. Education was very, very important since it's considered the key to achieving higher social ranks. In Haiti, boys were educated, they went to university, they earned graduate degrees in medicine, law, or accounting, but girls didn't get these opportunities. Boys were more valued than girls in the sense that boys were educated to assume their future functions as breadwinners and heads of family. Girls obeyed their fathers or brothers. As authority figures, boys were more protected than girls were. Girls only needed to do basic math and know to write their names because once they'd got married, they'd only need to supervise the household and the domestics' work. *Mum didn't want my brothers to enter the kitchen.* [italics added] She told them: "Kitchen isn't your place! This is not your place here. It's woman's work, not yours and stay away from the kitchen!" *Kitchen was a strictly feminine domain because parents were afraid to feminize boys by allowing them to perform domestic tasks.* [italics added] Cooking, housekeeping, cleaning, and all other domestic chores were seen as women's work. It was the same for raising the children or caring for the sick or the elderly. Domestic tasks were automatically attributed to girls since it was the custom.

She went on to explain how the women of her generation were socialized to fulfill their attributed roles in the Haitian society. These roles consisted of performing or supervising household duties, raising the children, and caring for the sick and the elderly. Another participant explained how women of her generation were socialized to perform or supervise household duties, "Grandmother used to say that only boys need to be educated and girls needn't. Girls must know how to write their names and do basic maths."

George, an 87-year-old man, described Haitian traditional men's and women's roles, as they were when he was raised in his native country. George performs domestic and housekeeping tasks due to his wife's illness. It can be assumed that despite

*All participants of the study were attributed various pseudonyms, to protect informants' confidentiality. As well, the identity of the number of children in some families and their gender were modified to further protect participants' confidentiality. Therefore, the reader must be aware that the number of pseudonyms exceeds the number of 16 caregivers.

their socialization, some Haitian Canadian men adapt to the changing conditions of their lives, especially when they care for their very ill wives at home. When life circumstances in the context of migration clearly indicate they cannot do otherwise, men enter the kitchen, a private and restricted women's domain. Nevertheless, this transition is difficult to figure out in the reality of everyday life, even for some adult children. For instance, George's eldest son could not understand how his father could achieve the planning of meals and do the cooking. George said:

> Oh, you know I have to live with this. I've to get used to it. I cook, do the laundry, the housekeeping, and I wash her clothes as soon as possible. I'll tell you something else. Yesterday, our eldest son came in to visit and asked me: "Hey dad, from which restaurant do you order in?" I replied: "I didn't order anything in. I cook everything that's on the table here, in this home. I manage your mother's diet because of her (name of the illness). Each day I change the menu.

George discussed Canadian society and the gaps between Haitian and Canadian cultural values as they pertain to women's role and family dynamics. He contrasted the differences that he had noticed since his arrival in Canada:

> First of all, women weren't liberated here before. In earlier times, women weren't as powerful as they are now. But when they started claiming their rights, then everybody went their own way. And since then, women are independent and challenge men's authority. They're independent. I see it like revenge. It wasn't like this before. It was like this almost all around the world. Wives were submitted to husbands. Wives obeyed their husbands. It was a submission since husbands were breadwinners and women stayed at home. Women stayed home to cook, to look after the children, to supervise housekeeping even if we had servants. These were women's duty. But Quebec's women are so different! They resist! They resist! [In the sense they oppose or challenge men's authority].

This interview excerpt also demonstrates that patriarchy was influential across the world and also had an impact on the lives of Western women. The participant says, "It was like this almost all around the world. Wives were submitted to husbands." Therefore the impact of patriarchy in defining women's roles is not only restricted to Haitian Canadian women. Canadian women were also affected by patriarchy like other women around the world. Doyal (1995) mentions that "despite cultural variations between communities, it is usually women who continue to be allocated responsibility for what is regarded as domestic work – the daily tasks of cooking, cleaning and caring for children and other dependants" (p. 28). This would tend to support the cross-cultural effect of gendering of caring activities among women of the South and of the North.

Subsequently, George shifted his comments back towards Haitian men and described how men were assuming their social role in his former homeland. Margaret's description of traditional Haitian women's educational and familial duties was confirmed. The participant explained:

> The Haitian husband is a guy who, once his studies are completed, gets involved in a certain area of work, a liberal work, as physician or lawyer, and with his family's background and education in hand, wants to get married. He seeks a wife and usually the bride's family must bring a dowry, for the girl to be accepted by the man's family. For instance, the bride's family can give a house or a piece of land as dowry. It helps the young couple to get started. The woman brings a dowry and the man brings his knowledge and good manners. They stay together and remain on the same wavelength regarding the education of their offspring. It's fundamental, the education of the children.

This is only George's perspective on how men and women ought to carry out their respective roles in Haiti. As pointed out earlier, George is a spouse caregiver and carries out all the domestic work previously realized by his wife. This interview excerpt shows the influence of Haitian traditional values in shaping mens' and womens' roles in the family and illustrates how these roles can be reshaped under the influence of immigration and new social and cultural contexts. The roles of men and women are thus seen to be socially and culturally constructed in specific historical, cultural, social, and economic contexts. George's interview excerpt also demonstrates that these roles may vary according to these contexts; roles are not fixed as static entities but are modelled according to the demands of immigration.

The Impact of Immigration on Family Dynamics

Immigration adds a layer of complexity to the existing issue of race, gender, and class in constructing Haitian Canadian men and women caregivers' ways of caring. For instance, immigration heightens Haitian Canadian women's awareness of their rights, and the development of this consciousness has a direct impact on Haitian Canadian men. As well, Haitian Canadian women's participation in waged-work represents another factor that puts pressure on the men to share in domestic tasks. The integration of women into the paid labor force is a means to achieve financial freedom and therefore, men can no longer be considered as the sole family breadwinners, as was the case in Haiti. In Canada, the higher cost of living pushes women into the workforce, though Quayson (2000) underlines that in accessing economic freedom, women risk becoming alienated subjects. His contention must be located in a particular context that may not necessarily apply to Canada:

Namely, this is in the peculiar condition of women taking their rightful place in modernity but having simultaneously to renounce "normality." Viewed another way, this could be described as the conundrum of attaining citizenship whilst becoming alienated subjects. This conundrum that afflicts women's lives is arguably greatly aggravated in the Third World, where women's existence is strung between traditionalism and modernity in ways that make it difficult for them to attain personal freedoms without severe sacrifices or compromises. (Quayson, 2000, p. 103)

Without implying that the Haitian Canadian women caregivers who participated in the research were alienated subjects, the findings demonstrate that family dynamics can be fluid and redefined to face the demands of a different social context. Family roles are not anchored in Haitian traditional values since they may be reconfigured into a hybrid model of Haitian Canadian family dynamics. Moreover, because women struggle to reconfigure family dynamics and their roles, they are not alienated but instead are challenging the status quo. Haitian Canadian women caregivers use their agency to integrate men into the private sphere of domesticity and modify a situation to provide better care for their aging parents. Women caregivers also want to have some free time for themselves, since they usually shoulder the triple-task issue, which can be draining. The major drawback is that women caregivers, in contrast to men caregivers, cannot dissociate their private lives from the public spheres. In other words, a boundary cannot easily be drawn to delineate caring activities and the work outside the home. For Haitian Canadian women, caring has an impact on the waged work and their full-time participation in the workforce also influences their caring. Doyal (1995) points out that "whatever their cultural differences, most societies give women ultimate responsibility for the well-being of their families, often at considerable cost to their own health" (p. 30).

The emphasis here is to present interviews and participant observation excerpts to illustrate how Haitian Canadian women caregivers manage the reconfiguration of family dynamics and to describe patterns of negotiation that are used to achieve this reconfiguration. The influence of immigration on Haitian traditional values is typically translated into the needs for Haitian Canadian women to enter the workforce to increase their family's wealth and meet the higher cost of living in the host society. When examining family patterns of negotiation, Haitian Canadian men's resistance to share the domestic chores is assumed to increase women's workload. Also, patterns of negotiation demonstrate the effect of immigration on Haitian Canadian men since they too need to adapt to a new way of living. While women struggle against the Haitian Canadian men's patriarchy, men must juggle the idea of equalizing or sharing power with women in the household. Men and women have different, but related, struggles that arise from the levelling of social classes and the soaring demands of Canada's free market economy. These two issues have impacts on women caregivers, especially when assuming the competing roles as wives, daughters, daughters-in-law, and workers in Canada.

Writer bell hooks (2000) emphasizes "consumer capitalism was the force leading more women into the workforce" (p. 50). The market economy and higher cost of living explains why Haitian Canadian husbands, like many other Canadian men, can no longer remain as the sole provider of the family's wealth. The transition from housewife to working-woman is the central issue upon which cultural clashes occur over the redistribution of domestic duties in some Haitian Canadian families. Negotiations to reconfigure the Haitian Canadian family dynamics have an important bearing on the issue.

Family Patterns of Negotiation

When referring to the fieldwork and to the literature, It is perceived that Haitian Canadians do not extensively differ from Haitian American families, especially in the examination of family dynamics and functioning. In this regard, the work of Stepick (1998) is relied on, he described Haitian American family dynamics and functioning. Stepick (1998) states: "Families (one's relatives) and households (with whom one lives) include not only parents and children, but also grandparents and grandchildren, uncles and aunts, cousins both near and far, and even nonrelatives from one's hometown back in Haiti" (p. 15). Despite immigration, family dynamics and functioning are maintained as much as possible to keep living arrangements close to the Haitian ways of living. The cultural shock of late immigration of aging parents may thus be alleviated, though an impact may be felt by the women caregivers who ask their partners to share in the domestic tasks to alleviate their workload. As discussed earlier, the reconfiguration of family patterns is not without problems, especially in the context of a Western society, where Haitian Canadian women must integrate into the workforce to financially support their family's subsistence. Some women caregivers are divorced and must look after a family of more than two children. In such cases, the woman is the sole family breadwinner, while acting as the single parent raising the children.

The levelling of social classes has an impact on the relations of men and women since most Haitian Canadian women participants had to join the workforce when they arrived in Canada. This role transition from housewife to working-woman is the central issue for clashes over the re-distribution of domestic duties that arise in some Haitian Canadian households. Accessing the workforce is a means for women to achieve economic freedom, but paradoxically, Haitian Canadian women are often overwhelmed since they must juggle multiple roles. They must work outside, raise the children, and care for aging relatives, a triple-task that could not be worked out without asking for their husbands' participation to carry out domestic tasks. Men's involvement in the domestic sphere is a key issue for alleviating women's workload and the negotiations focus on encouraging men to share in housekeeping tasks.

In a participant observation session, it is desired to validate the data that had been previously collected about the different roles that men and women assume in Haitian Canadian families. The question was: "Is this okay, the perception I have that Haitian men exert a kind of power relation over women?" The participant said: "For sure, it's the case." Then, she was asked if her husband was involved in sharing housekeeping chores. She said that she unsuccessfully tried to convince him to help her to do some tasks. For instance, she tried to teach him how to do a laundry load, but she said: "He didn't want to know about it; he even refused to push the button to start the washing machine. So now, I don't wash his clothes anymore. I sort them out and put them in a bag. I only wash my kid's, my mum's and my own clothes." I said: "So what is he doing with that?" She replied: "Well, he brings his clothes to his mother's and she washes them." Of the caregivers whom I met, she was the only one to provide this amount of direct, hands-on instrumental care in supporting activities of daily living, which included bathing, showering, combing, cutting nails, and changing her mother's positions in the bed at night. When Sonia asks her husband for help, he replies: "I'm too tired." She answers: "I'm tired too and I need your help." She has repeated her request many times in the many years of their marriage. For instance, if she asks him to sweep the floor, he gets upset, saying: "It shows we live in Quebec. It shows we live in Quebec for you to ask me to do that. In Haiti, it would have been a different story!"

On the other hand, another woman caregiver raised a different viewpoint in describing her perception of machismo and its impact on men's family roles. She says: "It's relative, since it depends on the men's and women's level of education. It's related to the level of education and to the social background. It really depends on the kind of education the man receives in his family. What I can tell you for sure, I'm not the one who accepts my husband's domination. I don't have the personality, the attitude for this. I mean you must develop this consciousness too, it's a process, and it takes some time. Women mustn't be passive, subdued, but it's true that some men are machos and dominants. He's upset but I make many of the decisions."

Laguerre (1984) also reports this asymmetrical power relationship among Haitian American couples but underlines the impact of immigration on changing the direction of the power relation. Laguerre (1984) asserts that this phenomenon occurs because of the need for men to participate in household tasks and because of the fact that women are now earning money. Immigration introduces a re-definition of the roles in Haitian American families, and determines a new family economy where women's participation in the labor force gives them the right to express their ideas. If husbands were not happy, then the only choice they would have would be either to quit or get a divorce. "Life in New York has a tremendous impact on the relations between husband and wife. He [the husband] is asked to help with household duties, sometimes to cook. This is a new ingredient in Haitian household life" (Laguerre, 1984, p. 76). The same author mentions that immigration and the subsequent re-patterning of family roles leads some couples to break up. At the time of study, divorce was rare among Haitian American families, since it would jeopardize the entry of relatives into the United States (Laguerre, 1984).

Haitian Canadian couples endure clashes over the distribution of household tasks since families may no longer be able to afford domestic services. In Haiti, many care-givers reported, for those who belong to the elite, and even for those of the middle-class, domestic aid was easier to access. Historically, some distant relatives or cousins came to the town from their villages to earn a living and were hired to work in these families. Domestic aid was affordable and the men did not need to get involved in domestic duties. Immigration determines a new family dynamic and economy, which paves the way to marital conflicts, especially if the husbands are unwilling to share in the domestic tasks.

Thus far, it can be assumed that the family is seen as a social unit where the socialization of boys and girls takes place. Family is a microcosm of the larger social world in that it reproduces the social and gender inequalities on a smaller scale. Race, gender, and class mutually construct or influence the definition of roles of men and women, as well as the family organization and functioning. Patricia Hill Collins (2000) states:

> Families are expected to socialize their members into an appropriate set of "fam-
> ily values" that simultaneously reinforce the hierarchy within the assumed unity
> of interests symbolized by the family and lay the foundation for many social hier-
> archies. In particular, hierarchies of gender, wealth, age, and sexuality within
> actual family units correlate with comparable hierarchies in the U.S. society. (p.
> 158)

This statement also applies to Canadian society, where members of families learn their respective roles constructed around race, gender, and social classes, within family units. Families may be compared to a social laboratory, where children learn social values that rule the broader social world within which the family interacts. Thus, the roles of some men or women are seen as being natural and the hierarchy is not questioned since social rules were integrated during their childhood. Children must comply with these relations of ruling in determining how men and women contribute in shaping the social world. As Collins (2000) states:

> Individuals typically learn their assigned place in hierarchies of race, gender, eth-
> nicity, sexuality, nation, and social class in their families of origin. At the same

time, they learn to view such hierarchies as natural social arrangements, as compared to socially constructed ones. Hierarchy in this sense, becomes "naturalized"
because it is associated with seemingly "natural" processes of the family. (p. 158)

Collins (2000) points to understanding how social hierarchies influence the attri-
bution of caring as women's work. As well, this difficult issue of negotiating the share
of domestic duties must be also examined from Collins's perspective, where the sexual division of work is aimed at maintaining a gender hierarchy. Therefore, patriarchy
still influences Haitian Canadian women's roles, as wives, daughters, daughters-in-law,
and mothers. Patriarchy also has an impact on the roles of other Canadian women and
would not be restricted to Haitian Canadian women, only. According to Hooyman and
Gonya (1995), the sexual division of work was introduced by capitalism at the time of
the industrial revolution. The gendered division of work, which introduces the binary
division between private and public spheres, was created to satisfy the needs of a capitalist market economy, but is pervasive across this transnational and translational
world. The gendered division of work is not a particular characteristic of the Haitian
Canadian community but affects women of the South and the North. These findings
partly contradict Laguerre's (1984) assertion, who said that immigration equalized the
power imbalance that influenced men's and women's traditional roles. Laguerre (1984)
points out:

Haitian women tend to become more assertive in New York, not only because of
their economic independence but also because they are immersed in a more plu-
ralistic environment. Husbands tend to be more willing to share household chores
with their wives. Consequently, the imbalance in the traditional roles of husband
and wife tends to diminish. (p. 86)

Fieldwork would rather suggest that Haitian women may be more assertive in the
North American context but the extent to which they have convinced husbands to take
on domestic chores is a debatable issue. A woman caregiver told me that she would
not tolerate her husband's domination, even if they would have stayed in Haiti. It
deconstructs the myth of the submissive Haitian Canadian woman and shatters stereo-
types of submissive so-called Third-World women. The gendered division of domestic
labor is an issue that is yet to be overcome among Haitian Canadian women and it is
also the case for other women, whether of the South or the North. The impact of globalization and the spreading of liberal capitalism are likely to influence women's paid and
unpaid work across the world, since the ideology of the sexual division of labor, rooted in the ideologies of capitalism (Hooyman & Gonyea, 1999) and this role of women
serves corporate interests but, to some extent, the health care system interests as well
(Wuest. 1993).

Results show that the cultural component of caring is fluid and hybrid, and brings
a redefinition of traditional family roles for adapting activities of caring to a new social

context, with the demands for women to participate in the paid workforce in Canada. Caring is defined as being culturally constructed and mediated by social forces according to contexts as well as to caregivers' positions in the social world. For instance, Haitian Canadian women caregivers must renegotiate and re-pattern family dynamics in the host society to implicate their husbands or spouses in sharing domestic tasks. Renegotiation of family dynamics sometimes generates clashes between spouses but nevertheless constitutes the basis upon which Haitian Canadian women caregivers can alleviate the triple-task of working outside, parenting children, and caring for aging parents at home. It is not intended to apply Wuest's theory (1998) of "precarious ordering and repatterning" to Haitian Canadian women caregivers; however, it is contended that the repatterning of family dynamics associated with immigration represents a strategy used by Haitian Canadian women to balance the competing demands of caring with those of the social world. Wuest (2000) defines the process of repatterning as a strategy aimed at "reorganizing caring activities, to reduce or overcome the negative effects of caring demands" (p. 393).

Influence of the Gendering of Caring on Caregivers' Familial and Social Life

We now turn to explore how the gendering of caring influences caregivers' familial lives. Results illustrate how gender expectations influence relationships within families and mother-daughter relations. For instance, daughters-in-law are expected to care for their in-laws and some mothers can control their daughters' lives precluding them to marry and having their own family. This is followed by an examination of the influence of gendering of caring on caregivers' social lives. Findings show that both men and women caregivers must cut down on social activities to care for their aging relatives at home. Working women, who juggle the triple-task issue, seem to be most vulnerable to social isolation. No boundaries between the private and public spheres (e.g., between working outside, performing domestic chores, looking after the family, and caring for aging relatives) can be clearly drawn. This situation not only applies to Haitian Canadian women caregivers. The cross-cultural effect of gender on caring activities and its effects on women caregivers' family lives and economic welfare have been documented in non-Western and Western societies (Atkin & Rollings, 1996; Bunting, 1992; Climo, 2000; Doyal, 1995; Guberman, Maheu & Maillé, 1993; Guberman & Maheu, 1997; Neufeld & Harrison, 2000; Neufeld & Harrison, 2003; Waxler-Morrison, 1990).

Atkin and Rollings (1996) report that in the UK, some Asian and Caribbean women experience a general sense of isolation, resulting from the lack of support from close relatives and the increasing level of their caring commitment. Waxler-Morrison (1990) emphasizes the impact of migration on families and ways of living among

Western Canadian ethnic and cultural groups. Finally, Neufeld and Harrison (2000; 2003) mention that issues located at the intersection of domestic work, labor market demands, and gender expectations related to caring activities, influence North American women caregivers' familial and social lives.

Influence of Gendering of Caring on Familial Life

Gender expectations influence relationships within families in the sense that sons often rely on their wives to look after their own parents. A woman who cares for both her mother and her mother-in-law illustrates that the sharing of domestic tasks coupled with caring activities becomes a sensitive issue, for the couple. Joy has a university degree but in her roles as woman, wife, daughter, and caregiver, few differences are perceived from other women. All of the women face the same issue when it comes to the sharing of domestic duties with their spouses. She said:

> Sometimes I came back from work, sometimes I came back home very late, and I'm good for nothing. I'm very tired. I can't do anything and I just want to go to sleep. I can only look after myself but then, my husband asks me: "Can you cook something tonight? Can you cook something for the supper? We need to eat." It's always the woman who is accountable for the meals.

Reconciling family life with caring can be difficult and especially straining for the working woman. It is also observed, in some participant observation sessions, that relations could be very tense between fathers-in-law and sons-in-law. Not only did the mothers-in-law seem to be uncomfortable living with their sons-in-law, but fathers-in-law can experience the same situation, as well. Presented now are some interview segments to illustrate how the gendering of caring influences relationships between daughters-in-law and mothers-in-law. A woman participant described the differences between caring for her mother as opposed to her mother-in-law:

> In general, women are held responsible for caring for the elderly. Women have a moral duty to care for the aging people. See for instance, my mother-in-law lives with us. My husband, sure, he cares for her and he thinks about her. It's sure but I've to think twice since if she needs something, she asks her son and then he passes this on me.

Another woman, who was also caring for her in-laws, expressed the same idea of feeling more committed to caring for her in-laws, than was her husband. For these caregivers, it seems the relations with mothers-in-law are more complex when it comes to affective caring. The situation is the same for sons-in-law who cannot get along with their mothers-in-law. This lends support to the results from studies on daughters (Mui, 1995; Pohl, Boyd, Liang & Given, 1995; Sheehan & Dornorfio, 1999), daughters-in-law (Globerman, 1996; Guberman, 1999), and sons' differences, in their caregiving roles

(Campbell, 2000), to name a few. Blood ties and the affective depth of the mother-daughter relationships have an impact on caring activities. Daughters seem more comfortable with their mothers and the mothers seem to be less at ease with daughters- or sons-in-laws.

Gendering of caring has an impact on women caregivers' social lives, and more specifically on working women, by restraining the women's and their spouse's involvement in social or leisure activities. Data also demonstrates that men caregivers appear to be socially isolated despite not having to face the triple-task issue, as do their female counterparts. For men and women caregivers, it seems that little or no time is left for them to engage in social activities. Caregivers must adapt their social lives to the needs of the cared persons.

Influence of Gendering of Caring on Social Life

The influence of caring for aging relatives at home on the caregiver's social life is apparent, especially when the researcher spends time with caregivers and their families. Nevertheless, caregivers adapt to their situations using two specific coping strategies. The first consists of bringing the aging parents with them to the restaurant or to visit relatives for religious holidays or birthday parties. The second strategy is to limit social activities and cut back on leisure time to stay with the aging relatives. Both women and men caregivers' interview excerpts are presented to demonstrate how the restriction on social life affects both genders.

Alexandra reported that caring limits her social activities. On weekends, she has a respite since her father goes to another daughter's home, allowing her to be by herself for a short time. She is a busy woman who works full-time and has to perform almost all of the domestic duties. She describes her social life:

> Fortunately, I get this respite during weekends. It helps a lot you know. Otherwise, I'd feel like a prisoner in that house, I'd feel like being jailed. When mummy was staying with me, well usually, my parents came with us. I've never been somewhere without bringing mum and dad with me.

Caring also impacts Kathleen's social life since the couple and the family must adapt their social activities to the needs of their aging mother:

> When we go dining out or attending social events, we need to come back home earlier to put her in bed. Otherwise, we would feel guilty to come back at 3 a.m. and let her moan for such a long time. We come back home as soon as possible. If we go to attend a family party, she comes with us. When she's tired, we must come back home earlier too. So this is the picture . . . it impacts at this level.

A young woman, who also works full-time, commented that her social life is important, too. She reported that she also must take into account her own needs, if she is to continue in her caring commitment:

> Sometimes I'm tired and I also want to breathe some air. I'd like to be free a bit, not feeling this obligation to come back home immediately after work. I'd like to go downtown, sit at a terrace, and enjoy life.

It seems this younger caregiver raises another issue, an issue of gendering: Is it easier for men caregivers to have a social life? The next interview excerpts show that men and women do not differ much in that regard. As mentioned earlier, men also report feelings of social isolation as a result from their caring activities.

Contrasting Women's and Men's Perspectives

In a first interview, a man caregiver reported that caring does not have an impact on his social life but other male caregivers reported not having an enjoyable social life. John discusses his social life and mentions that caring activities do not impinge on his social activities: "We never complain. It's in our culture. It's not something we're forced to do; it's natural. There's no obligation. It's cultural." He suggested that his work and working environment were also stressful and hindered him from enjoying a social life:

> I find life much more stressful here [in Canada]. Since I remember, when I was in Haiti, I was working from 6 a.m. to 7 p.m. and I was never tired. I came back home, took a shower, and could go to the theatre. However, here, once my day at work is over, I'm too tired to go out. It's so different. Here I work 8 hours and I'm already tired when my shift is over. I mean I'm more tired than the time when I was working 12 hours in a row. Then, after a day at work, I can't go out and I stay in. That's what I do. It's so different. It's so different. The way of living is stressful.

Edward, a man in his sixties, who was caring for aging relatives from Haiti also reported that he had no social life:

> Social life? I don't have any social life now but I really don't care about it. I can't get out of the house. I don't want to leave them alone here. I'd need to call somebody to keep them for a couple of hours. Most of the time, I stay here. I don't go out. As well, going out is expensive and I can't really afford it. On the weekends, my wife and I, we go to the market (name of the market). I go to the market or the grocery store. It's my social life.

A man caregiver spoke about his restricted social life saying that interactions between Haitian immigrants and mainstream men and women are very restricted. The impact of caring cannot be isolated as a major cause of social isolation among both men and women caregivers. Many contextual factors pertaining to the larger social world can be associated with the lack of social activities such as work and racial relations. For instance, this caregiver mentioned that he could not go to the bowling centre since very few Haitian Canadians would be present. It is like a perceived process of "othering" precluded this caregiver to enjoy social life. As well, economic factors can explain why some caregivers prefer to stay home since going out means an extra cost to caring. The economic factor should be further examined since caregivers need to pay a "keeper," therefore increasing the cost of an evening at the restaurant or theatre. Caring for an aging relative at home implies an economic cost of caring, which is often overlooked since it is invisible. These findings lend support to Waxler-Morrison (1990) who states that "the disruption of life associated with migration affects many people from different cultures in similar ways. Much has been lost; family ties, familiar language, community support, the comfort that comes from the general predictability of life" (p. 6-7). Again, this finding is not exclusive to Haitian Canadian caregivers. The impact of the lack of leisure time on women's health and unpaid caregiving experiences has been studies among a group of Caucasian women in Nova Scotia (Gahagan, Loppie, Rehman, Maclellan & Side, 2006) addressing the important component of self care activities among this group of caregivers.

The Impact of Paid Work on Caring

The impact of paid work on caring cannot be isolated from the opposite, which is the influence of caring on work, as these phenomena are intertwined and mutually influence each other. bell hooks (2000) points out "when women in the home spend all their time attending to the needs of others, home is a workplace for her, not a site of relaxation, comfort, and pleasure" (p. 50). Haitian Canadian women caregivers involved in paid work and caring activities are almost always on duty. For instance, Kathleen is a professional who works full-time on evening shifts. When she comes back home around 1:00 a.m., she goes to her mother. She needs to alternate her mother's position at least twice a night to prevent bedsores. She wakes up to prepare her children for school and then goes back to sleep. When I asked her if she encountered problems in caring for her mother, she immediately referred to her work. She said:

> Of course, it [caring activities] does not fit with my working hours. Sometimes, I simply run out of time, I don't have the time since I'm working outside the home. I have no choice. I must work. I told you before that I'm a (name of occupation), and I'm scheduled to work on shifts. I also have children and I must look after them too. And it takes . . . [Silence] . . . It takes a bit of my own comfort. It cuts my sleeping hours but I do it. The problem is having shorter hours of sleep.

Paula, like Kathleen, is one of the younger women caregivers who participated in the study (she was in her late 30s). The lack of sleep did not affect her health. It is not possible to talk of the burden of care in this situation, since Paula's teenaged daughter sometimes assists in caring for her grandmother. Nevertheless, this interview excerpt also illustrates that caring and paid work (private and public spheres) cannot easily be separated from each other. The situation is like a continuum where caring and working outside the home mutually influence each other and neither aspect can be dealt with in isolation. Then, the conversation was shifted to present a hypothetical situation to ask her what she would do if her mother felt acutely ill. She answered: "It would be economically, a little difficult, since it would be less money in our pockets. It would surely have an impact on the family's budget."

This woman's work is essential for bringing in money for the family and supports the soaring needs from a market economy, but it also covers expenses related to caring. Paula said that her husband would find it difficult if he were the only breadwinner in the family since Paula earns higher wages. The assumption seems to be valid in that the host country's economy and home care policies affect ways of caring since women have no choice but to enter the workforce and earn a living. Also, this example supports the notion of the devaluation of the unpaid work of caring, because it is women's duty. Caring must not affect workplace efficiency, but problems at the workplace affect caring activities.

During a participant observation in a woman caregiver's family, it was noticed how busy she was parenting her young children and caring for her aging mother. She works full-time and earns good wages but has to pay for the rent, groceries, children's kindergarten, and other utilities. The participant told me she was depressed. She said she felt overwhelmed and swamped by responsibilities, since she is accountable for doing so many tasks. Another caregiver reported the problems she was having in attempting to reconcile work outside of the home with her caring activities:

> When I come back home, it's already dark outside. It's past 5:00 p.m. I come back and change my clothes. I never sit down when I come back from work since I won't be able to stay up and prepare the meal. I go to the kitchen to cook and sometimes I'm so exhausted that I crouch down on the kitchen counter. I cook the meal, I serve the people, and then I sit down and eat. After, I must help the kids with their homework. Sometimes I do that in my bed since I can barely stand up.

This woman also reported being torn between her multiple roles as wife, mother, daughter, and worker. She found she was not doing enough for her aging mother; she would like to do more for her. So far, these women, who are both raising young children, seem extremely busy and feel they do not have much time to devote to their aging parents. They care for them, but not to the extent to which they would like. As well, they need to work and it has an impact on caring by decreasing the amount of time spent with the aging parents. Demands, related to housekeeping and parenting, are also high and add up to the already significant workload for these women.

Other events, which are directly associated with the workplace, also have an impact on men's and women's caring commitment. More specifically, racial discrimination and sexism at work and at school have an impact on caring activities and the decision made by caregivers to not utilize the health care system. Issues pertaining to the social world must not be overlooked since they account for a major part of the caregiver's subjective burden. It is not caring *per se*, or hands-on activities that induce sleeplessness, stress, fatigue, depression, and other physical and psychological manifestations. Sexual division of labor, the influence of a market economy, racial discrimination, and sexual harassment compose the larger social context within which caring activities occur. Thus far, results show that it is a challenge for women to clearly separate paid work and caring activities. It seems as if caring continues at work and work continues at home, influencing caring activities, caregivers and care-receivers. As Doyal (1995) points out:

> The most obvious characteristics of *domestic work* in all countries [italics added] are probably its open-endedness and its sheer volume. There is no limit to how much can be required in a given period, and no entitlement to holidays or even meal breaks. Very importantly there may be no obvious end to the working day, so that many find it difficult to separate work from rest or "leisure." Indeed those with young children may never really be "off duty" as working hours even extend to periods of snatched sleep. For many, this can lead to a punishing burden of both physical and mental labor. (p. 28)

A male caregiver reported that when he returned from work, he could relax. He clearly divides his paid work from his private life but does not share in the domestic tasks with his wife: "The working place is the working place. When I work, I think about my work. When I get back home, I forget the work."

Nevertheless, it may be assumed that the more likely men are to get involved in caring activities, the more likely they are to not be able to clearly divide their private and public spheres. Matthew, for example, cares for his wife and Harold looks after his cousins. In a participant observation session at Harold's home, it was observed that he was at the stove in the same way as are women. Harold, who is 65 years old, is now retired and does not need to go to work outside of the home and to care for young children. The similarity of the lived experiences that men caregivers, who do not share in household tasks or who are retired, have caring for their wives or aging mothers, is not comparable to the women caregivers' experiences. In general, men do not experience women's triple-task burden. The social context and the demands on men are different, though, Matthew's case is an exception.

A man caregiver clearly described the impact of caring on his work since he had decided not to apply for job promotions. Matthew said that he was already exhausted with the situation at home with his wife and his children and that he could not get any more stress in his life. He basically avoids all stressful situations, as a survival strategy, since he feels that he would reach his breaking point. He cannot do overtime work, which affects his family's finances, since Matthew is the sole breadwinner and his wife can no longer work outside of the home like she did before her illness. Furthermore, Matthew cannot stay later at his work since he must come home to look after his wife and work out any issues related to the five children or to her illness.

Conclusion

This chapter has demonstrated the expression coined by the late Michelle Rosaldo (as cited in Lugo & Maurer, 2000) "gender matters" when it comes to explaining women's struggle with issues related to the binary opposition of domestic and private spheres. Gender intersects with immigration to create difficulties in negotiating and redefining family dynamics while trying to preserve some cultural values inherited from the native country. For Haitian Canadian women caregivers, the gendering of caring activities is marked by a "double oppression," in that women are torn between the native and host country's patriarchy and the process of racialization that mediates ethnic groups relations in the host society. Gandhi (1998) posits that "third-world women," as victim *par excellence*, are "the forgotten casualties of both imperial ideology, and native and foreign patriarchies" (p. 83).

After examining the gendering of caring activities, it may be assumed that a reconfiguration of family dynamics can only be achieved if Haitian Canadian men show a willingness to share in the domestic duties with the women. A reconfiguration of family dynamics points to the equalization of the previously asymmetrical power relationships between men and women, in a community where domestic tasks are assigned to the private sphere, and designated as belonging to the women's domain. On the other hand, the involvement of Haitian Canadian men in accomplishing household tasks is a means to an end, and would alleviate the Haitian Canadian women's workload. Although progress has been noticed, the results demonstrate that a compromise and sharing of domestic tasks is yet to be achieved. Nevertheless, women also contribute to construct the gendering of domestic work and caring activities by keeping men away from the kitchen – a form of sexism, since aging Haitian Canadian mothers were afraid that their sons would be feminized if allowed to perform some domestic work. The situation is clearly changing as described by one woman who encourages her sons to cook and to get used to it, since third-generation Haitian Canadian women are less likely to act like their Haitian-born mothers.

The gendering of caring activities only represents the tip of the iceberg when examining the experience of caring for aging parents at home among the Haitian Canadian community. Race, gender, and class intersect with the process of "othering" to affect the relations with mainstream society. It is not without its impact on Haitian Canadian caregivers' everyday lives, ways of caring, and perceptions about home care services and mainstream health care providers.

The influence of immigration in redefining family dynamics of Haitian Canadian families was examined in providing a detailed description of the lived experiences of both men and women caregivers. Findings illustrate the social, cultural, and economic impact of caring among older immigrants. Immigration and late arrival of family members is not without influencing family dynamics when adapting to the culture and social norms of the new country. For instance, immigration makes it necessary for Haitian women to involve husbands or spouses in the sharing of domestic tasks and care giving activities. Rather than solely focusing on gender to explain inequities in caring for an aging Haitian parent in Canada, the use of a postcolonial theoretical lens accounted for the examination of the broader social and cultural context within which caring activities unfold in the new country as opposed to Haiti. A postcolonial feminist perspective addresses care giving issues to uncover the social, political, economic, and cultural determinants that underpin family caregivers' construction of experiences of caring for aging relatives at home. Results show the relevance of locating Haitian Canadian caregivers' experiences in a larger social perspective where caring is understood in all its layers of complexity. Without locating Haitian Canadian caregivers' experiences of caring in a broader social perspective, the contextual factors that structure caring activities may be overlooked or silenced.

References

Anderson, J.M. (2000a). Writing in subjugated knowledges: Towards a transformative agenda in nursing research. *Nursing Inquiry, 7*(3), 145.

Anderson, J.M. (2000b). Gender, "race," poverty, health and discourses of health reform in the context of globalization: A postcolonial feminist perspective in policy research. *Nursing Inquiry, 7*(4), 220-229.

Atkin, K. & Rollings, J. (1996). Looking after their own? Family caregiving among Asian and Afro-Caribbean communities. In W.I.U. Ahmad & K. Atkin. (Eds.), *"Race" and community care.* (pp. 73-86). Buckingham, UK & Philadelphia, PA: Open University Press.

Bunting, S.M. (1992). Eve's legacy: An analysis of family caregiving from a feminist perspective. In J. Thompson, D.G. Allen & L. Rodrigues-Fisher (Eds.), *Critique, resistance, and action. Working papers in the politics of nursing,* (pp. 53-68). New York: National League for Nursing Press.

Campbell, L.D. (2000). Caring sons: Exploring men's involvement in filial care. *Canadian Journal on Aging, 19*(1), 57-79.

Climo, J.J. (2000). Eldercare as "women work" in poor countries. *Journal of Family Issues, 21*(6), 692-713.

Covan, E.K. (1997). Cultural priorities and elder care: The impact of women. *Health Care for Women International, 18*, 329-342.

Collins, P.H. (2000). It's all in the family: Intersection of gender, race, and nation. In U. Narayan & S. Harding (Eds.), *Decentering the center. Philosophy for a multicultural, postcolonial, and feminist world.* (pp. 156-176). Bloomington & Indianapolis: Indiana University Press.

Doyal, L. (1995). *What makes women sick: Gender and the political economy of health.* New Brunswick, NJ: Rutgers University Press.

Gahagan, J., Loppie, C., Rehman, L., Maclellan, M. & Side, K. (2006). "Far as I get is the clothesline": The impact of leisure on women's health and unpaid caregiving experiences in Nova Scotia, Canada. *Health Care for Women International, 28*, 47-68.

Gandhi, L. (1998). *Postcolonial theory: A critical introduction.* New York, NY: Columbia University Press.

Globerman, J. (1996). Motivations to care: Daughters- and sons-in-law caring for relatives with Alzheimers' disease. *Family Relations, 45*, 37-45.

Guberman, N. (1999). Daughters-in-law as caregivers: How and why do they come to care? *Journal of Women & Aging, 11*(1), 85-102.

Guberman, N. & Maheu, P. (1997). *Les soins aux personnes âgées dans les familles d'origine italienne et haïtienne.* Montréal, QC: Éditions du Remue-Ménage.

Guberman, N., Maheu, P. & Maillé, C. (1993). *Et si l'amour ne suffisait pas . . .* Montréal, QC: Éditions du Remue-Ménage.

Hall, S. (1997). *Representation: Cultural representations and signifying practices.* London & Milton Keynes, UK: Sage & The Open University.

hooks, bell. (2000). *Feminism is for everybody:. Passionate politics.* Cambridge, MA: South End Press.

Hooyman, N.R. & Gonyea, J. (1995). *Feminist perspective on family care: Policies for gender justice.* Thousand Oaks, CA: Sage.

Laguerre, M.S. (1984). *American Odyssey:* Haitians in New York. Ithaca, NY & London, UK: Cornell University Press.

Lugo, A. & Maurer, B. (2000).The legacy of Michelle Rosaldo: Politics and gender in modern societies. In A. Lugo & B. Maurer (Eds.), *Gender matters: Rereading Michelle Z. Rosaldo.* (pp. 16-34). Ann Arbor, MI: The University of Michigan Press.

Massé, R. (1983). *L'émergence de l'ethnicité haïtienne au Québec.* Thèse de doctorat. Faculté des Sciences Sociales. Département d'anthropologie. Université Laval. Canada.

Meleis, A.I. & Im, E.O. (1999). Transcending marginalization in knowledge development. *Nursing Inquiry, 6*(2), 94-102.

Mui, A.C. (1995). Caring for frail elderly parents: A comparison of adult sons and daughters. *The Gerontologist, 35*(1), 86-93.

Neufeld, A. & Harrison, M.J. (2000). Family caregiving: Issues in gaining access so support. In M.J. Stewart (Ed.), *Chronic conditions and caregiving in Canada.* (pp. 245-273), Toronto: University of Toronto Press.

Neufeld, A. & Harrison, M.J. (2003). Unfulfilled expectations and negative interactions: Nonsupport in the relationships of women caregivers. *Journal of Advanced Nursing, 41*(4), 323-331.

Pohl, J.M., Boyd, C., Liang, J. & Given, C.W. (1995). Analysis of the impact of mother-daughter relationships on the commitment to caregiving. *Nursing Research, 44*(2), 68-75.

Quayson, A. (2000). *Postcolonialism: Theory, practice or process?* Cambridge, UK: Polity Press.

Racine, L. (2003). Implementing a postcolonial feminist perspective in nursing research related to non-Western populations. *Nursing Inquiry 10*(2), 91-102.

Racine, L. (2004). *The meaning of home care and caring for aging relatives at home: The Haitian Canadian primary caregivers' perspectives.* Unpublished doctoral dissertation, University of British Columbia, Vancouver, British Columbia, Canada.

Schutte, O. (2000). Cultural alterity: Cross-cultural communication in feminist theory in North-South contexts. In U. Narayan & S. Harding (Eds.), *Decentering the center: Philosophy for a multicultural, postcolonial, and feminist worlds.* (pp. 47-66). Bloomington & Indianapolis: Indiana University Press.

Sheehan, N.W. & Donorfio, L.M. (1999). Efforts to create meaning in the relationship between aging mothers and their caregiving daughters: A qualitative study of caregiving. *Journal of Aging Studies, 13*(2), 161-176.

Smith, D.E. (1987). *The everyday world as problematic: A feminist sociology.* Toronto, ON: University of Toronto Press.

Stepick, A. (1998). *Pride against prejudice: Haitians in the United States.* Needham Heights, MA: Allyn & Bacon.

Waxler-Morrison, N. (1990). Introduction. In N. Waxler-Morrison, J. Anderson & E. Richardson (Eds.), *Cross-cultural caring. A handbook for health professionals.* (pp. 3-10). Vancouver, BC: UBC Press.

Wuest, J. (1993). Institutionalizing women's oppression: The inherent risk in health policy that fosters community participation. *Health Care for Women International, 14,* 407-417.

Wuest, J. (1998). Setting boundaries: A strategy for precarious ordering of women's caring demands. *Research in Nursing & Health, 21,* 39-49.

Wuest, J. (2000). Repatterning care: Women's proactive management of family caregiving demands. *Health Care for Women International, 21,* 393-411.

Acknowledgments

I am grateful to Haitian-Canadians who participated in this study. I thank Dr. Joan Anderson from the School of Nursing at the University of British Columbia for providing me with her comments and support in writing my Ph.D. dissertation. I thank the National Health Research Program Development (NHRDP) and the Canadian Institutes of Health Research (CIHR) for their financial support.

18

An Exploration of the Factors Impacting Upon Elderly Ukrainian Immigrant Women

Nuelle Novik, (University of Regina)

The population of Canada is aging and this older population is predominantly female (Statistics Canada, 2007). Due primarily to the sheer force of demographics, the study of aging has necessarily become a women's issue (Ray, 1996). The total Canadian population over the age of 65 years also has a very high ethnic composition, meaning that many of these individuals were born outside of Canada (Ujimoto, 1995). It is currently estimated that one in every four Canadian seniors was born elsewhere.

In recent years, there has been more emphasis in the health, social service and social work literature on lifestyle and quality of life issues across the lifespan. This has resulted in an increase in the body of research which examines quality of life issues specific to older individuals. However, much of this research has been deficit-based and problems-driven, with a focus primarily upon issues related to physical health (Higgs, Hyde, Wiggins & Blane, 2003; Sarvimaki & Stenbock-Hult, 2000). This orientation has been questioned as recognition of the complexity of quality of life issues has increased (Higgs et al., 2003). This is not to suggest that health and health-related issues do not impact upon quality of life throughout the lifespan. However, it is important to recognize that there are other factors, in addition to physical health, which have an impact upon perceived life quality. Consequently, more recent research has highlighted the relevance of a variety of domains and determinants when evaluating the quality of life of older people.

Largely absent from the quality of life literature is an acknowledgement of the impacts that early life stage immigration might have for individuals as they age in place. There has been a marked increase in research studies which look at issues surrounding ethnicity and aging (MacLean & Sakadakis, 1989). However, these studies do not focus upon the possible impact that immigration may have had for older members of ethnic populations who have lived the majority of their lives in the country in which they settled.

The process of immigration can be very difficult (Djao & Ng, 1987; Rasmussen, Rasmussen, Savage & Wheeler, 1976; Stambrook & Hryniuk, 2000). The experiences that Ukrainian women have had in terms of immigration and settlement have impacted upon their life in Canada and upon their current quality of life as they have aged. The trauma associated with the original immigration, the struggles and hardships of assimilation and the experiences of aging over the life-span, in a place other than the country of one's birth, are important issues. It is almost impossible to assume that these events would not have some direct impact upon quality of life in old age (Kostash, 2000; Seiler, 1996; O'Connor, 2003; Swyripa, 1993). Ukrainian women continue to be an under-studied segment of the population. Although Swyripa (2000; 1993; 1978) has produced a significant body of research examining Ukrainian women in Canada, there has been little systematic study of the role of Ukrainian Canadian women, nor about their role in the immigration process (Stambrook & Hryniuk, 2000).

Ukrainian Canadians have a unique history. As one of the largest ethnic groups that came to Canada through planned immigration and nation-building policies, Ukrainian Canadians have lived in this country for more than four generations (Luciuk, 2000; Swyripa, 1978). Many of the Ukrainian women that came to Canada, especially during the second wave of immigration, continue to be active members of their families and their communities. Their experiences may be relevant to future immigrant populations who settle and age in this country.

This chapter focuses upon a research study that examined the factors impacting upon the quality of life of elderly Ukrainian first generation immigrant women from their own perspectives, as well as from the perspectives of a daughter and a granddaughter. While there is much written which documents the history of Ukrainian immigrants in Canada, this history has consistently not included a female perspective. The literature demonstrates that the female immigration experience can be quite different than the male experience (Omidvar & Richmond, 2005). These particular differences have impacted the lives of first generation Ukrainian immigrant women, as well as subsequent generations of their daughters and granddaughters.

This chapter will begin with a definition of relevant terms, and will then explore a brief history of Ukrainian immigration to Canada, as well as a more specific history of Ukrainian immigrant women. This history will include a focus upon gender based roles and the impact of relationships. A brief overview of the research methods will then be presented. The results of the research will be discussed, and the chapter will conclude with an examination of the implications for practice and service delivery.

Definition of Terms

Within social science and health research, terms referring to older members of society remain loosely defined (Cheal & Kampen, 1998). While the term *seniors* most often refers to older people aged 55 to 64, the term *elderly* refers to those aged 65 and over (Cheal & Kampen, 1998; Green, 1993; Hilleras, Pollitt, Medway & Ericsson, 2000). Other terms used within the literature include *older, elderly people,* and *older people* (Green, 1993). Within this chapter, the terms most often used will be *elderly* and *older*. The term used throughout this chapter to refer to the grandmothers is the Ukrainian term "Baba."

The term *first generation* refers to those foreign-born participants who immigrated to Canada. The term *second generation* refers to Canadian-born participants with at least one foreign-born parent (Hansen & Kucera, 2004). *Third generation* refers to Canadian-born participants with Canadian-born parents.

History of Ukrainian Immigration to Canada

The majority of Canadians of Ukrainian descent originally immigrated from the western provinces of Galicia and Bukovyna (Doroshenko, 1914; Kaye, 1964; Himka, 1982; Keywan & Coles, 1977; Lehr, 1983). At the time of initial immigration, Ukraine had been occupied by the Austro-Hungarian Empire (Keywan & Coles, 1977). Historically, while Ukraine had abundant and rich agricultural land, the country lacked geographical barriers against powerful invaders. As a result, Ukraine has been an easy target for invasions from all directions throughout history. Following the Mongol destruction of the original Ukrainian state in the 13th century, Ukrainian lands were largely dominated by Russia, Poland, Austria and Hungary (Doroshenko, 1914; Gerus & Rea, 1985). The Ukrainian aristocracy that survived the invasions over the years tended to assimilate quickly under the influence of the ruling and invading power. Consequently, the Ukrainian nation remained essentially peasant in character (Doroshenko, 1914; Luciuk, 2000; Woycenko, 1967). Ukraine became severely over-populated and the wealthy landlords who managed huge landholdings released little land for peasant people. With each passing generation, family property was divided amongst the children ensuring that individual family landholdings became progressively smaller (Keywan & Coles, 1977).

There were three main waves of Ukrainian immigration to Canada. The first wave occurred between 1890 and 1914, prior to the First World War (Barlow & Barlow, 2003; Woycenko, 1967; Yuzyk, 1967). Ukrainian immigrants during this first phase numbered approximately 170 000 with the majority coming from the two western provinces of the Austro-Hungarian Empire (Barlow & Barlow, 2003; Ostryzniuk, 2002; Yuzyk, 1967). This wave saw gender differences in new arrivals within both the peasant community and the Ukrainian intelligentsia. Although families were still encouraged to move together, men far outnumbered women at that time. This resulted in the male domination of community life in the bloc settlements and within the larger national picture (Lysenko, 1947; Swyripa, 1993).

The second wave of Ukrainian immigration to Canada occurred during the inter-war period between 1919 and 1939 (Barlow & Barlow, 2003; Yuzyk, 1967). This wave brought in approximately 68 000 settlers, almost all from the regions of western Ukraine (Barlow & Barlow, 2003). The reasons for coming to Canada at this time continued to centre upon economic and political motivations.

The period between 1947 and 1954, known as the third wave of Ukrainian immigration to Canada, brought approximately 34 000 Ukrainian refugees from camps across Europe following the Second World War (Barlow & Barlow, 2003; Cipko, 1991; Gerus & Rea, 1985; Woycenko, 1967). The biggest difference between these third wave immigrants and their predecessors lay in the fact that they had been forced from their homeland (Barlow & Barlow, 2003). As a result, many who came to Canada did so with the intent of someday returning home to a free Ukraine (Barlow & Barlow, 2003; Yuzyk, 1967). Their arrival raised some concern amongst the Ukrainian Canadians who had settled previously (Yuzyk, 1967). Although they were quick to welcome the newcomers, there was also a fear that they might resist or damage the gains that had been made towards assimilation. However, the postwar immigrants did manage to establish a strong presence in Canada while still valuing Ukrainian culture and reviving the use of Ukrainian language (Barlow & Barlow, 2003).

Ukrainians also found themselves in conflict with Anglo-Canadians upon their initial arrival in Canada. Known as "Ruthenians" or "Galicians" during the first half of the twentieth century, Ukrainians found their early attempts to establish themselves in Canada to be very difficult. This difficulty was largely due to high levels of unemployment and anti-foreign sentiment aroused by the First World War (Kaye & Swyripa, 1982; Ostryzniuk, 2002). Ukrainians were not only the largest group of immigrants to arrive in Canada at that time, they were also the most conspicuous in terms of appearance and behavior (Luciuk, 2000; Martynowych, 1983). Swyripa (1983) described a relationship in which Anglo-Canadians saw Ukrainian immigrants as individuals who were "desirable as laborers and agriculturalists but possessing questionable ideals and ways of life" (p. 47). Lysenko (1947) notes that Ukrainians were "systematically underpaid and provided a cheap source of labor for building up the Canadian west and the heavy industries of the east" (p. 109). Barlow and Barlow (2003) discuss the fact that "Ukrainians were viewed as the scum of Europe – physical and moral degenerates not fit to be classified as white" (p. 230). The hostile attitudes towards them persisted for decades in the memories of the Ukrainian pioneers (Kaye & Swyripa, 1982).

Each of the three waves of Ukrainian immigration produced three very different kinds of settlers based upon the different circumstances unfolding in both Ukraine and Canada at the time of immigration (Barlow & Barlow, 2003; Keywan & Coles, 1977; Woycenko, 1967; Yuzyk, 1967). The first group was overwhelmingly of peasant farmer origin with little education. They acquired homesteads and farms and established new communities across the prairies (Barlow & Barlow, 2003; Driedger, 1996; Yuzyk, 1967). The second group possessed higher levels of education and had been participants in the Ukrainian struggle for freedom at the end of the First World War. Although many still settled into the agricultural sector upon arrival, most Ukrainian immigrants who came to Canada during the second wave moved into urban centres during the Depression years (Yuzyk, 1967). The third wave, largely political refugees, was comprised of skilled tradesmen, professionals and scholars from the urban areas of Ukraine. Most of these individuals settled in urban centres with an industrial based economy (Yuzyk, 1967). Each of the three waves of Ukrainian immigration brought Ukrainian women to Canada. This next section will explore their unique history in this country.

History of Ukrainian Immigrant Women

In order to understand the history of Ukrainian immigrant women in Canada, it is helpful to examine their numbers upon arrival. The first wave of immigration brought approximately 41 000 females, the second wave brought 21 000, and the third wave brought approximately 13 000 Ukrainian women to Canada (Petryshyn, 1980). The general trends identified in terms of the characterizations of Ukrainian immigrants holds true for the female segment of that population as well. However, while the first wave of female immigrants was largely comprised of the wives of peasants, there is evidence that there were some single women who came as well (Petryshyn, 1980; Swyripa, 1993). The literature suggests that one of the motivations for these single women to come to Canada was the fact that there was a shortage of men available to them at home in Ukraine (Petryshyn, 1980; Romaniuk & Chuiko, 1999). Large numbers of men immigrated and many men had been killed during the wars. This had seriously diminished the number of males in Ukraine. Those women who did come on their own without spouses or families were often restricted to agricultural labor or domestic services (Rasmussen et al., 1976). These occupations coincided with the "entrance status" sought by the Government of Canada in bringing female immigrants into the country (Petryshyn, 1980).

The dependent and minority status of most Ukrainian women kept them isolated and hidden from active participation in Canadian society for many years (Swyripa, 1993). While the men were required to leave and seek work across the country for months at a time, the women were left to maintain the homestead on their own (Lehr, 1983; Luciuk, 2000; Smith, 1922; Swyripa, 1993). These long periods of isolation left the Ukrainian woman with "social contacts limited to those of her own nationality and language" (Kaye & Swyripa, 1982, p. 47). Although they received little recognition, these women did carry all of the necessary work at the homestead in their husband's absence. It is noted that these women were extremely hard workers and that "they proved they could wield an axe or a grub hoe as well as any man" (Keywan & Coles, 1977). However, conditions still reinforced patriarchy and the traditional role of the female within the family socioeconomic unit (Swyripa, 1993). There is a proverb which states "let a wife be like a cow so long as she is strong" (Bridger, 1992, p. 281). In examining the historical roles of women, Ostryzniuk (1997) states that "the Ukrainian woman's role was a traditional one of dependence and subordination in a patriarchal society, and this cultural baggage was brought to Canada" (p. 24).

The historic gender roles predominant in the Old Country found their way to Canada in other ways as well. For example, young Ukrainian Canadian women were expected to marry young and raise a family (Ostryzniuk, 1997; Swyripa, 1993). It was not uncommon for marriages to be arranged for girls as young as age 13 or 14 to men who were much older and who had immigrated to Canada earlier (Connor, 1909; Ostryzniuk, 1997; Wolowyna, 1980). In this way, many of the marital traditions of life as it had been in Ukraine took root on Canadian soil (Worobec, 1992). The nature of immigrant society in Canada, at that time, saw these young women mentored into their societal roles by their mothers and isolated within culturally contained Ukrainian communities (Seiler, 1996). This resulted in the further marginalization of these women as they continued to function within the restrictions of their peasant culture (Kirtz, 1996; Ostryzniuk, 1997; Stambrook & Hryniuk, 2000; Swyripa, 1993).

It was also the marginalization and the isolation of these women that brought them a great deal of attention from the host Canadian society. Observing the way that they lived, and the customs that governed their lives, Anglo-Canadians saw these women as backward and naive. With an overall goal of assimilation and with the Ukrainian intelligentsia taking the lead, the Ukrainian community began to recognize that they had to organize in such a way as to better meet the standards and values of the host society. They believed, that they had to demonstrate that they were equal to other Canadians (Ostryzniuk, 1997).

While the expectations to integrate and conform increased, so too did the pressure to maintain cultural identity. Anderson (1976) stated that "a higher proportion of Ukrainian Orthodox and Ukrainian Catholic females than males tended to favor identity preservation" (p. 101). Thus began an intensified campaign to feverishly protect Ukrainian culture. In essence, Ukrainian culture came to be represented by a wide variety of customs which contributed to the maintenance of a unique ethnic identity. These customs included Ukrainian foods, crafts, dress, and techniques for building homes, ways of decorating those homes, types of farming, performing arts, and kinship networks (Anderson, 1976). Women have always been the ones to transform tradition. It is what they learn from their mothers, fathers, their kin, and from their culture that they pass on to future generations. However, what they have learned, they inevitably reshape based upon their own experience (Alpern Engel, 1991).

While they still believed it necessary to preserve their language, culture and religion, Ukrainian Canadians quickly came to regard education as an effective way to improve their social and economic status (Ostryzniuk, 2002; Pivnenko & DeVoretz, 2003; Swyripa, 1993). Since women were largely responsible for the children and the education of children, much of the responsibility for the transition of Ukrainians into Canadian society fell to Ukrainian women (Swyripa, 1993). Even though few of the immigrant women learned English themselves, they did ensure that their children attended school for as many years as possible. The participation of Ukrainian children in the assimilation process of the Canadian school system contributed to overall integration (Swyripa, 1993). To this day, it is widely believed that this transition was one of the most successful in the history of Canada (Luciuk, 2000; Lupul, 1982; Martynowych, 1983; Stambrook & Hryniuk, 2000).

Today, many older Ukrainian women continue to reside in rural locations. This appears to be more predominant in the Prairie Provinces where initial settlement of Ukrainian immigrants was primarily in rural areas (Balan, 1984; Stambrook & Hryniuk, 2000; Swyripa, 1993). Although scholars and researchers have begun to document the strength and importance of more contemporary rural older women, much of the literature continues to frame them as "the sturdy, forward-looking, "sun bonneted helpmate" in partnership with her husband" (Osterud, 1988, p. 99). Although there remain gaps in the study of rural older women, the challenges that they face have been well documented (Butler & Kaye, 2003; Dorsch, 1995; Kenkel, 2003; McCulloch & Kivett, 1998). These women often report high rates of isolation and loneliness, both of which are seen as being detrimental to successful aging (Kenkel, 2003; Lubben & Gironda, 2003; Milne & Williams, 2000; Stevens, 2001). Statistically, women live longer than men (McCulloch & Kivett, 1998; McDonough & Strohschein, 2003; McLaughlin & Jensen, 1998; Milne & Williams, 2000). This reality has often dictated that these women are left behind to carry on alone long after their husbands have died (Health Canada, 2002; Kenkel, 2003).

Gender Based Roles

Gender, or the social organization of sexual difference, shapes the experiences of women (Malszecki & Cavar, 2005). Throughout much of Ukrainian history, being female meant being relegated to household and family. While men were entitled to participate in public life, women's relationships with the state and the larger society were mediated by men (Alpern Engel, 1991). For many Ukrainian Canadian women, this has continued to be the case. It is often not until the later stages of life, when these women have been widowed, that they first have an opportunity to make decisions about roles that they will occupy in their lives. However, even then, elderly women often turn to their adult children for direction and support.

Within the realm of successful aging, older women continue to be characterized within specific social roles. The two most important roles assigned are seen to be that of family member and wife (Zhurzhenko, 1999). Encompassed within the role of family member are included the titles of *mother, grandmother,* and *sibling.* Other roles that have been identified as having significance to the social identity of women include those associated with work, friends, leisure, and community membership (McCulloch & Kivett, 1998; Kestin van den Hoonard, 2003).

Research has shown that approximately 80% of older women have living children and approximately 94% of these women have grandchildren (Roberto, Allen & Blieszner, 1999). Most women, regardless of geographic proximity, report having frequent contact with both their children and grandchildren. This contact is seen as contributing to a sense of well-being and success in the lives of these women. First-generation Ukrainian women fifty-five years of age and over have tended to have a larger family size than Ukrainians in the same age group but who were of second or more generations. These first-generation women were among the immigrants who settled in the rural prairies and tended to have larger families (Wolowyna, 1980). As such, many elderly Ukrainian women have large numbers of grandchildren and great-grandchildren.

Religion and spirituality hold significance in the lives of Ukrainian Canadian immigrant women. As such, roles and work within the church are highly valued. Many of these now elderly women continue to be active in their church congregations and associated women's organizations and, in many cases, are the ones that continue to ensure the survival of the church (Ostryzniuk, 2002; Swyripa, 1993). These involvements are seen to provide important mutual support and a sense of personal belonging (Gessler, Arcury & Koenig, 2000; Magilvy & Congdon, 2000; Mitchell & Weatherly, 2000; Kestin van den Hoonard, 2003). However, even women that have been involved in the church for their entire lives have found that they most often tended to be involved through their husbands. Regardless, research has shown that Ukrainian women tend to be more regular churchgoers than their male counterparts (Anderson, 1976).

The concept of *caring* is almost inextricably linked to gender (Cancian & Oliker, 2000). Women most often find themselves in the role of informal care provider in their families. Due to their longer life expectancy, they care for children, grandchildren, spouses, and often their own parents. By the same token, they also end up being the care-receivers, especially in the older age groups (Aronson, 1998). Often it is their daughters and granddaughters who provide their care.

As discussed previously, women are often the ones who are the purveyors of culture through their demonstration and teaching of customs and traditions. This has been, and continues to be, a critical role occupied by Ukrainian Canadian women.

Impact of Relationships

Regardless of ethnicity, relationships are an important aspect of women's lives (Barnes & Parry, 2004; Chatters & Taylor, 1995). Of particular importance are family and marital relationships (Bengston, 2001; Burholt & Wenger, 1998; Roberto et al., 1999). Older women are most embedded in family and community and the relationships found within (Markson & Hess, 1997). Central to these relationships are the roles played by the women themselves, and the changing and fluctuating nature of those roles. It is not uncommon for women to talk about how they have come to know themselves as they are known through their relationships with others, especially their family members (Roberto et al., 1999).

Upon coming to Canada, high birth rates for Ukrainian women were common. This was not only a continuation of traditional practices it also reflected the reality of the living and working conditions experienced by the settlers (Bridger, 1992). Peasant tradition placed an enormous burden on women in the home and on the family's land, at the same time as it reinforced their subordination to men. However, the immense poverty that women experienced made marriage a matter of economic security and necessity (Bridger, 1992).

People of Ukrainian ethnic origin are very proud of their heritage and culture (Ewanchuk, 2000; Luciuk & Hryniuk, 1991; Woycenko, 1967). There have been countless books and articles published which document their collective struggles and accomplishments. Ukrainian women tend to have a profoundly strong connection to their children and grandchildren. This connection provides, not only a sense of personal and cultural pride, it also provides individual women with emotional support and validity. These connections have an impact on the quality of life of elderly Ukrainian women.

Research Methods

The epistemology framing this qualitative research study is post-modern feminism. A post-modern feminist approach draws upon elements of feminist research which emphasize openness to the fluid intentions and shifting contexts of the research question and accompanying variables (Nagy Hesse-Biber & Leckenby, 2004). Given the fact that qualitative research is an inductive process, the researcher is able to remain open to the possibilities of how research participants will impact the research question, the propositions, and the identification of research variables (Grinnell & Unrau, 2005).

Participants in this research study were drawn through a process of purposeful sampling. Qualitative in-depth interviews were conducted with a total of twenty women using a life history reminiscence approach (de Vries, Blando, Southard & Bubeck, 2001). Interest in a reminiscence approach to research has grown in recent years (Sheridan & Kisor, 2000; Webster, 2001). This technique involves the creation of a forum for the individual to share personal meanings of life experiences and can be conducted through the use of either structured or unstructured interview questions (Sheridan & Kisor, 2000). Older Ukrainian women, as is the case with many older people in general, enjoy the time to talk and visit and enjoy the opportunity to share their ideas and life experiences (Milne & Williams, 2000; Stevens, 2001). A reminiscence approach to research recognizes the time required to build and maintain the research relationship with the intent of increasing the depth and quality of information shared (de Vries et al., 2001; Webster, 2001). A laddered question approach was utilized in conducting all of the interviews for this study. Described as a technique for selecting the most appropriate level of inquiry, laddered questions are arranged in an order that "starts with the least invasive and proceeds to deeper matters if the other signals their readiness" (Price, 2001, p. 276). Consequently, laddered questions are presented at one of three levels beginning with questions about action, moving towards questions about knowledge, and eventually culminating with questions about philosophy (Price, 2001).

The twenty women who were interviewed represented seven distinct family units. As such, seven elderly first generation immigrant women were interviewed; six daughters were interviewed; and seven granddaughters were interviewed. All of the first generation women were immigrants who came to Canada from Ukraine as children or young adults and have aged in place. These women ranged in age from seventy-two to eighty-eight years at the time of interview. Of these women, two currently reside in an urban setting, and the remaining five live in small towns or rural locations. The ages of these women at the time of immigration ranged from one year to twenty-one years. The average number of years spent living in Canada following immigration was 73 years. The daughters who were interviewed ranged in age from forty-six to sixty-nine. Of these women, four were married at the time of interview. In total, three of the six participants from this group had been divorced, were divorced, or were proceeding with a divorce. Four out of the six women lived in close geographic proximity to their mothers. Of the daughters that participated in the study, four were employed outside of the home. The granddaughters ranged in age from seventeen to forty-five years old. Of the seven granddaughters, three were married and one was in a common-law relationship. Of the unmarried granddaughters, one lived independently and the remaining two granddaughters continued to reside in the parental home. Five of the granddaughters lived in fairly close proximity to their mother and/or Baba. Five of the seven granddaughters were employed outside of the home, and one was a high school student at the time of interview. Two of the granddaughters had children of their own.

In total, 64 hours of interviews were completed and transcribed. Once the interviews were transcribed, they were coded and re-coded thematically until patterns began to emerge.

There is some recognition within the literature that research techniques as applied when working within ethnic communities should be different than those which are applied to members of the general population (Consedine & Magai, 2002; Matsuoka, 1993; Nevid & Sta Maria, 1999; Quandt, McDonald, Bell & Acury, 1999; Torres, 1999). Techniques and strategies that do not take into account differences in perception due to experience and language barriers may not be the most helpful when either working with, or researching the lives of, individuals of various ethnic backgrounds (Consedine & Magai, 2002; Durst & Delanghe, 2003; Quandt et al., 1999). Researchers should take into account culture and the application of particular cultural meanings as important to the individual or cultural group being studied.

Discussion

This research has shown that individual perceptions about the quality of life of these elderly Ukrainian immigrant women appear to be impacted by how successful they feel they were in their life relationships. They seem to have defined their quality of life external to themselves and within three predominant categories. The categories that emerged within this theme are found in the way in which the Babas interviewed for this study viewed their entire lives within the context of three significant relationships: marital relationships, family relationships and community relationships. The daughters and granddaughters who were interviewed supported these same ideas through the information that they shared during the interview process.

The roles of the Babas within these relationships, and the ways in which they define their identities as situated within marriage, family and community relationships, have impacted upon the ways in which they perceive their quality of life. The experience of immigration, along with the settlement process, has also impacted upon the nature of these life relationships, as well as upon life quality. However, the impact of immigration and settlement appears to have lessened as these women have aged. That is, the process of immigration and settlement had a more significant impact on life quality for these women when they were younger and were considered to be newcomers. As these women have lived their lives and grown older in Canada, the lessening impact of the immigration experience has changed how they see themselves. For example, while these women still identify themselves as Ukrainian, they also identify themselves as citizens of Canada. They now view themselves in terms of having survived the experience of immigration, and the experience of immigration no longer solely defines who they are.

The way in which people see themselves is a direct result of the range of relationships in which they engage. The exploration of the factors that contribute to such self-identity and self-understanding is an essential aspect of post-modern feminism (Payne, 2005). While this self-identity is not seen to be static, it is constantly renegotiated based upon changing life experience and context. The notion of subjectivity refers to the processes that shape us as individuals, and ultimately determine how we see ourselves and how we situate ourselves in the world (Fawcett, 2000; Flax, 1990; Harting, 2008). Subjectivity is seen to be impacted by cultural, social, political and psychological processes (Harting, 2008). Historically, the concept of subjectivity developed in contrast to the notion of identity (Harting, 2008). Identity is seen to be much more determined by the individual (Flax, 1990).

The Babas interviewed for this study all described their early experiences in Canada as having been shaped by immigration and settlement in ways that included the impact of poverty, harsh living conditions, intense isolation, and trauma. They all spoke about the family members and friends left behind in Ukraine. For most, relationships with their own grandparents and extended family members, as well as relationships with the communities in which they were born, were completely severed when they immigrated to Canada. Of the seven Babas interviewed for this research study, only three had returned to Ukraine for one or two brief visits. All three were elderly when they made these trips, and they all spoke about how difficult and strange it was to return. Not only had the family and friends that they had known all passed away, but they barely recognized communities, landmarks, and a country that had changed so drastically. One of the Babas spoke about how her visit saddened her when she realized that she no longer had a connection with her homeland, and that her life and family was now solely situated in Canada. The Babas who did not return to Ukraine to visit talked about how little desire they had to do so since they knew that nothing there would have been the same as they had remembered it to be. Through the years, all of the Babas have renegotiated their identities and roles based partially upon their changing connections to their country of origin, as well as their changing connections to their adopted homeland.

The daughters and granddaughters recognized the many contradictions in the roles taken on by their own mothers or Babas as compared to what they perceived as expected roles found within relationships for women within traditional Ukrainian society. In many cases, the daughters in particular did not see their mothers as being the ones to carry on some of the traditional roles – specifically in regards to maintaining and teaching language and culture to subsequent generations. In four families, the daughters had taken on the role of maintaining and teaching language and culture in place of their mothers. However, all daughters recognized their mothers' roles as caregivers, and the specific duty to care for husbands throughout their lives and at the end of their lives. Two of the daughters had taken on these same roles with their own husbands. The granddaughters all tended to view their Babas as carrying on very traditional roles in terms of gender and cultural expectations.

A primary focus of this research related to how the Babas identified themselves and their roles within the relationships in their lives. Post-modern feminism regards identities and subjectivity as multiple and contradictory, and as always open to challenge (Fawcett, 2000). The data derived from the interviews were analyzed in terms of how the Babas positioned themselves within their stories, and also in terms of how they critiqued and renegotiated this positioning. A goal of post-modern feminism is to create openings for alternative interpretations of reality (Payne, 2005). Through the interview process, the Babas were encouraged to tell their life stories in whatever manner felt most comfortable to them. A process of laddered questioning encouraged them to take their stories to a deeper level and served to highlight the often contradictory roles that they identified for themselves within their marital, family and community relationships. Interviews with the daughters and granddaughters followed the same laddering techniques. The data gathered from the interviews with the daughters and granddaughters supported the data provided by the Babas. These marital, family and community relationships that were identified will be further discussed in terms of analysis within a post-modern feminist perspective.

Marital Relationships

All of the Babas who participated in this research study continued to identify their marital relationship as having pivotal importance in their life and in their interpretation of personal life qualit, even in situations where a spouse was deceased. The six Babas who were widowed all displayed intense emotions of grief and sadness when describing the loss of her husband. However, they all continued to identify themselves as wives of their late husbands during the interview process, and none of them used the term *widow* in relation to their personal situation or to their self-identity. From a post-modern feminist perspective, these choices in self-identification might represent a range of meanings. First, the absence of the term *widow* within the Baba's stories and self-descriptions might reflect an inherent denial of reality. This denial may represent personal coping mechanisms within the grief process. That is, refusal to use the term *widow* may serve to lessen the impact of the grief experienced by the loss of a spouse. Second, the term *widow* may carry connotations for the Babas that they simply do not relate. The word *widow* is mentioned in the Old Testament and widows are referred to as individuals that should be cared for, and specifically as those who are "poor, without support, and old" (Orr, 2008). Other sources suggest that the word *widow* comes from an Indo-European term meaning "to be empty, separated, to be destitute or lack" (Gilbert, 2001). The Babas may carry their own meanings of the term *widow* and may not personally identify themselves according the definitions of the term *widow* as out-lined above. Finally, it may be more important to focus attention, not on the absence of the term *widow,* but instead upon the continued use of the term *wife* in the absence of a husband. This might represent the absolute importance of the identity of the role of wife to the Babas. Clearly, these women continue to see themselves as wives, but they are essentially wives without husbands. Post-modern feminist theory focuses upon the construction of the subject. The experiences of these women contribute to the value that they place upon their roles and identities. That is, their roles may have changed following the death of their husbands, but their identity has not changed. The term *widow* is a label that has been applied to these women. However, they are not accepting this label, and instead are rebelling in their own silent way through a process of role renegotiation. None of the daughters or granddaughters identified their mother or Baba using the term *widow* during the interview process.

All of the Babas who were widowed also talked about their role as caregiver to their late husbands. In doing so, they all demonstrated the impact of gendered pat-terns of caregiving within our society. However, the text of the interviews was laden with contradictions when the Babas spoke about caregiving. All of these women talked about how happy they were to be able to provide such care for their husbands. In addition, all of the Babas interviewed had provided care and end-of-life care to multi-ple family members, including their own mothers, mothers-in-law, and children. They all placed a great deal of value on this caregiver role as they had experienced it, and all continue to identify themselves in that way. However, all of the Babas stated throughout the interviews that they did not expect their own daughters to provide care or end-of-life care for them. That is, while the Babas identified such care provi-sion for their own mothers and other family members as an important duty and responsibility, they did not express this as a reasonable expectation of subsequent generations of women. Again, within a framework of post-modern feminism, this could be interpreted in more than one way. First, these women may have come to recog-nize, through their own experiences, how it is often the women who tend to provide care within the family. They may not want their daughters to be burdened within these same social constructs. Second, these contradictions might also be interpreted as a demonstration that the Babas identify with a martyr role, and as such, they see their daughters as incapable of providing the same kind of care and demonstrating the same kind of selflessness as they themselves were able to demonstrate. Third, the Babas may recognize that they were able to establish very different and closer rela-tionships with their own mothers, mothers-in-law, and other family members than they see their daughters as having established. These different relationships may be due to the fact that many women now work outside of the family home, and that fam-ilies do not tend to live in close geographic proximity to one another as they had in the past. These different relationships may also be due to the fact that the Babas might be more interested in promoting their own independence than their own mothers had been. In other words, this is another example of how these women have renegotiated their roles. Previous generations of Babas expected their daughters to care for them in their old age. However, this research study suggests that this is no longer the case for these Ukrainian women.

Finally, only one of the seven Babas interviewed talked about how she thought that her own daughter would someday have to provide care for her own husband. The other six Babas did not address the issue of their daughters someday providing care to their spouses. This may reinforce the idea that they see their daughter's roles and relationships as being very different than their own. Two of the daughters interviewed identified themselves as caregivers for their own husbands. None of the granddaughters self-identified in this manner. However, this could be primarily due to age and life stage. Five of the daughters personally identified with the role of caregiver to their own mothers, while one daughter indicated that she was not willing to take on a caregiving role in relation to her mother.

As marital relationships were discussed during the interviews, there was not always a demonstrated congruency of interpretation between the generations. Half of the daughters and granddaughters described the relationship that they observed between Baba and Gido (grandfather) as being very different than what was described by Baba. In three families, the daughters and granddaughters described that relationship as close and loving, while the Baba in each family did not describe a loving relationship with her husband. In at least two families, the opposite was true and the daughters and granddaughters saw the relationship between Baba and Gido as unhealthy and conflictual, while Baba described the relationship as close and loving. This incongruence and inconsistency is welcomed within a post-modern feminist perspective in that it is seen to prove one of the basic beliefs of this theoretical perspective – the belief that there is no one universal truth. That is, everyone perceives things differently, and individuals will change their own perceptions over time.

The Babas who participated in this study enacted and maintained their roles as spouse and mother based upon the way that they saw these roles enacted by their own mothers. However, the Babas interviewed for this study did not have an opportunity to maintain relationships with their own Babas due to the fact that they all immigrated to Canada and had little contact with family left behind in Ukraine. Without role-modeling of the ongoing roles that a Baba should have in the lives of her grandchildren, these Babas may be different than the Babas that they themselves knew as young children. This will be explored further in an analysis of family relationships.

Family Relationships

In a post-modern era, the transmission of knowledge between generations loses its significance (Polivka & Longino, 2002). Within all societies, there was a time when intergenerational relationships were critical in order to transmit cultural and traditional symbols and practices. However, an overall loss of the importance of tradition has tended to diminish the relevance of the elderly as sole sources of knowledge and wisdom within western societies (Polivka & Longino, 2002). The findings of this research study support this aspect of a post-modern feminist perspective as reflected in the loss of Ukrainian language, a diminishment of the observance of Ukrainian religious holidays and Ukrainian cultural practices, and an overall decrease in the numbers of people of Ukrainian background who continue to be active members of Ukrainian faith communities. All of these noted changes are most prevalent among second and third generation Ukrainian Canadians. The Babas who participated in this study demonstrated intense pride if they were able to identify children and grandchildren who speak the Ukrainian language, and who continue to observe Ukrainian traditions, or at least have some interest in learning about them. All of the Babas had children and grandchildren who married outside of the Ukrainian Church. All of the Babas spoke about dwindling congregations in their own churches, and described the membership as elderly and largely female. The Babas did not identify relationships with their children and grandchildren to actively pass on Ukrainian cultural practices and traditions.

All of the Babas participating in this research study identified relationships with their families as being critically important to their well-being and to their overall quality of life. Of particular importance to all of these women was the identity of *Baba* in terms of relationships with grandchildren and great-grandchildren. In fact, they placed more value upon their role as *Baba* as opposed to their role as *mother*. As younger women, there was no time to enjoy and build relationships with their children. All time and energy focused upon physical survival, as this was the reality faced by immigrants to Canada at that time. Again, these constructed identities are seen to be very important within a post-modern feminist framework. Tthis preference for the role of *Baba*, as opposed to the role of *mother*, demonstrates the changing nature of roles based upon context and experience within a post-modern feminist perspective.

Community Relationships

In 1988, Martha Bohachesky-Chomiak published a comprehensive study of the history of Ukrainian women in Ukraine entitled *Feminists Despite Themselves: Women in Ukrainian community life, 1884-1939*. In this work she examines the rise of a Ukrainian feminist movement and chronicles the development of what she refers to as *community feminism*. She suggests that women were motivated, not within a context of sexual liberation, but within a context of community development (Bohachevsky-Chomiak, 1988). Ukrainian women were not as intent on freeing themselves from the conventions of their own society as they were intent on becoming active members of their own community. As demonstrated by Bohachevsky-Chomiak (1988), the influences of a very strong sense of nationalism are evident throughout their history. According to Bohachevsky-Chomiak (1988), "they stressed the special role of women in society and made opportunity, rather than equality, their goal" (p. xxii). She further suggests that "the Ukrainian women had no problems with identity . . . the realm of the private flowed into that of the public" (Bohachevsky-Chomiak, 1988, p. xxiii). For Ukrainian women, the years of the injustice of the suppression of Ukrainian culture was seen to be more important than the traditional discriminations faced by women. As such, feminism could not become a political goal early on (Bohachevsky-Chomiak, 1988).

The concept of community feminism did not effectively impact upon Ukrainian women who came to Canada during the earlier waves of immigration. These women found themselves living very isolated lives in what were often hostile, oppressive and competitive communities. While all of the first generation women described at least minimal involvement in the Ukrainian Women's Associations over the years, they describe this earlier membership as sporadic and task-oriented. The primary purpose of these Associations at that time was to raise money to send back to Ukraine in order to help towards the goal of freeing the Ukrainian people from an oppressive political regime.

Five of the seven Babas interviewed for this research study are currently members of various organizations, including the Ukrainian Women's Associations affiliated with the Ukrainian churches. Their description of their roles within these organizations today is decidedly different than they had been when they were involved as younger women. Now, they describe their participation as much more social in nature, and their opportunities to participate as being much more consistent. In addition, due to the lower rates of involvement of younger people in the Church, these women find themselves assuming leadership roles more often. Once again, these changes in role definition fit within a post-modern feminist theoretical framework by demonstrating the shifts in both the *construction of* and *constructing of* roles and identities within changing contexts.

Implications for Practice and Service

In terms of the implications for practice and service delivery, this study makes two main contributions: the production of applied knowledge and the production of process knowledge. Applied knowledge is context-specific and is useful for the solution of practical problems. Process knowledge is a relatively new term that refers to the development of knowledge which focuses upon the processes by which judgments are made in practice and research (Sheppard & Ryan, 2003). The core of process knowledge is found within the concept of reflexivity (D'Cruz, Gillingham & Melendez, 2007; Sheppard & Ryan, 2003). As utilized in this particular research study, reflexivity is defined as a self-critical approach which questions how knowledge is generated (D'Cruz et al., 2003; Sheppard, Newstead, Caccavo & Ryan, 2000). This research study creates process knowledge in terms of the steps that were followed in interviewing elderly Ukrainian women. What has been demonstrated is the value of an interview approach which encourages narrative, and is more unstructured, utilizing open-ended questions and a laddering technique of inquiry. This approach created an environment whereby the Babas felt comfortable to discuss and share deeper layers of personal information. This approach also created an opportunity for reflexivity on the part of all research participants. This type of reflexivity enables participants to process their own information and create knowledge which can build self-understanding and assist in making life choices (D'Cruz et al., 2003; Kondrat, 1999). Although this study has focused upon elderly Ukrainian immigrant women, these findings may also apply to other older ethnic women who also immigrated to Canada.

In regards to applied knowledge, previous research, although limited, has focused on specific roles for those individuals working with Ukrainian immigrants in terms of intervention strategies for helping newcomers make the transition into Canadian society (Barlow & Barlow, 2003). While it is commonly perceived that, as a cultural group, Ukrainians were successful in both the immigration and assimilation processes involved with their settlement in Canada, there are specific issues that must be still be considered and understood by social workers who work with members of this population. First, it is essential to understand the issues related to the religious, spatial and ethnic diversity amongst members of this group. Also critical is an understanding of the impact of the time of arrival and place of settlement (Barlow & Barlow, 2003). This study adds to an understanding of the issues necessary to focus upon by also drawing attention to the importance of marital, family and community relationships in the lives of elderly Ukrainian immigrant women.

There continues to be gaps in the general knowledge base specific to elderly Ukrainian women, as well as other older women of other ethnic backgrounds. Matsuoka (1993) calls for more focused and targeted studies which will help to build an understanding of the needs of the elderly which arise from ethnic differences.

Within a framework of post-modern feminism, the perspectives of clients take on a significant importance, and the focus of attention necessarily becomes the clients' narratives (Rossiter, 2000). Practitioners must listen to the stories of elderly ethnic women and familiarize themselves with the information that is most significant to such individuals, and the information that is most significant about such individuals. For example, even though each of the Babas interviewed for this study has lived in Canada for more than sixty years, the experiences of immigration and settlement continue to be a predominant part of their storytelling.

This research study has highlighted a number of other issues which were identified as having importance to the elderly Ukrainian immigrant women who were interviewed. First, all of the Babas identified multiple losses in their lives. It is important to acknowledge and recognize the impacts of such cumulative grief. Second, all of the Babas described trauma associated with the conditions that they experienced in Ukraine prior to immigration, and trauma associated with the conditions that they experienced during their settlement period in Canada. Again, the cumulative impact of unresolved trauma over long periods of time can be significant. Finally, all of the Babas described multiple roles within their marital, family and community relationships, and each demonstrated the changing nature of these roles as they are negotiated and renegotiated based upon life experience and context. It is important to acknowledge this role of multiplicity.

Practitioners must be aware of the importance of these issues when working with elderly Ukrainian immigrant women. Again, this knowledge may also be relevant when working with other elderly women of different ethnic backgrounds.

References

Alpern Engel, B. (1991). Transformation versus tradition. In B. Evans Clements, B. Alpern Engel & C. D. Worobe. (Eds.), *Russia's women: Accommodation, resistance, transformation.* (pp. 135-147). Berkeley: University of California Press.

Anderson, A. (1976). Ukrainian identity change in rural Saskatchewan. In W.W. Isajiw (Ed.), *Ukrainians in American and Canadian society.* (pp. 93-121). Jersey City: M.P. Kots Publishing.

Aronson, J. (1998). Dutiful daughters and undemanding mothers: Constraining images of giving and receiving care in middle and later life. In C.T. Baines, P.M. Evans & S.M. Neysmith (Eds), *Women's caring: Feminist perspectives on social welfare.* (pp. 114-138). Toronto: Oxford University Press.

Balan, J. (1984). *Salt and braided bread: Ukrainian life in Canada.* Toronto: Oxford University Press.

Barlow, C. & Barlow, A. (2003). Social work with Canadians of Ukrainian background: History, direct practice, current realities. In A. Al-Krenawi & J.R. Graham (Eds), *Multicultural social work in Canada: Working with diverse ethno-racial communities* (pp. 228 – 250). Don Mills: Oxford University Press.

Barnes, H. & Parry, J. (2004). Renegotiating identity and relationships: Men and women's adjustments to retirement. *Ageing & Society, 24,* 213-233.

Bengtson, V. (2001). Beyond the nuclear family: The increasing importance of multigenerational bonds. *Journal of Marriage and the Family, 63,* 1-16.

Bennett, K. (1997). A longitudinal study of well-being in widowed women. *International Journal of Geriatric Psychiatry, 12,* 61-66.

Bridger, S. (1992). Soviet rural women: Employment and family life. In B. Farnsworth & L. Viola (Eds.), *Russian peasant women.* (pp. 271-293). New York: Oxford University Press.

Bohachevsky-Chomiak, M. (1988). *Feminists despite themselves: Women in Ukrainian community life,* 1884-1939. Edmonton: Canadian Institute of Ukrainian Studies.

Burholt, V. & Wenger, G. (1998). Differences over time in older people's relationships with children and siblings. *Ageing and Society, 18*, 537-562.

Butler, S. & Kaye, L. (Eds.). (2003). *Gerontological social work in small towns and rural communities.* New York: The Haworth Social Work Practice Press.

Cancian, F. & Oliker, S. (2000). *Caring and gender.* Walnut Creek: Altamira Press.

Chatters, L. & Taylor, R. (1995). Social integration. In R. Neugebauer-Visano (Ed.), *Aging and inequality: Cultural constructions of differences.* (pp. 187-204). Toronto: Canadian Scholars' Press Inc.

Cheal, D. & Kampen, K. (1998). *Poor and dependent seniors in Canada.* Aging and Society, 18, 147-166.

Cipko, S. (1991). In search of a new home: Ukrainian emigration patterns between the two world wars. *Journal of Ukrainian studies, 16*(1-2), 3-28.

Connor, R. (1909). *The foreigner.* Toronto: Westminster Press.

Consedine, N. & Magai, C. (2002). The uncharted waters of emotion: Ethnicity, trait emotion and emotion expression in older adults. *Journal of Cross-Cultural Gerontology, 17,* 71-100.

D'Cruz, H., Gillingham, P. & Melendez, S. (2007). Reflexivity, its meanings and relevance for social work: A critical review of the literature. *British Journal of Social Work, 37*(1), 73-90.

de Vries, B., Blando, J., Southard, P. & Bubeck, C. (2001). The times of our lives. In G.Kenyon, P. Clark & B. de Vries (Eds.), *Narrative gerontology: Theory, research and practice.* (pp. 137-158). New York: Springer Publishing Company, Inc.

Djao, A. & Ng, R. (1987). Structured isolation: Immigrant women in Saskatchewan. In K. Storrie (Ed.), *Women: Isolation and bonding. The ecology of gender.* (pp. 141-158). Toronto: Methuen.

Doroshenko, D. (1914). *A survey of Ukrainian history.* Winnipeg: Humeniuk Publication Foundation.

Dorsch, J. (1995). "You just did what had to be done": Life histories of four Saskatchewan "farmers' wives". In D. De Brou, & A. Moffat (Eds.), *"Other" voices: Historical essays on Saskatchewan women.* (pp. 116-130). Regina: Canadian Plains Research Center, University of Regina.

Driedger, L. (1996). *Multi-ethnic Canada: Identities and inequalities.* Toronto: Oxford University Press.

Durst, D. & Delanghe, P. (2003). Culturally appropriate social work for successful community development in diverse communities. In A. Al-Krenawi, & J.R.Graham (Eds.), *Multicultural social work in Canada: Working with diverse ethno-racial communities.* (pp. 47-69). Don Mills: Oxford University Press.

Ewanchuk, M. (2000). *Vertical development: A new generation of Ukrainian Canadians.* Winnipeg: Michael Ewanchuk Publishing.

Fawcett, B. & Featherstone, B. (2000). Setting the scene: An appraisal of notions of post-modernism, post-modernity and post-modern feminism. In B. Fawcett, B. Featherstone, J. Fook & A. Rossiter (Eds.), *Practice and research in social work: Post-modern feminist perspectives.* (pp. 5-23). London: Routledge.

Flax, J. (1990). *Thinking fragments: Psychoanalysis, feminism and post-modernism in the contemporary west.* Berkeley: University of California Press.

Gilbert, S. (2001). *Widow. Critical Inquiry, 27*(4). Retrieved February 2, 2008 from http://criticalinquiry.uchicago.edu/issues/v27/v27n4.gilbert.html

Gerus, O. & Rea, J. (1985). *The Ukrainians in Canada.* Ottawa: Canadian Historical Association.

Gessler, W., Arcury, T. & Koenig, H. (2000). An introduction to three studies of rural elderly people: Effects of religion and culture on health. *Journal of Cross-Cultural Gerontology, 15*(1), 1–12.

Green, B. (1993). *Gerontology and the construction of old age: A study in discourse analysis.* New York: Aldine De Gruyter.

Grinnell, R. Jr. & Unrau, Y. (Eds.). (2005). *Social work research and evaluation: Quantitative and qualitative approaches.* Oxford: Oxford University Press.

Hansen, J. & Kucera, M. (2004). *The educational attainment of second generation immigrants in Canada: Evidence from SLID.* Retrieved August 2, 2007 from http://www.iza.org/en/webcontent/teaching/summerschool/7thsummer_school_files/ss2004_kucera

Harting, H. (2008). *Subjectivity.* (n.d.). Retrieved, March 23, 2008 from http://anscombe.mcmaster.ca/global1/glossary_print.jsp?id=CO.0036

Health Canada. (2002). *Canada's aging population.* Ottawa: Health Canada.

Higgs, P., Hyde, M., Wiggins, R. & Blane, D. (2003). Researching quality of life in early old age: The importance of sociological dimension. *Social Policy and Administration, 37*(3), 239-252.

Hilleras, P., Pollitt, P., Medway, J. & Ericsson, K. (2000). Nonagenarians: A qualitative exploration of individual differences in wellbeing. *Aging and Society, 20,* 673-697.

Himka, J. (1982). The background to emigration: Ukrainians of Galicia and Bukovyna, 1848-1914. In M. R. Lupul (Ed.), *A heritage in transition: Essays in the history of Ukrainians in Canada.* (pp. 11-31). Toronto: McClelland and Stewart Ltd.

Kaye, V. (1964). *Early Ukrainian settlements in Canada: 1895-1900.* Toronto: University of Toronto Press.

Kaye, V. & Swyripa, F. (1982). Settlement and colonization. In M.R. Lupul (Ed.), *A heritage in transition: Essays in the history of Ukrainians in Canada.* (pp. 32-58). Toronto: McClelland and Stewart Ltd.

Kenkel, M. (2003). Rural women: Strategies and resources for meeting their behavioural health needs. In B. Hudnall Stamm (Ed.). *Rural behavioural health care: An interdisciplinary guide.* (pp. 181-192). Washington: American Psychological Association.

Kestin van den Hoonard, D. (2003). Expectations and experiences of widowhood. In J. Gubrium, & J. Holstein (Eds), *Ways of aging.* (pp. 182-199). Malden: Blackwell Publishers Ltd.

Keywan, Z. & Coles, M. (1977). *Greater than kings: Ukrainian pioneer settlement in Canada.* Montreal: Harvest House.

Kirtz, M. (1996). Old world traditions, new world inventions: Bilingualism, multiculturalism, and the transformation of ethnicity. *Canadian Ethnic Studies, 28*(1), 8-19.

Kondrat, M. (1999). Who is the "self" in self-aware: Professional self-awareness from a critical theory perspective. *Social Service Review, 3,* 451-477.

Kostash, M. (2000). *All of Baba's great grandchildren: Ethnic identity in the next Canada.* Saskatoon: Heritage Press.

Lehr, J. (1983). Propaganda and belief: Ukrainian emigrant views of the Canadian west. In J. Rozumnyj (Ed.), *New soil – old roots: The Ukrainian experience in Canada.* (pp. 1-17). Winnipeg: Ukrainian Academy of Arts and Sciences in Canada.

Lubben, J. & Gironda, M. (2003). Centrality of social ties to the health and well-being of older adults. In B. Berkman & L. Harootyan (Eds.), *Social work and health care in an aging society.* (pp. 319-345). New York: Springer Publishing Company, Inc.

Luciuk, L. (2000). *Searching for place: Ukrainian displaced persons, Canada, and the migration of memory.* Toronto: University of Toronto Press.

Luciuk, L. & Hryniuk, S. (Eds.). (1991). *Canada's Ukrainians: Negotiating an identity.* Toronto: University of Toronto Press.

Lupul, M.(Ed.) (1982). *A heritage in transition: Essays in the history of Ukrainians in Canada.* Toronto: McClelland and Stewart Ltd.

Lysenko, V. (1947). *Men in sheepskin coats: A study in assimilation.* Toronto: The Ryerson Press.

MacLean, M. & Sakadakis, V. (1989). Quality of life in terminal care with institutionalized ethnic elderly people. *International Social Work, 32,* 209-221.

Magilvy, J. & Congdon, J. (2000). The crisis nature of health care transitions for rural older adults. *Public Health Nursing, 17*(5), 336-345.

Malszecki, G. & Cavar, T. (2005). Men, masculinities, war, and sport. In N. Mandell, (Ed.), *Feminist issues: Race, class, and sexuality, 4th edition.* (pp. 160-187). Toronto: Pearson Prentice Hall.

Markson, E. & Hess, B. (1997). Older women in the city. In M. Pearsall, (Ed.). *The other within us: Feminist explorations of women and aging.* (pp. 57-70). Oxford: Westview Press.

Martynowych, O. (1983). "Canadianizing the foreigner": Presbyterian missionaries and Ukrainian immigrants. In J. Rozumnyj (Ed.), *New soil – old roots: The Ukrainian experience in Canada.* (pp. 33-57). Winnipeg: Ukrainian Academy of Arts and Sciences in Canada.

Matsuoka, A. (1993). Collecting qualitative data through interviews with ethnic older people. *Canadian Journal on Aging, 12*(2), 216-232.

McCulloch, J. & Kivett, V. (1998). Older rural women: Aging in historical and current contexts. In R.T. Coward & J.A. Krout, (Eds.). *Aging in rural settings: Life circumstances and distinctive features.* (pp. 149-166). New York: Springer Publishing Company, Inc.

McDonough, P. & Strohschein, L. (2003). Age and the gender gap in distress. *Women & Health, 38*(1), 1-20.

McLaughlin, D. & Jensen, L. (1998). The rural elderly: A demographic portrait. In R.T. Coward & J.A. Krout (Eds), *Aging in rural settings: Life circumstances and distinctive features.* (pp. 15-44). New York: Springer Publishing Company, Inc.

Milne, A. & Williams, J. (2000). Meeting the mental health needs of older women: Taking social inequality into account. *Aging and Society, 20,* 699-723.

Mitchell, J. & Weatherly, D. (2000). Beyond church attendance: Religiosity and mental health among rural older adults. *Journal of Cross-Cultural Gerontology, 15*(1), 37–54.

Nagy Hesse-Biber, S. & Leckenby, D. (2004). How feminists practice social research. In S. Nagy Hesse-Biber, & M.L. Yaiser (Eds.), *Feminist perspectives on social research.* (pp. 209-226). New York: Oxford University Press.

Nevid, J. & Sta Maria, N. (1999). Multicultural issues in qualitative research. *Psychology & Marketing, 16*(4), 305-326.

O'Connor, D. (2003). Anti-oppressive practice with older adults: A feminist post-structural perspective. In W. Shera (Ed.), *Emerging perspectives on anti-oppressive practice.* (pp. 183-199). Toronto: Canadian Scholar's Press Inc.

Omidvar, R. & Richmond, T. (2005). Immigrant settlement and social inclusion in Canada. In T. Richmond & A. Saloojee (Eds.), *Social inclusion: Canadian perspectives.* (pp. 155-179). Halifax: Fernwood Publishing.

Osterud, N. (1988). Land, identity and agency in the oral autobiographies of farm women. In W.G. Haney & J.B. Knowles (Eds.), *Women and farming: Changing roles, changing structures.* (pp. 73-87). Boulder: Westview Press.

Ostryzniuk, N. (1997). *Savella Stechishin: A case study of Ukrainian-Canadian women activism in Saskatchewan, 1920-1945.* Regina: Unpublished Thesis.

Ostryzniuk, N. (2002). *75 years of service, friendship and commitment, 1927-2002,* Ukrainian Women's Association of Canada, Daughters of Ukraine Branch, Regina, Saskatchewan. Regina: University of Regina Printing Services.

Payne, M. (2005). *Modern social work theory, 3rd Edition.* Chicago: Lyceum Books, Inc.

Petryshyn, M. (1980). The changing status of Ukrainian women in Canada, 1921-1971. In W.R. Petryshyn (Ed.), *Changing realities: Social trends among Ukrainian Canadians.* (pp. 189-209). Edmonton: The Canadian Institute of Ukrainian Studies.

Pivnenko, S. & DeVoretz, D. (2003). *The recent economic performance of Ukrainian immigrants in Canada and the U.S. Research on Immigration and Integration in the Metropolis:* Working Paper Series. Vancouver: Vancouver Centre of Excellence.

Polivka, L. & Longino, C. (2002). Commentary: Aging politics and policy in a post-modern society. *Journal of Aging and Identity, 7*(4), 287-292.

Price, B. (2002). Laddered questions and qualitative data research interviews. *Journal of Advanced Nursing, 37*(3), 273-281.

Quandt, S., McDonald, J., Bell, R. & Arcury, T. (1999). Aging research in multi-ethnic rural communities: Gaining entrée through community involvement. *Journal of Cross-Cultural Gerontology, 14,* 113-130.

Rasmussen, L., Rasmussen, L., Savage, C. & Wheeler, A. (1976). *A harvest yet to reap: A history of prairie women.* Toronto: The Women's Press.

Ray, R. (1996). A post-modern perspective on feminist gerontology. *The Gerontologist, 36*(5), 674-680.

Roberto, K., Allen, K. & Blieszner, R. (1999). Older women, their children, and grandchildren: A feminist perspective on family relationships. In J.D. Garner (Ed.), *Fundamentals of feminist gerontology.* (pp. 67 – 84). Binghamton: The Haworth Press.

Romaniuk, A. & Chuiko, L. (1999). Matrimonial behaviour in Canada and Ukraine: The enduring hold of culture. *Journal of Comparative Family Studies, 30*(3), 335-361.

Rossiter, A. (2000). The post-modern feminist condition: New conditions for social work. In B. Fawcett, B. Featherstone, J. Fook & A. Rossiter (Eds.), *Practice and research in social work: Post-modern feminist perspectives.* (pp. 24-38). London: Routledge.

Sarvimaki, A. & Stenbock-Hult, B. (2000). Quality of life in old age described as a sense of well-being, meaning and value. *Journal of Advanced Nursing, 32*(4), 1025-1033.

Seiler, T. (1996). Including the female immigrant story: A comparative look at narrative strategies. *Canadian Ethnic Studies, 28*(1), 51-63.

Sheppard, M., Newstead, S., Caccavo, A. & Ryan, K. (2000). Reflexivity and the development of process knowledge in social work: A classification and empirical study. *British Journal of Social Work, 30,* 465-488.

Sheppard, M. & Ryan, K. (2003). Practitioners as rule using analysts: A further development of process knowledge in social work. *British Journal of Social Work, 33*(2), 157-176.

Sheridan, M. & Kisor, A. (2000). The research process and the elderly. In R.L. Schneider, N.P. Kropf, & A.J. Kisor (Eds.), *Gerontological social work: Knowledge, service settings, and special populations, 2nd edition.* (pp. 97-135). Belmont: Wadsworth/Thomson Learning.

Smith, W. (1922). Building the nation: *The churches' relation to the immigrant.* Toronto: The Ryerson Press.

Stambrook, R. & Hryniuk, S. (2000). Who were they really? Reflections on east European immigrants to Manitoba before 1914. *Prairie forum, 25*(2), 215-232.

Statistics Canada. (2007). *2006 Census.* Ottawa, ON: Government of Canada. (No. 97-551-XWE20060010.)

Stevens, N. (2001). Combating loneliness: A friendship enrichment programme for older women. *Aging and Society, 21,* 183-202.

Swyripa, F. (1978). *Ukrainian Canadians: A survey of their portrayal in English language works.* Edmonton: The University of Alberta Press.

Swyripa, F. (1983). The Ukrainian image: Loyal citizen or disloyal alien. In F. Swyripa & J.H. Thompson (Eds), *Loyalties in conflict: Ukrainians in Canada during the great war.* (pp. 47-68). Edmonton: Canadian Institute of Ukrainian Studies.

Swyripa, F. (1993). *Wedded to the cause: Ukrainian-Canadian women and ethnic identity 1891-1991.* Toronto: University of Toronto Press.

Swyripa, F. (2000). Negotiating sex and gender in the Ukrainian bloc settlement: East central Alberta between the wars. In C.A. Cavanaugh & R.R. Warne (Eds.), *Telling tales: Essays in western women's history.* (pp. 232-260). Vancouver: UBC Press.

Torres, S. (1999). A culturally-relevant theoretical framework for the study of successful aging. *Aging and Society, 19,* 33-51.

Ujimoto, K. (1995). The ethnic dimension of aging in Canada. In R. Neugebauer-Visano (Ed),. *Aging and inequality: Cultural constructions of differences.* (pp. 3-29). Toronto: Canadian Scholars' Press Inc.

Webster, J. (2001). The future of the past: Continuing challenges for reminiscence research. In G. Kenyon, P. Clark & B. de Vries (Eds.), *Narrative gerontology: Theory, research and practice.* (pp. 159-185). New York: Springer Publishing Company, Inc.

Wolowyna, J. (1980). Trends in marital status and fertility of Ukrainians in Canada. In W.R. Petryshyn (Ed.), *Changing realities: Social trends among Ukrainian Canadians.* (pp. 161-188). Edmonton: The Canadian Institute of Ukrainian Studies.

Worobec, C. (1992). Temptress or virgin? The precarious sexual position of women in postemancipation Ukrainian peasant society. In B. Farnsworth, & L. Viola (Eds), *Russian peasant women.* (pp. 41-53). New York: Oxford University Press.

Woycenko, O. (1967). *The Ukrainians in Canada.* Winnipeg: Trident Press, Ltd.

Yuzyk, P. (1967). *Ukrainian Canadians: Their place and role in Canadian life.* Toronto: Kiev Printers.

Zhurzhenko, T. (1999). Gender and identity formation in post-socialist Ukraine: The case of women in the shuttle business. In R. Bridgman, S. Cole & H. Howard-Bobiwash (Eds.), *Feminist fields: Ethnographic insights.* (pp. 243-263). Peterborough: Broadview Press Ltd. .

19

Filial Piety, Financial Independence, and Freedom: Explaining the Living Arrangements of Older Korean Immigrants

Ann H. Kim (York University)

Introduction

The adaptation of Korean immigrants in Canada has received very little consideration in the literature. Yet, for several reasons, the integration experiences of this group, and their older members, warrants greater research attention. First, changes in Canadian immigration policy since the 1960s opened the borders to different immigrant groups and to their extended families through sponsorship provisions. With a foreign-born contingent of approximately 83 percent, understanding the integration experiences of the Korean community can be informative for understanding the integration experiences of other ethnic communities. More specifically, Korean seniors are overwhelmingly foreign-born with little knowledge of either of the official languages, and they are likely to share similar challenges and issues as other immigrant seniors.

Second, a report by Statistics Canada (2005) projects Koreans to be the second fastest growing visible minority group – after West Asians – doubling their numbers by 2017. Their high growth rate can be attributed to immigration and not to their fertility rate, suggesting that immigrant settlement will continue to be an important issue for the community for some time.

Third, compared to other ethnic groups, Koreans have the highest rate of self-employment at over 34 percent of the working population aged 15 and older (2001 Canadian Census of Population). As self-employment in small business is often a family affair (Yoon, 1997) and business owners can work well past retirement age, this has important implications for family life, aging and senior care.

Finally, the living arrangements and senior care of Korean immigrants lie at the intersection of traditional culture and modern Western socio-political philosophies and structural and ecological conditions. Traditional Korean culture based on Confucian moral teachings dictates the responsibility of family members, particularly adult children and eldest sons (and their wives), in housing and caring for seniors. Filial piety is demonstrated and experienced through living with aging parents. This is generally reflected in the social welfare state in Korea, as housing and care for seniors is considered a family issue, not a social one (Palley, 1992; Song, 1998). Given this context, it is not surprising that about three quarters of elderly Koreans live with their children (Martin, 1989). In Canada, Korean families must adapt to different social and economic circumstances and there is a need to understand how they navigate between the Confucian moral code and the Canadian social system and institutions, and how this manifests as household arrangements.

This chapter begins to address the gap in the literature on Korean immigrants by examining the housing options and living arrangements of Korean seniors. Housing issues are an important part of the aging adjustment process and affects seniors' quality of life (Bryant et al., 2004; Health Canada, 2002). In general, transitions through the stages of the life course are associated with shifts in housing needs, preferences and economic resources. A sequence of mobility decisions is made, otherwise known as a housing career or housing trajectory (Clark, Deurloo and Dieleman, 2003; Murdie, 2002; Özüekal and van Kempen, 2002), and at each stage of the trajectory, decisions about housing type, tenure, and living arrangements are determined by a combination of structural, cultural and individual factors (Foner, 1997; Phua, Kaufman & Park, 2001). These factors are more salient than for immigrants in later life.

Since little is known about Koreans across Canada, the first part of the chapter provides a brief overview of immigration from Korea and of the current community as a backdrop for understanding the housing issues faced by seniors. Following this is a section describing the research design. Then, a statistical profile of Korean seniors is offered, comparing their current socio-demographic and household characteristics to Charter Group seniors. Structural and cultural and individual explanations for changes in expectations around living arrangements, housing and elder care are highlighted next. This final section explores issues of access to different types of housing for older Korean immigrants, including barriers within institutional settings, and the degree to which the shift in living arrangements can be explained by shifts in cultural beliefs.

Immigration and the Korean Community

Migration from Korea to Canada dates back to the late 19th century, consisting of Christian missionary students on temporary visas and transient visitors (Yoo, 2002). Large numbers of permanent residents began to arrive only in the recent period, after the Canadian government eliminated national origins as a basis for admissions in its immigration legislation in 1962. Coincidentally, in that same year, the South Korean government enacted an emigration policy, encouraging population dispersion (Yoon, 2006).

Members of the current Korean community can be distinguished by their period of settlement (Kwak, 2004). A large wave of early permanent migrants moved to

Canada in the mid-1970s, after growing up in a politically and economically unstable Korea. Some were born into a country that had been recovering from 35 years of Japanese colonial rule, which ended with World War II, and the Korean War, 1950-1953. Others have lived through one or both wars as young children. Many were admitted to Canada with their high levels of educational and occupational attainment but they brought little financial capital. Upon arrival, they faced barriers in the Canadian labor market and as a result, many turned to self-employment (Yoon, 2006).

Migration rates fell after this first large wave and began to increase gradually a decade later in the late 1980s. This period marked a turning point in South Korea's position in the global economy; the first democratic elections took place in 1987 after decades of military rule, the 1988 Seoul Olympic Games attracted international attention, and many individuals and families benefited from Korea's aggressive economic strategies (Pae, 1992). Subsequently, Korean immigration to Canada peaked in 2001, in the aftermath of the Asian financial crisis. Like their predecessors, these more recent migrants also had high levels of educational and occupational attainment, but they differed in the economic resources they brought with them. And unlike their predecessors, many were admitted under the business class program, and they came expecting to be self-employed.

Based on the 2006 census, there are currently 146 545 ethnic Koreans in Canada. As previously stated, the Korean community is highly foreign-born, highly educated – with more than a third of the community having a university degree or higher, and characterized by a high level of self-employment in the retail trade and accommodation and food sectors. Similar to other immigrant groups from Asia, Koreans also tend to be highly urbanized, with the largest concentration in Toronto (39.1 percent), followed closely by Vancouver (31.4 percent).

Korean seniors, 65 years and older, comprise approximately 6 percent of this population and for the most part, their composition reflects the two migration waves identified above. Some of the seniors arrived in Canada as working adults with young children and have had years of exposure to the host society. Others arrived as seniors, under the sponsorship of their immigrant adult children, and are dealing with the aging and immigrant settlement processes simultaneously. The distinct migrating experiences of these two groups have a direct impact on how structural factors, cultural norms around family relationships and responsibilities, and personal preferences shape housing and living arrangements.

The Research Design

Both census data and semi-structured interviews were used to obtain a more comprehensive picture of Korean seniors in Canada. The use of secondary data permitted a detailed socio-demographic and economic profile of the community to be developed and it enabled a comparison of their characteristics to others, in particular, to native-born Charter Group seniors. For insight into issues related to the cultural and structural dynamics of living arrangements and housing, interviews with community leaders were conducted.

Data on ethnic Korean seniors and Canadian-born Charter Group seniors were obtained from the 2001 Public Use Microdata File of Individuals (PUMF-I), which is based on a 2.7 percent sample of the Canadian Census of Population, which omits the institutional population. Korean and Canadian-born Charter group respondents were selected based on their response to the question on ethnic origin and the sample includes only seniors with either Korean as a single ethnic origin or Canadian, English, French, Irish, or Scottish as a single ethnic origin.

The senior population has been defined as individuals who are 60 years and older. This age threshold was selected for three reasons: to maximize the sample size; to maintain consistency with past studies on seniors; and due to the significance and meaning of the 60th birthday for Koreans. Turning 60 is the greatest event in an individual's life (Pang, 1991) as the sexagenarian is celebrated as having lived a full life after a 60-year cycle of 5 elements (wood, fire, earth, metal, water) by 12 zodiac signs (rat, ox, tiger, rabbit, dragon, snake, horse, sheep, monkey, rooster, dog, pig).

Once the statistical profile of Korean seniors was compiled, interviews with 9 community leaders, 5 females and 4 males, were conducted in January and February of 2008. These leaders represented 7 community organizations in the Greater Toronto Area that either served only Korean seniors or served Korean seniors as part of their mandate, which ranged from providing housing information and referrals to providing Long-Term Care (LTC) services. In addition to working with these organizations, 6 were seniors themselves – 3 males and 3 females – and they were able to speak from personal experience as well as from their work or volunteer experience with the Korean community.

A Profile of Korean Seniors: A Distinctive Population

A comparison of the demographic, social and economic portraits of Korean and Canadian-born Charter Group seniors in Table 1 reveals that they share a few characteristics but differ in significant ways. First, Korean seniors were much more likely to be found in Toronto and Vancouver than seniors belonging to the Charter Groups. In terms of age groups, those 75 years and older formed a smaller percentage of each group compared to the younger 60-74 age grouping. For both groups, the majority were female and married. Yet, Korean seniors were less likely to be single, or divorced, separated or widowed compared to seniors belonging to the Charter Group members born in Canada.

Table 1 A Socio-Demographic Profile Comparing Korean and Charter Group Seniors		Korean	Charter Groups
Age Groups	60-74	73.2	67.4
	75+	26.8	32.6
Gender	Male	46.0	44.6
	Female	54.1	55.4
Marital Status	Single	1.3	6.2
	Married	74.6	59.1
	DSW	24.1	34.7
Immigrant Status	Native-born	1.3	100
	Immigrant	98.7	0
Timing of Arrival	Before 1991	81.7	–
	1991-2001	18.3	–
Age at Immigration	<25 years old	1.4	–
	25-59 years old	80.7	–
	60+ years	18.0	–
Citizenship	Citizen	82.6	100
	Non-citizen	17.4	0
Language	English and/or French	66.1	100
	Neither English nor French	33.9	0
Religion	Catholic	25.9	55.7
	Protestant	38.4	36.5
	Other	20.1	1.1
	None	15.6	6.8
Education	HS or less, PS Diploma/Certificate	77.2	94.0
	University degree	17.0	3.8
	Postgraduate degree/certificate	5.8	2.2
Employment	Unemployed or not in laborforce	73.7	86.6
	Employed, paid	12.5	9.2
	Employed, self-employed	13.9	4.2
Individual Income	<$15 000	79.9	68.1
	$25 000-$49 000	12.1	23.6
	$50 000+	8.0	8.2
CMAs	Toronto	50.5	6.9
	Vancouver	24.1	3.5
	Others (incl. non-CMAs)	25.4	89.6
Total		224	41 971

Table 1 Notes:

Data source: 2001 Public use Microdata Series – Individuals from the Census of Canada

A chi-square test shows statistically significant differences at p<.001 for all variables with the exception of age and gender. Immigrant status, timing of arrival, age at immigration, citizenship, and language variables are not applicable.

Weighted data.

Moving onto immigrant characteristics, nearly all Korean seniors were born outside of Canada and close to one fifth were not Canadian citizens. Moreover, over 18 percent were recent arrivals, arriving within the 10-year period prior to the census and 18 percent arrived as seniors, (60 years or over). With respect to language, a full third of the Korean senior population could not speak either of the two official languages.

A look at their religious characteristics demonstrates that Korean seniors were significantly less likely to be Catholic than their Canadian-born Charter Group counterparts. They were affiliated with Protestantism more so than any other religion, although there was a substantial percentage of other religious groups represented (i.e., Buddhism). While similar levels of Charter Group seniors identified as being Protestant, they were less likely to have no religion than Korean seniors.

Korean seniors present a further contrast to Charter Group seniors when socioeconomic traits are considered. Korean seniors appeared to be more educated and economically integrated but less affluent than Charter Group seniors based on their education, employment and income characteristics. Over 22 percent of Korean seniors reported having a university degree, over 25 percent reported being employed (in either paid or self-employment), and almost 79.9 percent reported incomes of less than $25 000. For Canadian-born Charter Group seniors, the levels reported were 6 percent, 13.4 percent and 68.1 percent, respectively.

Older Korean Seniors: Low Incomes and Social, Political and Linguistic Isolation

Some important differences surface when Korean seniors are disaggregated by age. Not surprisingly, the percentage of females increased to 63.4 percent in the 75 years and older group due to the longer life expectancy of women compared to men (Table 2). The percentage of those divorced, separated or widowed was also significantly higher in the older age group compared to those in the 60-74 age group, primarily as a result of the death of a spouse as opposed to divorce or separation.

There is no difference between the two age groups in their immigrant status and timing of arrival as nearly all members of both were immigrant and they were more likely to have arrived before 1991 than in the more recent period. But the older group of Korean seniors is distinctive compared to their younger counterparts on a number of other important traits that underscore their levels of isolation, such as their age at immigration, citizenship and language.

Table 2 Selected Characterisitics of Korean Seniors by Age Group			
		60-74 years	75+ years
Gender	Male	49.4	36.6
	Female	50.6	64.4
Marital Status	Single	0.6	3.3
	Married	84.8	46.7
	DSW	14.6	50.0
Immigrant Status	native-born	1.2	1.7
	Immigrant	98.8	98.3
Timing of Arrival	Before 1991	82.6	89.3
	1991-2001	17.4	10.7
Age at Immigration	<25 years old	1.9	0
	25-59 years old	90.7	51.8
	60+ years old	7.5	48.2
Citizenship	Citizen	86.0	73.3
	Non-citizen	14.0	26.7
Language	English and/or French	75.6	40.0
	Neither English nor French	24.4	60.0
	Total	164	60

Notes: 1. Differences between age groups are statistically significant ($p<.05$) for all variables, with the exception of immigrant status and timing of arrival.
2. Weighted data.

Nearly half of Korean seniors in the older age group immigrated to Canada as seniors as shown in Table 2. Over a quarter did not have Canadian citizenship and 60 percent could not "carry on a conversation of some length on various topics" in either official language, English or French. This profile of older Korean seniors raises serious questions regarding their low levels of social, political and linguistic integration as such isolation can be detrimental to their health and well-being (Hurh,1998; Mui et al., 2007; Pang, 1991; Song & Moon, 1998).

The two groups of Korean seniors reveal an interesting contrast in economic profiles. An examination of the levels and sources of income reveals that the older group of Korean seniors had a lower median income ($12 316) compared to younger Korean seniors, aged 60-74 ($15 070). Still, neither group had higher median incomes than

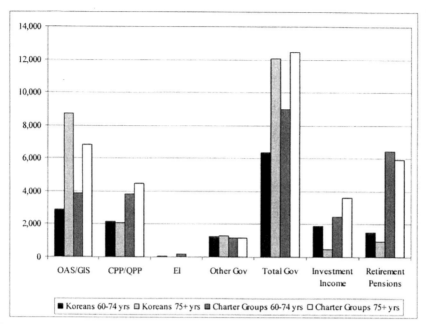

Notes:
1. Other government sources include assistance received from federal, provincial or munici-pal programs not already specified such as social assistance payments, veterans' pensions, GST/HST/QST refunds, etc.
2. total government transfer payments are the sum of OAS/GIS, CPP/QPP, EI, Canada Child Tax Benefits and other government sources.
3. Retirement pensions include superannuation and annuities, such as those from RRSPS and RRIFs.
4. Weighted data.

Figure 1. Other types of income by age group, means

Charter group seniors in either of the age groups ($16 953 and $17 342, respective-ly). Moreover, older Korean seniors appeared to depend more on government assis-tance for financial support than the younger Korean group and Canadian-born Charter group seniors, who had higher mean levels of investment income and private retire-ment pensions (Figure 1). These differences could be explained by their high levels of self-employment in small businesses where there are no pension funds and by their older ages at immigration for nearly half of this older age group.

Levels of government support reported were similar to Charter group seniors in the same age category, although the oldest Korean seniors appeared to rely more on Old Age Security and the Guaranteed Income Supplement (OAS/GIS) and less on CPP/QPP. The younger group of Korean seniors, aged 60-74, reported the lowest mean levels of government assistance overall, which is not surprising given that over 25 percent of them were still in the labor force. While they reported more investment income and retirement pensions than the group of older Korean seniors, they still had less compared to Charter group seniors in the same age category.

This snapshot of older Korean seniors, those aged 75 plus, highlights a high level of financial dependence on government since income from private investments and retirement pensions were generally very low. Financial support from adult children to their elderly parents has also been identified as a source of support in the interviews with community leaders and in past research (Ishii-Kuntz, 1997), although it is not known how many Korean seniors receive money this way or how much is provided. For some who immigrate as seniors under the family sponsorship program; however, they are almost entirely dependent on their adult children for financial support as they are ineligible for OAS/GIS based on residency requirements, which includes a minimum of 10 years in Canada. This dependence often also leads to co-residence.

Households and Living Arrangements

In general, the type of living arrangement has a considerable impact on a senior's quality of life and happiness (Statistics Canada, 2006). Compared to those who live alone, seniors living with others, with family in particular, are more likely to have people and resources available in times of need. While seniors in collective dwellings or institutions such as retirement or nursing homes may have access to health-related services, they may not have access to adequate social and emotional support. As a result, living arrangements, either in private or institutional settings, have important implications for seniors' well-being.

While the type of living arrangement on its own is an important indicator of the structural and cultural dynamics of families within an ethnic group, household resources must also be taken into account. In Table 3, a comparison of Korean and Canadian-born Charter Group seniors on a number of household features is provided. The most common type of living arrangement for both groups of seniors aged 60 and over was as a couple, living without children. For Charter Group seniors, this held for the 60-74 age group as well as for older seniors, 75 years and older. For Koreans, this type of arrangement was also the most common for those in the younger age group (38.4 percent). However, the percentage of older seniors living as a couple without children, dropped to 23.3 percent. This also coincided with a decrease in the percentage of older seniors living with unmarried children and increases in those living alone and those living with other relatives, which include married children.

As expected, Koreans had a greater likelihood of living with family members (either unmarried children or other relatives) than Canadian-born Charter Group seniors across all age groups. Due to data limitations it is not possible to distinguish the percentage of seniors living with married children or in 3-plus generation households. However, the large drop in the percentage living with unmarried children combined with the large jump in the percentage living with other relatives for the older Korean group suggests that much of the increase may be due to moving in with married children.

This translated into higher household sizes. Close to 90 percent of Charter Group seniors, across all age groups, had a household size of two or less, while this characterized about half of Korean seniors. The tendency for larger household sizes also appeared to translate into higher household incomes. There were a higher percentage of Korean seniors in private homes with a household income of $100 000 or greater compared to Charter Group seniors.

However, despite higher household income levels and larger household sizes, Korean seniors were more likely to be renting than Charter Group seniors across all age categories. Moreover, the homes of Korean seniors were less likely to need regular maintenance and more likely to need minor repairs compared to Charter Group seniors. Yet, the need for major repairs was somewhat similar across the two ethnic groupings, with the exception of the oldest age group.

In the data presented in Table 3, Korean seniors were more likely to live with their unmarried children or with other relatives (including married children), than Charter Group seniors. To explain ethnic differences in living arrangements, both cultural and structural explanations have been offered (Foner, 1997; Ishii-Kuntz, 1997; Phua, Kaufman & Park, 2001). In terms of cultural explanations, the values and norms surrounding family relationships, and associated responsibilities and duties, have been important factors for understanding why some ethnic groups have a tendency to live in extended family and intergenerational households more so than others. However, for immigrant families in North America, cultural orientations are insufficient to explain decisions regarding housing and living arrangements and they do not fully account for the differences observed between groups. Family relationships and dynamics are as much determined by social and economic factors as by the cultural precepts that underlie them.

In the next section, the results of the interviews with community leaders are discussed. Interview questions focused on two related issues regarding living arrangements and housing. Respondents were asked to explain why some Korean seniors live with married children and why some live alone or as a couple, as well as reasons for placing seniors in institutional care when Korean culture obliges adult children to care for them. The common underlying premise is that according to tradition, elderly parents should not be living on their own or in an institution. Co-residence with adult children is believed to reflect the degree of filial piety, one of most essential maxims of Confucian ideology. Responses to these questions underscore how the living arrangements of older Korean immigrants lie at the junction of cultural conventions and structural conditions.

		Korean			Charter Groups		
		60+ yrs	60-74 yrs	75+ yrs	60+ yrs	60-74 yrs	75+yrs
Living Arrangement	Alone	12.9	8.5	25.0	28.0	22.2	39.8
	Couple, no children	34.4	38.4	23.3	52.3	57.3	42.1
	W/unmarried children	25.5	32.3	6.7	7.5	9.2	4.0
	W/other relatives	23.2	16.5	41.7	5.6	5.1	6.4
	Other arrangement	4.0	4.3	3.3	6.7	6.2	7.7
Household Size	Two or less	49.1	48.2	51.7	86.6	85.1	89.6
	Three or more	50.9	51.8	48.4	13.4	14.9	10.4
Household Income	<$25 000	31.3	26.8	43.3	33.8	30.2	41.2
	$25 000-$49 999	29.5	31.7	23.3	36.3	36.9	34.9
	$50 000-$99 000	22.8	23.2	21.7	23.5	25.8	18.8
	$100 000+	16.5	18.3	11.7	6.5	7.1	5.0
Housing Tenure	Owner, non-condominium	48.7	53.0	36.7	65.7	69.3	58.1
	Owner, condominium	11.2	12.8	6.7	6.9	6.3	8.3
	Renter	40.2	34.2	56.7	27.4	24.4	33.6
Housing Condition	Regular maintenance	62.1	64.6	55.0	74.8	73.8	76.8
	Minor repairs	32.1	28.7	41.7	19.3	20.1	17.6
	Major repairs	5.8	6.7	3.3	5.9	6.1	5.6
	Total	224	164	60	41 971	28 279	13 692

Table 3
Housing and Household characteristics by Age Group

Notes:
1. For the variable on living arrangement, respondents have been classified as living alone, as a married or common-law couple without children, as a married or common-law couple or a loneparent living with unmarrid children as living with other relatives including married children, or as living in some other arrangment such as with non-relatives.
2. Differences between age groups within ethnic categories are statistically significant (p<.05) for all variables, with the exception of household income and housing condition for Koreans.
3. Weighted data.

Determinants of Intergenerational Living Arrangements and Explaining the Decline

A number of factors can explain the living and household arrangements of Korean immigrant families in addition to composition and geography (i.e., the availability and proximity of children): culture, i.e., the tenets of Confucianism and the increasing diffusion of Western socio-political ideals; financial ability; age at arrival and immigrant class; the availability and quality of institutions and social housing; and intergenerational relationships and the circumstances and needs of seniors and adult children.

Cultural Considerations: Confucianism and the Ideals of Individualism and Egalitarianism

Confucian doctrine, adopted by Korean rulers for nearly five centuries prior to Japanese annexation in 1910, continues to dominate Korean social systems and guide social and interpersonal relationships, even for emigrants living abroad. It dictates that the basic unit of society is the family, not the individual, and that a hierarchical order in all social relationships (e.g., between parent and child, husband and wife, old and young, etc.) is key to harmony and to building a moral society (Hurh, 1998; Kim, 1998). Two of the central tenets of Confucianism, and hence, Korean culture, have lead to extended family living arrangements and they are filial piety and the ideal woman.

Filial piety means more than respect for elders and ancestors and is the cardinal virtue (Hsu, 1998; Hurh, 1998; Jo, 1999; Pang, 1991). It entails subservience, absolute and unquestioning obedience, dependence and loyalty. The underlying premise for filial piety is that parents, especially mothers, suffer enormously in childbearing, childrearing and caring for children. As adults then, children must repay parents by serving them unconditionally in their old age and Korean seniors are supposed to enjoy status, prestige, and advising younger generations. Most of the responsibility for the housing and caring of aging parents is shouldered by the eldest son and his wife as in the patrilineal system, the eldest son becomes head of the family after the passing of the father.

The image of the ideal woman, as a submissive wife and sacrificial mother, also has a significant bearing on the living arrangements of Korean seniors. Women, no longer considered a member of her family of origin after marriage, join her husband's family and are expected to serve and care for them. In her subservient role, she is a full-time homemaker and must adhere to the decisions made by the husband. Both filial piety and this paragon of the ideal woman translate into intergenerational co-residence since the independent or institutional living of aging parents implies a serious lack of filial piety or a contumacious daughter-in-law, and brings shame upon the family. Failure to perform filial duties to the in-laws is considered to be a "deadly sin" and a socially sanctioned cause for divorce (Rhee, 1998).

In the interviews, four respondents referred to Confucianism, culture or tradition as an explanation for understanding the living arrangements of Korean seniors and the barriers they face to institutionalized housing. They shared how many Korean seniors still hold expectations of co-residence with their adult children. A male respondent who is the eldest son in his family, spoke of his sisters' expectations for him to care for their ill mother in his own place, until her death. Another male participant stated that as a result of pride, Koreans are apprehensive of seniors' institutions. That is, to send elderly parents to an institution is to avoid responsibility, and they hide this from other members of the community.

While Confucian values prevail in Korean society and among immigrants, a number of interrelated macro-social and economic changes associated with modernization are believed to be gradually shifting the structure of the kinship system in Korea from extended families to nuclear ones. These include increased globalization, industrialization, urbanization, international migration, demographic changes in fertility and the compression of the childbearing years, longer life expectancy and improved health, female labor force participation, and the on-going diffusion of Christianity (Hurh, 1998; Jo, 1999; Kim, 1998; Lee, 1998; Palley, 1992). Along with these changes is the diffusion of Western values and ideals, in particular those associated with individualism and egalitarianism. These have had a significant influence on Korean immigrant family members, both adult children and seniors, on their social roles and social control, shifting the focus to individual achievement, individual life satisfaction, and gender and status equality.

The disruptive nature of the migration process, on lifestyles, patterns of role relationships and social identities, also leads to shifting values and behaviors (Pang, 1991). First, both internal and international migration not only leads to increased geographic distance between kin, it also results in declining social control. Decreased contact between neighbors increases anonymity offering protection to those who do not adhere to the Confucian ideal of filial piety. Second, most immigrants arrive with spouses and children only, and families undergo a process of nuclearization, with a greater emphasis on the conjugal tie than on the consanguineous one (Kim, Hurh & Kim, 1993). Sponsored parents are viewed not as advisors to be revered and served, but as sources of domestic help for adult immigrants still attempting to establish themselves in the local labor market. This role reversal comes as a cultural shock to older Korean immigrants and drives them towards independent living.

This role reversal is as significant as longer life expectancy for the shift in living arrangements. Korean seniors in Canada now enjoy a longer life span and can remain socially and physically active longer. These Korean seniors place value on their own pursuits and interests, and discourage one another from living with adult children and from making further sacrifices for their children. For contemporary immigrants, to live with an adult child is to live as a domestic servant and to live independently is to be "free." Some would rather live independently and pay for services than ask their children for assistance.

Economic Circumstances

Despite the cultural directives regarding filial piety and women's roles and shifts toward individualism and egalitarianism, financial circumstances often dictate whether any of these ideals can be achieved in housing and living arrangements. In some cases, having the financial resources leads to co-residence, as adult children or seniors are able to support the larger household. In reality, however, co-residence most often depends on the economic situation of adult children and the inability of adult children to maintain an intergenerational household was cited as a reason for independent living for those who desire to live together.

In other cases, sufficient economic resources results in independent living, most especially for those seniors who desire residential independence. However, in contrast to co-residence, the maintenance of a separate home depends in large part on seniors' financial circumstances, not the adult children's. For many seniors, costs associated with separate dwellings and private retirement homes are prohibitive. Thus, the low levels of income observed in the Korean senior population in the statistical data partly explains the high levels of shared accommodations. Yet, the increasing likelihood of financial self-sufficiency of longer-term immigrants, i.e., those who arrived as working adults, is leading to increasing residential independence. These Korean seniors are enjoying their retirement phase with some degree of accumulated wealth and property, which influences how they perceive the rest of their lives to play out. For example, an older female respondent commented that "for the first time, Korean seniors have things of their own."

Age at Arrival and Immigration Policy

For many immigrants, the age at migration and the category of admission influenced living arrangements. Korean immigrants arriving as seniors (18 percent of those aged 60 plus, and 48 percent of those 75 years and older) are highly likely to have arrived under the Family Class, having been sponsored by their adult children. According to the sponsorship provisions in the immigration policy, these adult children are required to provide their dependents with financial support for up to 10 years and this financial support often translates into co-residence as seniors' housing options are limited. They not only lack the information needed to live independently, they are ineligible for government assistance and social services such as social housing. It is only once they meet eligibility requirements for social assistance that those who clearly desire residential separation are able to move out on their own, if they do not already have the financial means (Pang 1991).

In addition to immigration policy effects on seniors' living arrangements, the age at arrival is also important in terms of the degree of adaptation to the host society. Those who become seniors after immigrating should be expected to have different orientations than those who arrive as seniors. Immigrants who arrived in Canada as working adults are not only better equipped to navigate the institutional structures related to housing and health care, they are also more likely to espouse views of freedom, individualism and independence. This positive effect of the age at immigration on family co-residence for seniors is consistent with past research (Boyd, 1991; Ng, Northcott & Abu-Laban, 2007).

Formal Services and Institutional Care: Perceptions, Availability, Accessibility, Quality

A key factor that influences co-residence among seniors in any given location is the existence of community level services and other types of housing (Burr & Mutchler, 2007; Kim & Lauderdale, 2002) and the perceptions associated with each. Alternatives to intergenerational co-residence include social housing, supportive housing, retirement homes and long-term care facilities. The proximity, availability, accessibility and quality of facilities and services geared to the elderly set the structure within which housing decisions and arrangements are made.

Until the recent decade, there were very few formal services sensitive to Korean seniors in Canada, particularly in regards to institutional living. This lack of ethno-specific services or lack of sensitivity to ethnic minorities has serious impacts on a senior's aging process and adjustment. Past research by MacLean and colleagues (1986, 1989) of immigrant seniors in mainstream long-term care facilities demonstrates how their loss of family, culture and community negatively influenced motivation, health and interpersonal relations.

It is in the context of mainstream institutions that several interview respondents had contact with a family member, friend or client that inspired their paid or volunteer work with seniors and senior care. They identified three key barriers to supportive housing, formal institutions and independent living for those who require some degree of home support services, and they were language, food, and staff attitudes.

Two respondents recounted separate stories of visiting an elderly friend or relative in a long-term care home in the late 1980s. Each respondent spoke of the challenges the resident faced in communicating their needs and receiving sensitive and appropriate care. Respondents felt that the inability to communicate in English had resulted in the improper treatment of elderly Korean residents. For example, a female respondent witnessed the senior calling for assistance and being deliberately ignored. In an unrelated experience, a male respondent recalled finding his mother "tied to a wheelchair" upon one visit and was told by staff it was to prevent her from falling. They told him she had been yelling and screaming but, according to him, she had been talking in Korean; to staff, he argued, she "must have seemed like a crazy person" when she had been trying to tell them she had to use the restroom. Several days later, he received a phone call from the home telling him his mother had a bladder infection and, as he expressed it, she had to wear "adult diapers." An experience he felt was painful and degrading.

Although sharing a language does not prevent miscommunication and misunderstanding, not sharing a language exacerbates the feeling of disadvantage and mistreatment for immigrants and ethnic minorities. Communication difficulties do not only have the potential to lead to the misinterpretation of a resident's behavior among staff and result in mistreatment, but they can also lead to the misinterpretation of staff behavior among a resident and his/her family.

Respondents identified Korean seniors' distaste for non-Korean food as another significant barrier and this is consistent with past studies (Pang 1991). For seniors in any kind of institutional care, food preferences have implications for health, nutrition and psychological well-being. Another older male respondent indicated that some Korean residents have refused to eat and argues that the strict Western nutritional guidelines are a barrier to bringing in Korean food for residents. For this reason, many seniors are not comfortable with the idea of going into nursing homes, using meals-on-wheels programs, and other formal services.

Staff attitudes were also identified as a barrier to social programs and formal care. Many respondents felt some staff in institutions were insensitive toward Korean seniors, and this perception was heightened by difficulties in communication. Due to such barriers, many Korean families are reluctant to have older members live in supportive housing or in a more formal group setting and they take on the responsibility of caring for older members in their own homes. Moreover, language and cultural barriers do not only affect the living arrangements of Korean seniors and their utilization of formal services, but can also lead to health problems and poor quality treatment (Mui et al., 2007; Pereira & Lazarowich, 1996). For example, there was a feeling among respondents that institutional residents were over-medicated; they were drugged if they "acted up." But, as one younger male respondent put it, "you need to be able to understand what they're trying to express, not increase their dose to calm them down."

Yet, the increasing availability and accessibility of these institutions suggest that Korean seniors will be more visible within them. First, health care officials often instruct Korean families and seniors to enter long-term care facilities without discussing other options such as home support services or recruiting a paid caregiver. Second, increased life expectancy has been associated with a longer burden of care for seniors (Quah, 2003), whose families are more likely to turn to institutions. Third, there is a growing number of housing options tailored for Korean seniors in Canada. In the Toronto region alone, there are two retirement homes (Hancajok Maxome Centre and Pleasant Valley Rest Home) and two long-term care facilities (Castleview-

Wychwood Towers and the Rose of Sharon). The Rose of Sharon, a 60-bed facility with life lease condominiums, will be the first long-term care facility in Canada operated by Koreans. When interviewees were asked whether sending seniors to a Korean-run nursing home would be more tolerable to Korean families, they all agreed that it would make a difference. According to an older male respondent, "we need it desperately."

The availability of social housing also shapes rates of intergenerational co-residence (Kim & Lauderdale, 2002). A number of non-profit apartments are available to Korean seniors who meet the criteria and wish to live independently. Although none of the buildings are specifically for the Korean community, several of them have clusters of Korean senior residents. One in particular, Calvary Manor, was initially built as non-profit housing for Korean seniors in 1992 but is currently low-income housing and open to others. However, the majority of residents are Korean, mostly elderly women who benefit from the shared location; as the same older male respondent put it, "they stick together, entertain one another and are comfortable." Camaraderie and companionship develop among Korean seniors in seniors' apartments such that friends become family (Pang, 1991). However, the current wait list for a senior's apartment in the City of Toronto is 8 to 10 years. As a result, seniors either remain in the homes of their adult children or for those who wish to live independently, they find market rent housing. This lack of affordable rental housing, coupled with limited financial resources, makes older Korean immigrants dependent on their family members.

The growth of Korean services and facilities will accommodate many Korean families who do not or are not able to live up to the traditional expectation of filial piety in living arrangements. While many have a difficult time utilizing mainstream services, where they are perceived to fall through the cracks, they are likely to have less difficulty using Korean-based services. This is captured in the comment by a female respondent, "If Koreans don't look after Koreans, who will?" Having access to services not only in the Korean language but sensitive to the needs of Korean seniors and their families will have a significant impact on their adjustment, health and well-being.

Intergenerational Relationships and the Circumstances and Needs of Seniors and Adult Children

An additional theme in the living arrangements of Korean seniors is intergenerational relationships and the needs of seniors and/or adult children, which has also emerged in past research (Crimmins and Ingegneri, 1990). This includes aspects such as adult children's work and family needs, seniors' fears and health, and intergenerational conflict and elder abuse.

Some seniors in good health live with their adult children to help out with the family business, with domestic chores and/or childcare. In fact, previous studies found that elderly immigrants were sponsored by and lived with their adult children to help in these areas (Hurh, 1998; Pang, 1991). However, for many seniors, especially those who have resided in Canada for some time, the needs of their adult children drive them in the opposite direction, toward residential independence. This is in order to escape from becoming domestic servants for their children.

For seniors in poorer health, business ownership as well as female labor force participation prevent adult children from providing direct care to aging parents. Business owners spend long hours away from home, and the stress and uncertainty of entrepreneurship leads Korean immigrants to have one of the highest rates of problems in self-employment (Teixeira, Lo & Truelove, 2007). This affects their ability to manage additional responsibilities in the home, and their degree of integration within the family and their extended family.

In terms of working women, daughters and daughters-in-law in many Korean families are also unlikely to be at home full-time to provide hands-on care to seniors (and increasingly so with rising divorce rates). While women's increasing involvement in paid economic activities play a large role in the changing conceptions of women's roles and responsibilities, it also contributes to a heavy double burden with duties at work and at home (Hurh, 1998; Kim, 1998). To avoid adding to that "burden," Korean seniors are reluctant to live with adult children. In addition, caring for children often takes precedence over caring for elders, which goes against traditional norms and can lead to conflict between seniors and their adult children as aging parents may feel as if they are not being treated respectfully.

Actual and the potential for conflicts – often between mothers-in-law and daughters-in-law – are common reasons for maintaining separate households. Korean seniors with adult children belonging to the second generation face an increased potential for conflict or misunderstanding due to cultural gaps, particularly if children are in exogenous marriages. As a result, to preserve a close relationship with their adult children, many Korean seniors choose to live on their own. one senior male expressed this best with "sometimes distance makes you closer."

Conflict can also manifest as elder abuse, although due to traditional ideals of filial piety this has not received much attention in the community. Yet, one younger female respondent, in particular, had seen several cases of elder abuse by adult children in her work. Abuse was mostly financial although there had been instances of physical, emotional and mental abuse, and neglect. These abused seniors move into independent housing or to supportive housing. At the other extreme are those adult children who are sensitive to the fears of their elderly parents, fears related to living alone, and will accommodate them in their homes.

Summary and Discussion

Cultural explanations are insufficient for elucidating ethnic group differences in the context of immigration. This analysis underscores how changes in the social and economic structure, the impact of immigration, ethnic resources and networks, family dynamics, human capital, and individual situations and preferences all play a role. In particular, the living arrangements of Korean seniors and their use of institutionalized care sit at the junction between traditional and modernizing Korean cultural ideology and structural opportunities and constraints. This highlights Barth's argument that it is "inadequate to regard overt institutional forms as constituting the cultural features which at any time distinguish an ethnic group – these overt forms are determined by ecology as well as by transmitted culture" (1969, p. 13).

On the one hand, values regarding filial piety and women's roles, individualism and egalitarianism, and the social consequences of behavior (i.e., stigma and shame) shape the extent to which multiple generations of families share housing space. On the other hand, these decisions take place in the context of structural circumstances, either in terms of financial resources and women's labor force participation or in terms of the resources available in the larger local community such as social housing and Korean-based retirement homes and long-term care homes.

As in all cultures, some Korean immigrants adhere to traditional norms and mores more steadfastly than others. These individuals are more likely to live in intergenerational households. However, additional factors contribute to the decision to co-reside: being a newcomer to Canada and/or sponsored by children, having limited incomes or savings, having adult children who could use additional labor in the home, and the lack of social housing or Korean-operated services and facilities. In contrast, those who are likely to live independently are those who have adopted a more individualistic orientation, have had a longer residence in Canada, have the financial means, and access to appropriate housing. In fact, several respondents in this study stated that many seniors want to live on their own and would, if they had the financial resources to do so. However, Korean seniors in institutions are likely those who have been placed there by healthcare professionals, and come from families where both husband and wife participate in the labor force, and predominantly in small family businesses.

While Korean seniors have a higher level of intergenerational living compared to Charter Group seniors, past studies have noted a declining trend in multi-generational households in Asia and among Asian immigrants (Hurh, 1998; Kim & Rhee, 1997; Martin, 1989; Palley, 1992; Quah, 2003). The results from this study emphasize that the declining trend in multi-generational households among Korean immigrants cannot be attributed solely to cultural shifts. The increase in the independent or institutional living among Korean seniors is not simply reflective of a devaluation of filial piety in the

Korean community. Rather, filial piety continues to remain firmly entrenched in the psyche of most Koreans and other Asians (Hurh, 1998; Kim, Hurh & Kim, 1993; Pang, 1991; Thomas, 1990). Yet, if filial piety is no longer demonstrated and experienced through extended family households, the more important question is in what ways is it manifested? In other words, how will the "traditional" concept endure rapid social change, be subject to new interpretations, and be demonstrated in subsequent generations (Kuo, 1998; Thomas, 1990)? These are important issues in light of the research that has shown co-residence itself is not the most beneficial for the well-being of older immigrants (Gee, 2000). This is attributed to harmonious, mutually respectful, meaningful and frequent social interaction with adult children and friends (Hurh, 1998; Pang, 1991).

Two issues remain open for further investigation. First, data from the census and interviews suggest there are two distinct groups of Korean immigrant seniors – those who became seniors in Canada, after being in the labor force, and those who arrived as seniors. Whether systematic differences exist between these groups in their cultural orientations, housing and integration patterns will be relevant for understanding the association between life cycle stage and adaptation. This study touched on some of their issues with respect to sponsorship obligations and financial dependence but more could be done in the future. A second area for further exploration is the degree to which there are gender differences in cultural and structural characteristics, in their responses to family and external conditions, and in their perceptions of the different types of housing arrangements. This was discussed only briefly in several of the interviews and should be addressed in-depth in a future study.

Korean seniors are a highly immigrant population, concentrated in Toronto and Vancouver, and distinctive for their linguistic and political isolation, high levels of education and employment – particularly in self-employment – and lower levels of income. In addition to financial assistance and social and emotional support, many Korean seniors also rely on their children for housing, regardless of whether they live together or apart.

References

Barth, Fredrik (Ed.). (1969). *Ethnic groups and boundaries: The social organization of culture difference.* Prospect Heights, IL: Waveland Press, Inc.

Boyd, Monica. (1991). Immigration and living arrangements: Elderly women in Canada. *International Migration Review 25*:4-27.

Bryant, Toba, Brown, Ivan, Cogan, Tara, Dallaire, Laforest, Clemence, McGowan, Sophie, Patrick Raphael, Dennis Lucic, Thompson, Richard, Loraine & Young,. Joyce (2004). What do Canadian seniors say supports their quality of life?: Findings from a National participatory research study. *Canadian Journal of Public Health 95*:299-303.

Burr, Jeffrey A. & Mutchler,. Jan E. (2007). Residential independence among older persons: Community and individual factors. *Population Research and Policy Review 26*:85-101.

Clark, William A.V., Deurloo, Marinus C. & . Dieleman, Frans M (2003). Housing careers in the United States, 1968-93: Modelling the sequencing of housing states. *Urban Studies 40:*143-160.

Crimmins, Eileen M. & Ingegneri, Dominique G. (1990). Interaction and living arrangements of older parents and their children: Past trends, present determinants, future implications. *Research on Aging 12*:3-35.

Foner, Nancy. (1997). The immigrant family: Cultural legacies and cultural changes. *International Migration Review 31*:961-974.

Gee, Ellen M. (2000). Living arrangements and quality of life among Chinese Canadian elders. *Social Indicators Research 51*:309-329

Health Canada. (2002). *Canada's aging population.* Ottawa: Division of Aging and Seniors. p. 43.

Hsu, Francis L.K. (1998). Confucianism in comparative context. In Walter H. Slote and George A De Vos . (Eds.) (pp. 53-71).*Confucianism and the famil.y* Albany: State University of New York Press. Hurh, Won Moo. (1998). *The Korean Americans.* Westport, CT: Greenwood Press.

Ishii-Kuntz, Masako. (1997). Intergenerational relationships among Chinese, Japanese and Korean Americans. *Family Relations 46*:23-32.

Jo, Moon H. (1999). *Korean immigrants and the challenge of adjustment.* Westport, Ct: Greenwood Press.

Kim, E.l-Hannah. (1998). The social reality of Korean American women: Toward crashing with the Confucian ideology. In *Korean American women: From tradition to modern feminism,* Young I. Song and Ailee Moon. (Eds.) (pp. 23-33). Westport, CT: Praeger Publishers.

Kim, Cheong-Seok & Rhee, Ka-Oak (1997). Variations in preferred living arrangements among Korean elderly parents. *Journal of Cross-Cultural Gerontology 12*:189-202.

Kim, Jibum & Lauderdale,. Diane S. (2002). The role of community context in immigrant elderly living arrangements: Korean American elderly. *Research on Aging 24*:630-653.

Kim, Kwang Chung, Hurh & Shin Kim, Won Moo. (1993). Generation differences in Korean immigrants' life conditions in the United States. *Sociological Perspectives 36:*257-270.

Kuo, Eddie C.Y. (1998). Confucianism and the Chinese family in Singapore: Continuities and changes. In Walter H. Slote and George A. De Vos. (Eds). (pp.231-247). *Confucianism and the family, .* Albany: State University of New York Press. pp. 231-247

Kwak, Min-Jung. (2004). *An exploration of the Korean-Canadian community in Vancouver.* Working paper series 04-14. Vancouver: CERIS. p. 35.

Lee, Kwang Kyu. (1998). Confucian tradition in the contemporary Korean family. In Walter H. Slote & George A. De Vos. (Eds.). (pp. 249-264). *Confucianism and the family,* Albany: State University of New York Press.

MacLean, Michael J & Bonar, Rita (1986). Ethnic elderly people in long-term care facilities of the dominant culture: Implications for social work practice and education. *International Social Work 29*:227-236.

MacLean, Michael J. & Venes Sakadakis. (1989). Quality of life in terminal care with institutionalized ethnic elderly people. *International Social Work 32*:209-221.

Martin, Linda G. (1989). Living arrangements of the elderly in Fiji, Korea, Malaysia, and the Philippines. *Demography 26:*627-643.

Mui, Ada C., Suk-Young Dooyeon, Kang,Kang & Domanski, Margaret Dietz . (2007). English language proficiency and health-related quality of life among Chinese and Korean immigrant elders. *Health & Social Work 32:*119-127.

Murdie, R.A. (2002). The housing careers of Polish and Somali newcomers in Toronto's rental market. *Housing Studies 17*:423-443.

Özüekal, A. Sule & Kempen, Ronald van (2002). Housing careers of minority ethnic groups: Experiences, explanations and prospects. *Housing Studies 17*:365-379.

Pae, Sung Moon. (1992). *Korea leading developing nations: Economy, democracy and welfare.* Lanham, MD: University Press of America, Inc.

Palley, Howard A. (1992). Social policy and the elderly in South Korea: Confucianism, modernization, and development. *Asian Survey 32:*787-801.

Pang, Keum-Young Chung. (1991). *Korean elderly women in America: Everyday life, health and illness.* New York: AMS Press, Inc.

Pereira, Irene & Lazarowich, N. Michael (1996). Ethnic content in long term care facilities for Portuguese and Italian elderly. *Canadian Ethnic Studies 28*:82-88.

Phua, Voon-Chin, Kaufman, Gayle & Park, Keong Suk. (2001). Strategic adjustments of elderly Asian Americans: Living arrangements and headship. *Journal of Comparative Family Studies 32*:263-281.

Song, Young I. (1998). Life satisfaction of the Korean American elderly" In Young I. Song and Ailee Moon. (Eds.) (pp. 193-206). *Korean American women: From tradition to modern feminism,* Westport, CT: Praeger Publishers.

Song, Young I. & Moon, Ailee. (Eds.). (1998). *Korean American women: From tradition to modern feminism.* Westport, CT: Praeger Publishers.

Statistics Canada. (2005). *Population projections of visible minority groups, Canada, provinces and regions: 2001-2017.* Ottawa: Demography Division. 91-541-XIE. pp. 78.

Statistics Canada. (2006). *A portrait of seniors in Canada.* Ottawa: Social and Aboriginal Statistics Division. 89-519-XIE. pp. 301.

Teixeira, Carlos, Lo, Lucia & Truelove, Marie (2007). *Immigrant entrepreneurship, institutional discrimination, and implications for public policy: A case study in Toronto.* Environment and Planning C: Government and Policy 25:176-193.

Thomas, Elwyn. (1990). Filial piety, social change and Singapore youth. *Journal of Moral Education 19*:192-205.

Yoo, Young-sik. (2002). Canada and Korea: A shared history. In R.W.L. Guisso and Young-sik Yoo.*Canada and Korea: Perspectives 2000,* Toronto, ON: Centre for Korean Studies, University of Toronto. pp. 9-43.

Yoon, In-Jin. (1997). *On my own: Korean businesses and race relations in America.* Chicago: The University of Chicago Press.

Yoon, In-Jin. (2006). Understanding the Korean diaspora from comparative perspectives. In *Asia Culture Forum.* Gwang-ju, South Korea. pp. 1-21.

20

Predicting Cultural Adaptation of Elderly Chinese Immigrants within a Bidirectional Model of Acculturation: Canadian Acculturation and Chinese Identification

Ben Kuo, (University of Windsor)

Introduction

Recent scholars have strongly recommended theory driven studies (Iwamasa & Sorocco, 2002; Lai, 2004a) and the use of culturally sensitive and empirically validated measures (Mui, 1998; Shibusawa & Mui, 2001) for the advancement of research with elderly Asian immigrants. The theory of acculturation, as an empirically tested conceptual framework of cultural change, has been nominated as a promising candidate to advance this research agenda (Iwamasa & Sorocco, 2002). By definition, acculturation occurs when firsthand contact between two autonomous cultural groups results in changes on either or both of the groups (Redfield, Linton & Herskovits, 1936). As such, acculturation is particularly useful in understanding individuals or groups undergoing cultural transitions or cross cultural adjustment, such as immigrants and international students (Kuo & Roysircar, 2004). As Berry (1997) posited, acculturation serves to explain changes in language, behavioral outcomes, cognitive styles, personality, identity, attitudes, stress, and psychological well being among those undergoing cultural transition. As a comprehensive model of cultural adaptation (Berry, 1997), acculturation is a fitting theoretical framework to study the cross-cultural experiences of immigrant older adults, including Asians in North America (Iwamasa & Sorocco, 2002; Kuo & Guan, 2006).

Migration poses unique adjustment difficulties for Asian immigrant elderly in the host country, often because of the compounded strains associated with cultural changes and with growing older (Gelfand & Yee, 1991; Wong & Ujimoto, 1998). Evidence indicated that acculturation related difficulties such as language and cultural adjustment concerns are among the most common life stressors identified by elderly Chinese immigrants (Tsai & Lopez, 1997). In fact, a recent review of late-life depression studies among older Asian immigrants in U.S. and Canada has linked the acculturation level of this population to depressive symptoms (Kuo, Chong & Vanessa, 2008). The phenomenon of the "health immigrant effect" further points to the potential long-term adverse impact of migration on the physical and mental well-being of immigrants (Ali, 2002). This effect dictates that while more recent foreign-born immigrants might be healthier than their native-born (e.g., Canadian-born) counterparts, this health advantage diminishes over time as immigrants become more acculturated to the behaviors, life styles, beliefs and attitudes of the host society. In fact, a recent large scale Canadian study has revealed that immigrant elderly in Canada who were 65 and older reported poorer overall health than their Canadian-born counterparts (Gee, Kobayashi & Prus, 2004).

Thus, researchers have observed that cultural orientations, in terms of both acculturation and cultural identification, have broad implications for the adjustment and well being of immigrant elderly (Tran, Fitzpatrick, Berg & Wright, 1996). However, a review of the literature showed that the discussion on acculturation and cultural identity of Asian immigrant elderly is often limited and cursory in nature (Iwamasa & Sorocco, 2002), and the measures of these cultural constructs frequently lack psychometric rigor (Kuo & Guan, 2006). Therefore, the purpose of the current study is to integrate acculturation theory into the investigation of the cultural adaptation experience of community dwelling elderly Chinese immigrants in Toronto, Canada. To this end, the specific purposes of the study are: a) to test two predictor models of Canadian Acculturation and Chinese Identification, respectively with various demographic, psychosocial, and health variables; and b) to offer recommendations for future research and service/intervention provisions for elderly Chinese immigrants based on the findings.

Acculturation Related Issues Among Elderly Chinese Immigrants

A review of the existing literature on Chinese immigrant older adults provides some clues to acculturation's link to a wide variety of demographic, psychosocial, and health variables. For instance, several studies found that a longer stay in the host country led to more depression (Lai, 2000a; Lam, Pacala & Smith, 1997; Wu, Tran & Amjad, 2004). Stokes, Thompson, Murphy and Gallagher-Thompson (2001) showed particularly high risks for depression among older Chinese immigrants those who lived in the United States for less than five years. Other studies had pointed to lack of English proficiency as a negative predictor of depression among older Chinese immigrants in the U.S. and Canada (Casado & Leung, 2001; Lai, 2000a; Lam et al., 1997).

One the other hand, in a large scale study of elderly Chinese immigrants across Canada, Lai (2004a) found that while participants' Chinese cultural identity (the involvement of Chinese elderly in cultural activities and affiliation with Chinese community) served as a protective factor against depression, adherence to traditional Chinese norms and beliefs in fact put them more at risk for depressive symptoms. Gee's (1999) study of 708 Chinese elderly on the west coast of Canada found Chinese ethnic identity to be negatively associated with perception of life quality, social support, and health. A study by Kuo, Chong, & Joseph (2008) reviewed 24 empirically-based studies examining the psychosocial correlates of depression study among older Asian immigrants in North America, including older Chinese immigrants. The authors reported that in nine of these studies acculturation and acculturation-related factors were investigated in relation to depression. The results across the majority of these studies suggested that overall a weak cultural identification with the host culture is associated with more reported depressive symptomatology among older Asian immigrants.

The quality of interpersonal resources and social support has also been found to be negatively affected by cultural transition (e.g., Mui, 1996; Shibusawa & Mui, 2001). Acculturation difficulties often cause immigrant elderly to feel profoundly estranged, isolated, and excluded from the mainstream society (Cheung, 1989; Tsai & Lopez, 1997) and to eventually develop internal psychological distress (e.g., depressive symptoms) (Lai, 2000b; Tran et al., 1996). Furthermore, it is noted that acculturation and cultural orientation of older immigrants also affect their utilization of community, social, and mental health services and their perception of service barriers (Abramson, Trejo & Lai, 2002; Kuo & Torres Gil, 2001). For example, Lai (2004a) found that elderly Chinese immigrants who held strong Chinese cultural and health beliefs were more likely to perceive greater cultural barriers in the current service system.

Theoretical Perspective on Acculturation and Its Correlates

The review above suggests that acculturation levels of older Chinese immigrants might be closely associated with a number of critical adjustment-related variables. These preliminary results are, in fact, consistent with the prevailing theory of acculturation. Acculturation theory dictates that cultural adaptation is affected by a whole host of demographic and psychosocial factors occurring prior to, during, and after an immigrant's migration experience. According to Berry and his colleagues (Berry, 1997; Berry & Sam, 1997), the critical moderating factors for acculturation before migration include immigrants' demographic (e.g., age, gender, education), cultural (e.g., language), economic (e.g., financial status), and personal (e.g., health status, knowledge of the host society) characteristics, and their migration motivation and expectations. This model further posits that moderating factors critical during acculturation encompass immigrants' acculturation strategies, length of stay in the host culture, degree of contact and participation with co-ethnic and host members, perceived social support, coping strategies, and experiences of discrimination. This framework also implicates that acculturation might lead to certain negative heath and psychological consequences, such as acculturative stress and psychopathology (e.g., depression). However, successful acculturation can also facilitate improved family and community relations, and positive inter-group interaction and participation in the host society (i.e., also known as socio-cultural adaptation) (Berry & Sam, 1997).

On the basis of this acculturation theory, several studies have examined the demographic and psychosocial correlates of acculturation with Asian samples in the U.S. and Canada (Farver, Bhadha & Narang, 2002; Kuo & Roysircar, 2004, 2006; Sodowsky, Lai & Plake, 1991). However, these studies were conducted with younger Asian populations (e.g., adolescents, college/university students). To the author's knowledge, no published studies have systematically and simultaneously investigated a constellation of critical correlates of acculturation in an integrated model among older immigrants in North America. Henceforth, the present study adopts the above acculturation theory as the guiding framework to identify the research questions and to direct the analyses of the data.

Bidirectional Measurement of Acculturation

Conceptually, there are two dominant perspectives in construing acculturation: the unilinear and the bilinear (bidirectional) positions (Kim & Abrue, 2001). Earlier acculturation theorists had conceptualized acculturation as a unidirectional construct that rests on a continuum with high and low scores for acculturation at opposite poles of the same continuum. Although researchers have noted the advantage of this unilinear approach for being parsimonious in defining acculturation, it is nevertheless conceptually limited (e.g., unable to distinguish between bicultural individuals and marginalized individuals) (Ryder, Alden & Paulhus, 2000).

Recent advancement in acculturation theory, however, supports a bidirectional model of acculturation (Kim & Abrue, 2001), which construes acculturation in terms of two separate (orthogonal) processes on two continua. Under this model, individuals' adaptation to the host culture's values, attitudes, and behaviors occurs independently from the maintenance of cultural characteristics associated with the cultures of origin; accordingly, the two processes are assessed separately. An empirical example of this bidirectional conceptualization is Ryder et al.'s (2000) development of the Vancouver Index of Acculturation (VIA). The VIA measures individuals' associations with the predominant cultural environment and their cultures of birth or upbringing in two corresponding subscales, which Ryder et al. named the mainstream identification and heritage identification subscales, respectively.

Examples of the items on the mainstream identification subscale of the VIA include: "I often participate in Canadian cultural traditions" or "I believe in mainstream

Canadian values." The items on the heritage identification subscale are parallel statements that are phrased in the direction of one's heritage culture: "I often participate in
my Chinese cultural traditions" or "I believe in traditional Chinese values." This model
allows a better account of biculturalism, because individuals can be high on their identification with both the host and the heritage culture simultaneously. It is within this
framework that the acculturation of elderly Chinese immigrants in the present study is
conceptualized and assessed.

Research Questions of the Present Study

The present study is an attempt to assess the cultural adaptation of elderly
Chinese immigrants in Canada in terms of Canadian Acculturation and Chinese
Identification by identifying key demographic and psychosocial predictors corresponding to each of these two constructs. As such, the present study will test two hypotheses corresponding to each of the two cultural orientations. First, it is hypothesized that
being a woman, being younger in age, having a higher educational attainment and
income, being in Canada for a longer period of time, using more English at home and
with others, having less involvement with co ethnic peers, having a more positive evaluation of one's physical health, having more positive relationships with adult children,
perceiving more social support, being less depressed, utilizing more services, perceiving fewer services barriers, greater participation in community programs, and greater
voting participation will be related to higher levels of Canadian Acculturation. Second,
it is hypothesized that being a man, being older in age, having lower education and
income, being in Canada for a shorter period of time, using less English at home and
with others, having more involvement with co ethnic peers, having a more negative
evaluation of one's physical health, having more negative relationships with adult children, perceiving less social support, being more depressed, having utilizing less services, perceiving more services barriers, less participation in community programs, and
less voting participation will be related to higher levels of Chinese Identification.

Method

Participants

The present sample consisted of 213 Chinese immigrant adults who were 60
years of age or older. The gender distributions of the sample were 64.8% (n = 138)
women and 34.7% (n = 74) men; one respondent did not provide gender information
(see Table 1). The mean age of the sample was 72.09 (SD = 8.94), and the participants' ages ranged from 60 to 98. All of the participants in the study were born outside of Canada. Among them, participants identified seven different countries through-

Table 1			
Demographic Characteristics of Elderly Chinese Immigrants (N = 213)			
		N	%
Gender	Men	74	34.7
	Women	138	64.8
	Not reported	1	0.5
Age	60-69	96	45.9
	70-79	65	30.1
	80-89	39	18.7
	90 and above	9	4.3
Marital Status	Married	119	56.1
	Widowed	83	39.2
	Divorced	6	2.8
	Separated	2	0.9
	Never Married	2	0.9
Level of Education	Elementary School	47	22.2
	High School Diploma	70	33
	College Diploma/Univ Degree	79	37.3
	Masters Degree	13	6.1
	Doctoral or Professional Degree	3	1.4
Monthly Income	under $1 000	90	49.2
	$1 000-$1 999	49	26.8
	$2 000-$2 999	17	9.3
	$3 000-$3 999	11	6
	$4 000-$4 999	6	3.3
	$5 000 or above	10	5.5
Place of Birth	Mainland China	93	43.7
	Taiwan	89	41.8
	Hong Kong	12	5.6
	Other	6	2.9
Primary Language Spoke at Home[a]	Mandarin	88	41.5
	Taiwanese	92	43.2
	Cantonese	84	39.6
	English	26	12.3
	Other	21	9.9
Current Living Arrangement[a]	Alone	50	23.7
	With Spouse/Partner	106	50.2
	With children	98	46.4
	With Grandchildren	40	19.0
Types of Residence/Dwelling	Own House	108	51.2
	Children's/Friends' Place	68	32.2
	Rental Unit	5	2.4
	Senior Apartment	30	14.2

out East and Southeast Asia as their places of birth. The participants' mean length of residence in Canada was 18.61 years (SD =11.14). In terms of socioeconomic status, 44.8% of the participants reported having completed university or college and higher degrees, and the remaining 55.2% reported elementary or high school education (see Table 1). According to an estimate based on the 2001 Census Public Use Microdata (Statistic Canada, 2006), the proportion of Chinese Canadian older adults 65 and over who received a university and above education was 15.4%. In comparison, the percentage of the current sample with a university and above education was 44.8%, significantly higher than the national figure. This might be attributed to the fact that nearly half of the present sample was consisted of immigrants originated from Taiwan and Hong Kong, who initially migrated to Canada as educated entrepreneurs or international students seeking higher education in Canada. Nearly half (49.2%) of the elderly indicated a monthly income below $1 000 (Canadian), and more than one quarter (26.8%) reported monthly income in the $1 000 to $1 999 range. Almost one quarter (23.7%) of the sample lived alone.

Procedure

The study employed grass roots, culturally appropriate recruitment strategies to achieve a sizable, diversified, and well represented sample of Chinese elderly. First, the researcher worked in close collaboration with Chinese and Taiwanese religious leaders, directors of community programs and organizations, and public senior service coordinators and social workers in Toronto to establish the recruitment plan. In the end, the participating organizations included one large scale senior community agency, two Chinese senior recreational clubs, and four Taiwanese churches in the Greater Toronto Area. Second, the snowball technique was used, that is, participants were asked to recruit other potential participants through their personal contacts.

Given the variability in degrees of literacy, reading ability, and physical mobility among Chinese elderly, the questionnaires were administered in three different formats: a) a group format facilitated by the researcher or a social worker with a paper-and-pencil questionnaire; b) unassisted self completion of a paper-and-pencil questionnaire; and c) face to face individual interviews conducted by a trained bilingual (Chinese and English) interviewer. All research sessions and interviews were conducted in the Chinese dialects appropriate for the respondents. Comparisons across the methods of data collection showed that those participants who completed the study via face-to-face interviews were significantly less acculturated and more strongly identified with Chinese values than those with the other methods. This was likely due to the fact that the individuals in the first category were most likely to be represented by older adults residing in government-sponsored seniors' apartments, and that they were considerably older and less literate than the other participants. In all cases, the partici- pants read and completed a signed consent form before responding to the question- naires. The resultant sample consisted of elderly Chinese immigrants who lived in the community as well as those who lived in government sponsored seniors' apartments. At the end, a total of 227 questionnaires were distributed, and 213 were completed and returned to the researcher.

Measures

The research materials were administered entirely in Chinese. To ensure the equivalence of the Chinese version of the questionnaire to its original English version, two bilingual scholars (one economics professor and one business professor at the author's university) independently rated the translated questionnaire. The two judges reported the linguistic accuracy of the translated questionnaire to be 95% and 98%, respectively. In addition, a pilot test of the questionnaire and the consent form was conducted, involving a number of elderly Chinese immigrants. The following section provides information on the measures used in the present study besides the demo- graphic sheet.

Canadian Acculturation and Chinese Identification: The VIA (Ryder et al., 2000) is a measure a bidirectional measure of acculturation based on a 7-point Likert scale. In the present study, only items that are developmentally relevant to Chinese elderly were included. This resulted in 5 items pertaining to the mainstream (Canadian) cul- ture, and 5 items pertaining to the heritage (Chinese) culture. The score of the for- mer was named *Canadian Acculturation* and the score of the latter *Chinese Identification.* In the study, the internal consistency of the Canadian Acculturation and the Chinese Identification items were α = .83 and .78, respectively. *Perceived social support:* Six items on the Multidimensional Scale of Perceived Social Support (MSPSS; Zimet, Dahlem, Zimet & Farley, 1988) associated with social support from friends and significant others were adopted to assess participants' perception of interpersonal support and resources. The scale uses a 7 point Likert type response and yielded α = .83 in the current study.

Relationship with adult children: Ten questions scored on a 7-point Likert were adopted from Yu's (1983) study of behavior and belief in filial piety among Chinese Americans. The internal consistency of the scale was α = .84. Depression index: The participants' mental health well being was represented by their scores on the Geriatric Depression Scale (GDS; Yesavage, Brink, Rose, Lum, Huang & Leirer, 1983). The cur- rent study adopted the 30 item Chinese GDS, translated by Stokes et al. (2001). Responses to the GDS items are in a *Yes* vs. *No* format. A depression score is calcu- lated based on the summation of all responses to the 30 GDS items. The GDS yielded an internal consistency of α = .89 in the present study. Self rated health: Three questions on 7-point Likert were used to determine participants' perception of their physical health and yielded an α of .80. *Perceived service barriers:* Five questions scored on a 7-point Likert scale asked participants about the degree to which they agreed with statements regarding expectations of facilities and programs for Chinese seniors, and with statements regarding the need for more culturally responsive servic-es and Chinese speaking service providers. These items produced α = .86. *Co ethnic peer involvement:* One question asked participants the proportion of ethnic Chinese represented in the typical social and organization groups in which they participated reg-ularly. The five response choices ranged incrementally from 1 = *all of them* to 5 = *none of them.* Service utilization: Two questions were presented to the participants. One question concerned the degree of the respondents' knowledge and familiarity with sen-ior serving community services and government agencies. The other question solicited the extent to which the participants utilized social services. Community program par-ticipation: In a checklist that included a list of community, recreational, and volunteer activities, the respondents indicated the activities in which they had participated in the past 12 months. The total number of the check marks was added up to form the par-ticipants' community program participation score. Voting participation: In a checklist format, the participants were asked to check off their previous participation in federal, provincial, and municipal elections in Canada. The number of check marks was summed up to represent the respondents' voting participation scores.

Findings

Prior to running the analyses, the data were screened for missing data, outliers, and were tested for multivariate statistical assumptions (i.e., normality, linearity, and multi-collinearity). The results indicated that the data and the analyses were robust against these assumptions. Following these steps, the relationships of the key variables examined in the present study were first tested with Pearson correlations.

The distribution of elderly Chinese immigrants, in terms of the two dimensions of cultural orientation, is presented in Table 2. Based on the median scores for Canadian Acculturation and Chinese Identification, the participants were split into the High vs. the Low categories on each dimension. This resulted a 2 x 2 (4) groupings of cultural orientation. As the Table 2 indicates, approximately one-third of the elderly Chinese participants fell into each of the High (Canadian Acculturation)-High (Chinese Identification) and the Low-Low groups. Another quarter fell into the Low-High group, while only slightly over a tenth of the participants fell into the High-Low group.

The Pearson correlation between Canadian Acculturation and Chinese Identification was tested and yielded a correlation of r = .25, p < .001. This result sug

Table 2
Distribution of participants in the Four Acculturation Groupings

		Chinese Identification (M=25.54; SD = 5.30)	
		High	Low
Canadian Acculturation (M=19; SD=5.94	High	69	29
	Low	53	62

Note: The means and standard deviations for Canadian Acculturation and Chinese Identification were baswed on the total score of the corresponding subscale on the VIA. The median scores for each of the two cultural dimensions (20 and 26 for Canadian Acculturation and Chinese Identification, respectively) were used to mark the high vs low groups.

gested a very weak relationship (i.e., a shared variance of $r^2 = .06$) between the two variables (Hinkle, Wiersma, & Jurs, 1998), supporting the notion that Canadian Acculturation and Chinese Identification are two distinct constructs (Ryder et al., 2000). Subsequently, two predictive models – one for Canadian Acculturation and one for Chinese Identification – were tested in two separate hierarchical regressions. Only those variables found significant in the correlational analyses were entered into the corresponding regression model. Given that no prior studies have examined the similar set of acculturation predictors, a rational approach was used to determine the entry sequences of these predictors into the regression equations, in consideration of Berry's (1997) acculturation theory, prior related literature, and the research interests of this study. As such, the acculturation-related demographics variables were submitted in the early steps of the regression, followed by the interpersonal relationship variables in the middle steps, and the adaptation indexes (i.e., community and service participation and health/mental health factors) in the later steps.

For Canadian Acculturation, gender, age, income, and education level were subjected to the regression as a block in the first step of the analysis to determine and to control the effect of demographic variables on acculturation (see Table 3). English usage which has been found to predict acculturation for the Chinese immigrant population as a proxy variable to acculturation (e.g., Lai, 2000a; Kuo & Roysircar, 2004; Stokes et al., 2001) was introduced in the second step. The affiliation variables, consisting of co-ethnic peer involvement and perceived social support, were entered into the analysis together in the third step. On step 4, community-based variables, in terms of community service and program utilization and voting participation, were entered. Lastly, self rated health and the depression index, as acculturation-related outcome indicators of well-being for elderly Chinese, were entered as a block in the final step.

Table 3
Result of Hierarchical Multiple Regression Analysis for the Predictor Variables of Canadian Acculturation (N=213)

Predictor Variable	*B* value	*SE B*	β	R^2	ΔP^2	*F*
Step 1				0.20	0.20***	9.20***
Gender	-2.33	0.94	-0.19*			
Age	-0.09	0.05	-.014			
Income	-0.53	0.33	-0.13			
Education Level	1.10	0.61	0.17			
Step 2				0.20	0.00	7.31***
English Usage	-0.36	0.75	-0.14			
Step 3				0.29	0.10***	8.72***
Co-etjmoc Peer Involvement	-1.11	0.50	-0.15*			
Perceived Social Support	0.12	0.07	0.13			
Step 4				0.38	0.09***	9.08***
Services Utilization	0.55	0.15	0.24***			
Community Program Participation	1.05	0.34	0.21**			
Voting Participation	0.13	0.34	0.03			
Step 5				0.41	0.03*	8.46***
Self-rated Health	0.20	0.11	0.13			
Depression Index	-0.14	0.07	-0.14			

Note: *B* values represent the unstandardized coefficients. b values represent the standardized coefficients. Predictor variables within each step were entered simultaneously into the regression as a block. * p<.05   ** p<.01   *** p<.001

The overall predictor model yielded a significant result, $F(12, 144) = 8.46$, $p <.001$, and accounted for 41% of the variance in Canadian Acculturation scores (see Table 3). This constitutes a statistically large effect size (Cohen, 1988). At step 1, gender, age, income, and educational level of Chinese elderly explained 20% of the variance in Canadian Acculturation scores, $R^2 = .20$, $F(4, 152) = 9.20$, $p < .001$. In the third step, co ethnic peer involvement and perceived social support significantly increased the prediction on Canadian Acculturation by accounting for an additional 10% of the variance, $R^2 = .29$, $F(7, 149) = 8.72$, $p < .001$. At step 4, service utilization, community program participation, and voting participation further accounted for 9% of the variance in Canadian Acculturation, $R^2 = .38$, $F(10, 146) = 9.08$, $p <.001$. At the final step, the self rated health and the depression index explained an additional 3% of the variance in Canadian Acculturation. Overall, four variables made significant, unique contributions to the prediction of Canadian Acculturation: gender ($p < .05$), co-ethnic peer involvement ($p < .05$), services utilization ($p <.001$), and community program participation ($p < .01$). It should be noted that the depression index fell short of reaching the significant level only slightly ($p = .055$).

In terms of the predictor model for Chinese Identification, a comparable ration-ale for the last model was adopted in this regression as well to determine the entry sequences of the predictors. The two demographic, socioeconomic indicators – income and educational level – were entered into the equation in the first block (see Table 4). In step 2, length of stay in Canada and English usage were introduced into the regres-sion. The affiliation variables of relationship with adult children, co ethnic peer involve-ment, and perceived social support were entered together in step 3. Services utiliza-tion and perceived service barriers were included in the final step of the equation.

Table 4
Results of Hierarchical Multiple Regression Analysis for the Predictor Variables of Chinese Identification (N=213)

Predictor Variables	β value	SE B	β	R^2	ΔR^2	F
Step 1				0.07	0.07**	6.17**
Education Level	0.06	0.46	0.01			
Income	-0.10	0.30	-0.03			
Step 2				0.16	0.09**	7.31***
Length of Stay Canada (years)	0.01	0.00[a]	-0.21**			
English Usage	-0.48	0.65	-0.06			
Step 3				0.32	0.16***	10.06***
Relationship with Adult Children	0.10	0.04	0.17*			
Co-ethnic Peer Involvement	1.04	0.48	0.16*			
Perceived Social Support	0.10	0.06	0.12			
Step 4				0.42	0.10***	11.85***
Services Utilization	0.4.3	0.14	0.22**			
Perceived Service Barriers	0.22	0.08	0.22**			

Note: B values represent the unstandardized coefficients. β values represent the standardized coefficients. Predictor variables within each step were entered into the regression simultaneously as a block.
a actual value = .003   * p<.05 ** p<.01 *** p<.001

The overall regression model for Chinese Identification was significant, $F(9, 150) = 11.85$, $p < .001$, and accounted for 42% of the variance in Chinese Identification scores. Again, this prediction of the current regression represents a large effect size (Cohen, 1988). At step 1, income and educational level accounted for 7% of the vari-ance in the Chinese Identification score, $R^2 = .07$, $F(2, 157) = 6.17$, $p < .01$. In the second step, with the inclusion of length of stay in Canada and English usage in the regression, an additional 9% of the variance in Chinese Identification was explained,

$R^2 = .16$, $F(4, 155) = 7.31$, $p < .001$. At step 3, relationship with adult children, co-ethnic peer involvement, and perceived social support further accounted for 16% of the variance in the criterion variable, $R^2 = .32$, $F(7, 152) = 10.06$, $p < .001$. In the final step, the entry of service utilization and perceived service barriers into the model increased the variance explained in Chinese Identification by an additional 10%. In total, five significant, independent predictor variables emerged from the regression model of Chinese Identification: length of stay in Canada ($p < .01$), relationship with adult children ($p < .05$), co ethnic peer involvement ($p < .05$), services utilization ($p < .01$), and perceived services barriers ($p < .01$).

Discussion

The results of the present study provided preliminary support for the bidirectional model of acculturation as it was applied to elderly Chinese immigrants, and substantiated the usefulness of adopting empirically validated acculturation measures to assess the adaptation experiences of this population. The results also evidenced the relationship of acculturation to a broad number of demographic, psychosocial, and health variables in the present sample.

In terms of Canadian Acculturation, the study showed that Chinese elderly who were men, who accessed community and government senior services more frequently, who were more actively involved in a variety of community based activities and programs, and whose social interaction had included non Chinese individuals were more likely to report higher levels of acculturation. While the immediate reason for the gender effect on acculturation is not clear, the t-test results revealed significant differences between Chinese elderly men and women in terms of income, English speaking ability, and the overall SES score (all $p < .001$). Chinese elderly men reported significantly higher levels in all these domains than did Chinese elderly women. This divergence in Canadian Acculturation between genders might be attributable to male - female differences in participants' language competencies and financial and economic factors.

Evidently, being more acculturated was related to being more knowledgeable and aware of community-based and government-based senior programs available to them, and to a greater utilization of these services. In other words, immigrant elderly who were more enthusiastic and active in accessing community resources were those who identified more strongly with Canadian traditions, values, and entertainment, and preferred friendship and social activities with Canadians. The opposite findings were true for Chinese elderly who were less acculturated. This result is consistent with Tsai and Lopez's (1997) finding of Chinese elderly immigrants in California; those who had the most acculturation difficulties (e.g., having poor English ability, lacking physical mobility), and feeling inferior owing to their minority status were also the most socially iso-lated and estranged from the mainstream society and the resources it offers.

The results suggest that the long term adaptation of elderly Chinese immigrants and their participation in the larger host community are at least in part contingent upon their knowledge and familiarity with the culture and the language of the domi-nant society, in this case English in Ontario. While generic services for immigrant sen-iors are available in some major cities across the United States and Canada (see Lai, 2001), currently few programs are specifically designed to address older immigrants' acculturation related concerns. Therefore, in order to promote older immigrants' pos-itive cultural adaptation in the host community, social service and government agen-cies would be well advised to vigorously implement ongoing language training and intercultural training for older immigrants. Through these interventions, older immi-grants would be given appropriate opportunities to develop the necessary working knowledge and adaptive skills to buffer them against the stresses and challenges aris-ing from immigration and acculturation (Kuo et al., 2008).

Furthermore, the results suggest that facilitating actual cross-cultural interaction between elderly Chinese immigrants and non-Chinese individuals (e.g., Canadian or other ethnic elderly or volunteers) might be critical in helping to break down the social and cultural isolation of immigrant elderly. The present study showed that Chinese eld-erly who were more likely to rely on and associate exclusively with other Chinese indi-viduals to meet their social needs were found to be less acculturated. Therefore, broadening of the social contacts of elderly Chinese immigrants to include White Canadians and other ethnic Canadian individuals may eventually contribute to a bet-ter adaptation of these immigrant elderly in Canada, the host society.

In terms of Chinese Identification, the present results showed that stronger iden-tification with Chinese cultural values was associated with older Chinese immigrants who were more recent immigrants (with a shorter time of residence) in Canada, who reported having more positive relationships with their adult children, who socially interacted with other Chinese peers more frequently, who utilized community and gov-ernment senior services more frequently, and who perceive more barriers in the exist-ing service delivery system. The fact that more recently arrived Chinese elderly were likely to have more immediate ties to their home cultures might, in turn, motivate them to seek similar cultural connections within the local Chinese communities in Canada. These tendencies might serve to reinforce their affinity and identification with Chinese values, traditions, and beliefs. This interpretation finds support in the evi-dence that elderly Chinese immigrants in the present study who had strong Chinese Identification also reported having more social interactions with other Chinese. Acquiring support from co-ethnic peers and adhering to one's cultural identity have been said to have buffering effects for older immigrants against difficulties arising from immigration and acculturation (Wong & Ujimoto, 1998). In a study of younger Chinese in the United States, Ying and Liese (1994) showed that the social ties Taiwanese international students maintained with their fellow Taiwanese students acted to enhance their emotional well-being. The Taiwanese peers aided their adjustment by offering much needed psychological and emotional support in coping with the strains of acculturation. It is suspected that a similar process was in operation with older Chinese immigrants. Future research would benefit from identifying the nature and the precise mechanism through which co-ethnic peers and community interact with the adjustment of older immigrants.

In addition, the present results also suggest that elderly Chinese immigrants who held more Chinese beliefs and values were also more likely to deem their parent–child relationships more satisfying and positive. This observation stands in contrast to the common notion that traditional values and cultural identity of immigrants contribute to intergenerational conflict between the less acculturated immigrant parents and the more acculturated immigrant children (Sung, 1985). It might be that Chinese traditions and values (i.e., having a strong Chinese Identification) held by immigrant elderly had acted as a unifying force within the Chinese family to ensure familial harmony and cohesion across generations. The elderly immigrants' belief in Chinese cultural values would have likely reinforced the principle of filial piety (i.e., an emphasis on extending respect, honor, and obligation to the elderly) with their children (Cheung, 1989). The observance of these familial principles and expectations on the part of their children, in turn, would have drawn them closer to their elderly parents and subsequently yielded a more satisfying parent–child relationship. The present findings suggest that Chinese traditional beliefs and values might still be an important governing force in familial and intergenerational relationships among contemporary Chinese immigrants.

Finally, it was found that having a strong Chinese Identification was related to increased awareness of available services and more frequent use of community programs. Ironically, a strong Chinese Identification was also associated with the perception of greater barriers in accessing services. This showed that while the immigrant elderly were willing users of social and community resources designed for seniors, these more traditional immigrant elderly clearly felt the adverse effects associated with the structural and cultural obstacles (e.g., the lack of linguistically appropriate and culturally responsive services) in the existing service system. Thus, the present study concurs with the calls made by previous researchers who advocated for the funding, recruitment, and training of more linguistically and culturally competent service providers and programs in the current system (Cheung, 1989; Lai, 2000a, 2001)

The results emerging from the present study deserve cautious interpretation in view of the following limitations. In the present study, the nonprobability sampling approach, the recruitment of elderly Chinese immigrants from only one urban locale, and the relatively high educational levels of the sample could not assure the generalizability of the findings to elderly Chinese immigrants elsewhere. In addition, the cross-sectional nature of the present study was also a limitation in that potential cohort effect on cultural adaptation among the participants was not controlled. Future research into acculturation of elderly Chinese immigrants would profit from extending the present study to a broader and more representative sample of this population. Ideally, a longitudinal design would be desirable to track and evaluate acculturation changes for older Chinese immigrants over time. Moreover, the measures used in the present study were carefully selected and administered to maximize the cultural and linguistic validity of these measures, but it was necessary to adapt some measures (e.g., the MSPSS and the VIA) from their original forms to make them developmentally appropriate for an elderly sample. While the adapted measures showed evidence of sound internal consistencies (i.e., strong Cronbach's alphas), the extent to which the psychometric structure of these measures might or might not have changed as a result of the modifications has not been ascertained. In this regard, it is recommended that future studies develop and utilize measures designed specifically for elderly populations.

Implications for Practice and Research

The results of the current study bear implications at the research as well as the service provision fronts. First, the present finding supports Iwamasa and Sorocco's (2002) assertion that acculturation and ethnic identity are cultural variables critical to the understanding of adaptation experiences of older Asian immigrant adults. The two predictor models hypothesized in the present study were significant, and they were efficacious in providing fine grained analyses and explanations for Canadian Acculturation and Chinese Identification in the present sample. In line with prevailing knowledge on acculturation (Sodowsky et al., 1991; Ward, 2001), the present study demonstrated that the acculturation experiences of elderly Chinese immigrants have a broad and complex association, with a wide variety of demographic, psychosocial, and health correlates. Future research of Chinese and other ethnic immigrant older adults would profit from adopting rigorous acculturation frameworks to further examine the antecedents of acculturation, (e.g., the predictor or correlate of acculturation) or the consequences of acculturation (e.g., the various health and psychosocial outcomes in terms of psychological indexes or quality of life indexes) in older immigrant adults (Ward, 2001). As such, acculturation theory offers a rich and comprehensive framework for advancing aging research with culturally diverse elderly (Iwamasa & Sorocco, 2002; Tran et al., 1996).

Second, with respect to gerontological practices and interventions, clinicians and service providers working with elderly Chinese immigrants should engage in an assessment of Chinese older immigrants' acculturation level and their knowledge of the host culture early in the helping relationship (Kim & Abrue, 2001; Sue & Sue, 2003). As revealed in the study, a considerable amount of information can be gleaned about the nature of older immigrants' relationship with their own children and with co-ethnic friends, their perception and awareness of social and community services, and their involvement with the community, from evaluating and ascertaining their acculturation experiences and cultural identity.

In regard to older immigrants' engagement with services and the larger community, the present results find support in Liao, Rounds, and Klein's (2005) recent study of help seeking attitudes of Asian American college students. Liao et al. found that the participants' degree of acculturation to the United States and their enculturation to Asian cultural values were the two key determinants of their receptiveness and willingness to acquire outside help such as counselling services for personal problems. Hence, a careful assessment of older immigrants' acculturation levels would give clinicians and service providers clues to clients' attitudes toward receiving professional psychological help and assistance. Attuning more closely to immigrant elderly clients' acculturation experiences and cultural identity would guide clinicians and service providers to eventually devise culturally responsive services and interventions for immigrant elderly.

References

Abramson, T.A., Trejo, L. & Lai, D.W.L. (2002, Spring). Culture and mental health: Providing appropriate services for a diverse older population, *Mental Health and Mental Illness in Later Life: 21*-27.

Ali, J. (2002). *Mental health of Canada's immigrants.* Supplement to Health Report, 13. 1-12. (Statistic Canada, Catalog 82-003). Ottawa: Health Canada.

Berry, J.W. (1997). Immigration, acculturation, and adaptation. *Applied Psychology: An International Review 46*: 5 34.

Berry J.W. & Sam, D. (1997). Acculturation and adaptation. In J.W. Berry, M.H. Segall, & C. Kagitcibasi (eds.). *Handbook of Cross-Cultural Psychology: Social Behavior and Applications* Volume 3, 2nd ed. (pp. 291-326). Needham Heights, MA: Allen & Bacon.

Casado, B.L & Leung, P. (2001). Migratory grief and depression among elderly Chinese American immigrants, *Journal of Gerontological Social Work 36:* 5-26.

Cheung, M. (1989). Elderly Chinese living in the United States: Assimilation or adjustment? *Social Work 34:* 289 384.

Cohen, J. (1988). *Statistical power analysis for the behavioral sciences.* (2nd ed.). Hillsdale, NJ: Lawrence Erlbaum Associates, Publishers.

Farver, J.A.M., Bhadha, B.R. & Narang, S.K. (2002). Acculturation and psychological functioning in Asian Indian adolescents. *Social Development, 11,* 11-24.

Gee, E.M. (1999). Ethnic identity among foreign born Chinese Canadian elders, *Canadian Journal on Aging 18*: 415-429.

Gee, E.M., Kobayashi, K. & Prus, S.G. (2004). Examining the healthy immigrant effect in mid to later life: Findings from the Canadian Community Health Survey. *Canadian Journal on Aging* (Suppl.): S55 S63.

Gelfand, D. & Yee, B.W.K. (1991). Influence of immigration, migration, and acculturation on the fabric of aging in America, *Generations. 15:* 7-10.

Hinkle, D.E., Wiersma, W. & Jurs. S.G. (1998). *Applied statistics for the behavioural sciences.* 4th ed. Boston, MA: Houghton Mifflin.

Iwamasa, G.Y. & Sorocco, K.H. (2002). Aging and Asian Americans: Developing culturally appropriate research methodology. In G.C.N. Hall & S. Okazaki (eds.). *Asian American psychology: The science of lives in context.* (pp. 105 130). Washington, DC: American Psychological Association.

Kim, B.S.K. & Abrue, J.M. (2001). Acculturation measurement: Theory, current instruments, and future directions. In J.G. Ponterotto, J.M. Casas, L.A. Suzuki & C.M. Alexander (eds.), *Handbook of Multicultural Counselling,* 2nd ed. (pp. 394 424). Thousand Oaks, CA: Sage Publications.

Kuo, B.C.H., Chong, V., & Joseph. J. (2008). Depression and its psychosocial correlates among older Asian immigrants in North America: A critical review of two decades' research. *Journal of Aging and Health.*

Kuo, B.C.H. & Guan J. (2006). Sociocultural predictors of depression for Chinese immigrant elderly in Canada: Acculturation, relationship with adult children, social support, and perceived services barriers. In D. Zinga (Ed.), *Navigating Multiculturalism: Negotiating Changes.* (pp. 379-398). Cambridge Scholars Press, Newcastle, U.K.

Kuo, B.C.H. & Roysircar, G. (2004). Predictors of acculturation for Chinese adolescents in Canada: Age of arrival, length of stay, social class, and English reading ability, *Journal of Multicultural Counseling and Development 32:* 143 154.

Kuo, B.C.H. & Roysircar, G. (2006). An exploratory study of cross cultural adaptation of adolescent Taiwanese unaccompanied sojourners in Canada, *International Journal of Intercultural Relations 30:* 159 183.

Kuo, B. & Torres Gil, F.M. (2001). Factors affecting utilization of health services and home and community based care programs by older Taiwanese in the United States. *Research on Aging. 23:* 14 36.

Lai, D.W.L. (2000a). Depression among the elderly Chinese in Canada. *Canadian Journal of Aging 19*: 409 429.

Lai, D.W.L. (2000b). Measuring depression in Canada's elderly Chinese population: Use of a community screening instrument. *Canadian Journal of Psychiatry 45*: 279-284.

Lai, D.W.L. (2001). Use of senior center services of the elderly Chinese immigrants. *Journal of Gerontological Social Work 35:* 59-79.

Lai, D.W.L. (2004a). Impact of culture on depressive symptoms of elderly Chinese immigrants, *Canadian Journal of Psychiatry 49*: 820-827.

Lai, D.W.L. (2004b). Health status of older Chinese in Canada, *Canadian Journal of Public Health 95*: 193-197.

Lam, R.E., Pacala, J. T. & Smith, S. L. (1997). Factors related to depressive symptoms in an elderly Chinese American sample. *Clinical Gerontologist 17*: 57-70.

Liao, H.Y., Rounds, J. & Klein, A.G. (2005). A test of Cramer's (1999) help seeking model and acculturation effects with Asian and Asian American college students. *Journal of Counselling Psychology 52:* 400-411.

Mui, A.C. (1996). Depression among elderly Chinese immigrants: An exploratory study, *Social Work 41:* 633-635.

Mui, A.C. (1998). Living alone and depression among older Chinese immigrants. *Journal of Gerontological Social Work 30:* 147-164.

Redfield, R., Linton, R. & Herskovits, M. (1936). Memorandum for the study of acculturation, *American Anthropologist. 38:* 149-152.

Ryder, A.G., Alden, L.E. & Paulhus, D.L. (2000). Is acculturation unidimensional or bidimensional? A head to head comparison in the prediction of personality, self identity, and adjustment. *Journal of Personality and Social Psychology. 79:* 49-65.

Shibusawa, T. & Mui, A.C. (2001). Stress, coping, and depression among Japanese American elders. *Journal of Gerontological Social Work. 36:* 63-81.

Sodowsky, G.R., Lai, E.W. & Plake, B.S. (1991). Moderating effects of sociocultural variables on acculturation variables of Hispanics and Asian Americans. *Journal of Counseling and Development 70:* 194 204.

Stokes, S.C., Thompson, L.W., Murphy, S. & Gallagher Thompson, D. (2001). Screening for depression in immigrant Chinese American elders: Results of a pilot study, *Journal of Gerontological Social Work.. 36*: 27-44.

Sue, W.S. & Sue, D. (2003). *Counselling the culturally diverse: Theory and practice* (4th edn.). New York: John Wiley & Son.

Sung, B.L. (1985). Bicultural conflicts in Chinese immigrant children. *Journal of Comparative Family Studies 16:* 255-269.

Tran, T.V., Fitzpatrick, T., Berg, W. & Wright, Jr., R. (1996). Acculturation, health, stress, and psychological distress among elderly Hispanics. *Journal of Cross Cultural Gerontology. 11*: 149-165.

Tsai, D.T. & Lopez, R.A. (1997). The use of social supports by elderly Chinese immigrants, *Journal of Gerontological Social Work. 29*: 77-94.

Ward, C. (2001). The A, B, Cs of acculturation. In D. Matsumoto (ed.), *Handbook of culture and psychology.* (pp. 411 445). New York: Oxford University Press.

Wong, P.T.P. & Ujimoto, K.V. (1998). The elderly: Their stress, coping and mental health. In C.L. Lee & N.W. Zanc (eds.). *Handbook of Asian American Psychology.* (pp. 165-209). Thousand Oaks, CA: Sage.

Wu, B., Tran, T.V. & Amjad, Q. A. (2004). Chronic illness and depression among Chinese immigrant elders, *Journal of Gerontological Social Work. 43:* 79-95.

Yesavage, J.A., Brink, T.L., Rose, T.L., Lum, O., Huang, V. & Leirer, V.O. (1983). Development and validation of a screening scale: A preliminary report. *Journal of Psychiatric Research. 17*: 37-49.

Ying, Y.W. & Liese, L.H. (1994). Initial adjustment of Taiwanese students in the United States: The impact of post arrival variables, *Journal of Cross Cultural Psychology. 25*: 466-477.

Yu, L. C. (1983). Patterns of filial belief and behaviour within the contemporary Chinese American family, *International Journal of Sociology of the Family. 13*: 17-36.

Zimet, G.D., Dahlem, N.W., Zimet, S.G. & Farley, G.K. (1988). The Multidimensional Scale of Perceived Social Support, *Journal of Personality Assessment. 52:* 30-41.

21

The Punjabi Elderly: Reflections on Culture, Background and Emerging Issues.

Gurnam Singh Sanghera, (Retired, Vancouver)*

In recent decades, Canada's population has ethnically, culturally, religiously and linguistically been radically transformed. Its demographic and social fabric is quietly undergoing a substantial change through a growing population via immigration from different countries. Waves of immigration from different countries are changing Canada's ethno-cultural composition. The sources of immigrants to Canada have changed in recent years, with increasing numbers from non-European countries such as China, India, Philippines, Pakistan, and the Middle East and Africa.

The visible minority population of Canada is increasing faster than its general population: 25% growth from 1996 to 2001 versus 4% growth in the general population. From 2001 to 2006, ten of the top twenty source countries for Canadian immigration were located in Asia or the Middle East; with China continuing to top the list by sending more than 155 000 migrants and India being the second sending more than 129 000 persons. The majority of the Indian immigrants come from Punjab and their mother tongue is Punjabi (though many of them are conversant in English as well). The evolving linguistic portrait (2006 Census) shows more than 200 languages in response to the Census question on mother tongue. Though the number of Canadians who can speak both English and French grew to 17.4% across the country, the other prominent top five mother tongues in Canada are Chinese - 16%, Italian - 7%, German - 7%, Punjabi - 6% and Spanish - 5%. Punjabi is the fourth most frequently reported mother tongue and its rate is up 34% from 2001. The German, Italian, Polish and Ukrainian language group – showing the largest data in 1971 – are no longer among the top immigration sources; most of the children and grand-children of these immigrants have listed French or English as their mother tongue.

> * The findings of this research are based upon general readings, library research, personal experiences in the Indo-Canadian community and through my participant observations. I am a Punjabi immigrant person and a social activist in the Indo-Canadian community.

Most immigrants (and mostly all Punjabis) believe that teaching their mother tongue (or heritage language) to their children is significant. Apart from cultural value, it imparts children with knowledge of another language, a powerful and healthy ethnic identity and assists/enables participation in their own ethnic socio-religious life. Punjabi immigrants are to a greater extent more likely than the overall population to be children or young adults. Generally, sponsored parents are over the age of 60 but not "very old." According to the 2006 Census, total seniors of Indian origin (ages 65-74) are 18 495. The Punjabi elderly could be around 12 000 and most of them are still capable of performing their activities of daily living (ADL). A substantial number of Punjabi immigrants are of working age, productive and of child bearing age. These Punjabis are also active in Canadian society, especially in political parties and religious institutions.

Punjabis (majority Sikhs) are all the more visible due to their unique dress (turban and long beard), religion and cultural activities (religious celebrations such as Baisakhi, sports such as Kabbaddi, and entertainment such as Bhangra). Punjabi seniors have a strong sense of belonging to Canada and all the Punjabi elderly have strong feelings of attachment to their own ethnic or cultural group.

Old age is a universal phenomenon and aging is part of the development sequence of life. Neugarten (1976) distinguished the aging population as the "young old" and the "old-old." Riley and Riley (1986) have identified the "young old" (aged 65 to 74), the "old-old" (74 to 84) and the "oldest old" (over 75 years of age). Pathak (1978) distinguished between aging or normal deceleration of activity, and senescence, which is age debility accelerated by disease, malnutrition, stress and strain.

There are genetic, non-genetic, cellular and physiological theories of aging. Although there is no single, unified and comprehensive theory of aging, each theory does suggest some important factors that may be related to aging and thus serves as a guide for possible intervention in the aging process. India's four ancient Ashrams have a distinct order in socio-religious life: (1) Studentship, (2) House holder's life, (3) Withdrawal from family obligations and relegating the house holder's stage to background and (4) Complete withdrawal to enable "mental integration." This mental integration transcends all prior stages and amounts to the opposition and renunciation of worldly activity. This scheme and procedure of life expresses a kind of differential disengagement that is distributed with growth and advancement throughout a life time. It inhibits the meaninglessness of life. Worldly life is to be understood as an engagement and renunciation may be perceived as disengagement. So, there is a delicate and indistinct interchange/interplay of both engagement and disengagement in the Indian "stages of life."

In Canada, however, the "stages of life" become blurred. The Punjabi elderly have remained engaged in family and social life by continuing to help in baby sitting, taking children to school, volunteering in Gurdwara (Sikh Temple) and Hindu Mandirs (Temple). Disengagement in the West is also seen as not only normal but desirable. Disengagement ultimately leads to institutionalization, social isolation and the logical completion of disengagement is death. Yet even in the West, the elderly remain engaged and active through travel, volunteer work and via interaction with others in community centres and so on. The West's mechanical, individualistic approach model is essentially on par with the bio-medical model in which only a diseased part is looked at and the rest of the person (cultural aspects and the totality) is more or less ignored. In Punjabi culture, since there is no complete disengagement, such a model or theory is not healthy as the aged could then be considered useless, undesired and to be put away in a secluded or isolated place - reminiscent of the late 1970s movie Blade Runner. People are generally healthier and active today and will not be content to disengage totally.

For Punjabis, old age is still considered a distinct stage of life with its own unique meaning and purpose. According to the Dharam Sastra (Hindu religious books and philosophy) and Gurbani (Word of the Guru-holy Sikh scripture, Sri Guru Granth Sahib) there are definitive and articulated stages of life. Gurbani states, "Remembering Him (God) in meditation, the fear of birth, old age and death will not trouble you" (Sri Guru Granth Sahib, p. 526). The third Guru (Amar Dass) pronounces, "Your consciousness shall remain attached to the Lord, there shall be no fear of old age, and the supreme status shall be obtained" (Sri Guru Granth Sahib, p. 490).

Modernization theory (Cowgill, 1972) suggests that as societies increase their level of modernization (industrialization and consumerism), the social status of older people declines. Urbanization also affects the family system. In India, there is no old age security or Guaranteed Income Supplement. So India's Parliament (Lok Sabha) passed a bill aiming to protect senior citizens and making neglect of parents above 60 years of age punishable by a fine and imprisonment, or both. It makes it obligatory on those who inherit property of their aged relatives to maintain them. This bill also aims to make provisions for setting up old age homes. The legislation is aimed at helping India's 76 million elderly citizens above 60 years of age who will reach 173 million by 2026 (Seniors World Chronicle, December 5, 2007). India's Minister for Social Justice and Empowerment commented, "In our tradition we take pride in serving the elderly – but with the joint families withering, the elderly are being abandoned. The bill is in response to the concerns expressed by many members over the fate of the elderly" (Seniors World Chronicle, December 5, 2007).

The elderly in Punjab still remain somewhat engaged after retirement (professionals) or when they are simply unable to work (due to old age) in an agricultural or agriculture related setting. Even when they become immobile, they carry on the role of advising their families. The immobile elderly meet at common "sitting" and "gathering" places or in Gurdwaras (Sikh Temple) for daily social talk and to share past experiences. Punjabi culture actively emphasizes age related socially ascribed roles and the elderly attempt to adjust to some age related theory (Cottrell, 1942). Among Punjabis, chronological age is used to determine activities, eligibility for various social positions, to evaluate the suitability of different roles and to shape expectations of people in social situations. Generally, individuals also hold norms about the appropriateness of their own behavior at any particular age, so that social roles become internalized and age norms operate to keep people on their time track (Hagestad & Neugarten, 1985). Roles are the basis of an individual's self concept. Punjabi seniors assume an elderly person's "role" which bestows higher status, giving of guidance and advice in socio-religious affairs of the family and the community: a role that is the symbol of experience and wisdom. Norms that exist for older adults in North American society tend to reflect "middle age" and "middle class" standards related to independence and social activity (Bergston, 1973). The Punjabi elderly are similar to Chinese seniors and Hsu's (1970) statement is most applicable: "In Chinese families, grandparents, as originators of the parents, fill the elevated role of super parents" (p. 319). Accordingly, Punjabi seniors become disengaged from their former role in order to assume a new one; thereby, still remaining an active participant in family and to some extent in community affairs.

Most of the Punjabi (elderly and young) immigrants are Sikhs from rural areas (majority) and a significant number of Sikh seniors owned land/property and were engaged (part time, full time or absentee landlords) in agriculture or allied occupations. Many Punjabi (Sikh) seniors were teaching (schools, colleges and universities), in administration (government revenue and banking) and security (police and army officers). A few were practicing law in India. Many of them are conversant in English but they naturally like to talk in Punjabi in their own gatherings and in daily social inter-action. The joint family system does prevail – having three or up to four generations living together in one household and the same pattern is being followed in North America. But, that is also creating tensions and, at times, conflicts. The family system itself is changing and the position and status of the elderly are being undermined by factors such as changing values, growing individualism, consumerism, rising aspirations for material gains, competitions and ballooning desires due to the impact of industrialization, urbanization and westernization. However, though the elderly no longer are a "patriarch" as in the past, they still get respect and are cared for by the families in Punjab and North America.

From a socio religious perspective, Bhai Gurdas, Sikh theologian exegete of Gurbani, narrates a family's account in which the married son, misguided by his wife, "leaves his parents, and forgets their blessings and benevolence and starts living away from them. Now the modus operandi of the world has become very unethical" (Bhai

Gurdas, 1982, p. 12). So parental and elderly parents/grandparents' neglect can be considered sinful.

The fourth guru of the Sikhs (Guru Ram Dass) says, "Why, O' son, you quarrel with your father? It is a sin to quarrel with him who begot you and brought you up." (Sri Guru Granth Sahib, p. 1200).

A Sikh believes in one God, the ten Gurus and their preaching and the Sri Guru Granth Sahib. Sikhs are to accept their Holy Scripture as the "living Guru." The first Guru (Nanak Dev) was born in 1469 and the last (tenth Guru Gobind Singh) expired in 1708. Guru's Word is called Gurbani and espoused a brother (sister) hood of humankind, equality, harmonious relations and religious pluralism. The third Sikh Guru (Amar Dass) says, "The world is on fire. Shower thy benedictions and save it through whatever portal it may be saved" (Sri Guru Granth Sahib, p. 853). Religion is also an important source of community identity, internal solidarity and cohesion (Basran & Bolaria, 2003). Sikh Temples provide space for the seniors to meet and socialize. They provide free tea, snacks and food. Some Gurdwaras have a senior's centre, a library, computer room and exercise room for the seniors on the premises. The Gurdwara is centred on religious preaching but has also become a pivot (for mainly religious and important social functions, such as marriage and funeral ceremonies) for the community and is a place of solace for the Punjabi Sikh seniors.

The Punjabi elderly desire that their own children and grandchildren retain religious and cultural values, marry within their community, visit Gurdwaras regularly, learn Punjabi along with English and French, stay with in the joint family system and perform filial piety towards parents and grandparents. Some Punjabi elderly are not prepared to adapt and make adjustments. Stubbornness of some elderly people in their habits, behaviors, values and the inability or unwillingness of some children not to accommodate an elderly person sometimes causes friction and a split in the family. Working age people living with their elderly parents and with their own young children are a "sandwich generation" who, at times, are caught between often conflicting demands of caring for children and caring for seniors. Some Punjabi seniors' alcohol drinking habits or sending a portion of their OAS and GIS money to India also engender friction and discord within the family.

The Punjabi elderly in Canada are a growing population for identifiable reasons. First, an increasing number of Punjabi Canadians are sponsoring their elderly parents and grandparents. Second, the percentage of age distribution in the 25/30 to 45 years of age group will bring a natural increase in the number of Punjabi seniors. Those in the Independent immigration category above the age of 40/45 will also contribute to this expansion. These seniors are not a homogeneous group as they are diverse in cultural values, social class, education and their length of stay in Canada. Punjabi seniors in Canada are of four broad categories: a) pre 1950's immigrants, 2nd and 3rd generations, b) those who came in the late 1960s and became seniors, c) those who immigrated in late 1970s/80s and "turned into" seniors, and, d) sponsored seniors. All such categories face racism and religious discrimination. The implementation of multiculturalism and its policies to combat racial discrimination, as well as immigration policies designed to replenish a decreasing population become instrumental to help vanquish overt racism and unequal treatment based on colour, ethnicity and religion, etc.

The migration of Punjabi seniors to Canada is a process of uprooting oneself from Punjab, leaving economic assets, social networks, and social status behind and replanting in an unknown and strange society. This is traumatic for some and joyful for others. But what is certain is that they are coming to settle with their children in a new country. In Punjab, the newly married daughter-in-law moves into the in-law's (or seniors) house. But, when the in-laws (or seniors) from India migrate (unless in the independent category) to Canada, the situation is reversed. They are now moving into their son's and daughter-in-law's house. For a time they become wholly or partially dependent upon their children for meeting their needs from transportation to money. Even retired officers, educated teachers and other professionals become de-skilled as they have no knowledge or information about transport (buses, trains), roads, post office, banks, hospital, the workings of police and the education system. They require assistance from their own family at the outset. Many seniors confide their despair in others which underscores the silent struggle/strife that takes place within some Punjabi homes. They face problems related to mobility, transportation, language (English), isolation and feelings of social dislocation.

Sponsored, dependent Punjabi seniors face "multiple jeopardy." This describes a situation that arise from old age, ethnicity (Marshall, 1987), religious discrimination and economic/financial dependence – thus losing various types of freedoms and choices. As sponsored immigrants, they are dependent, (financially and socially) on their children for up to ten years. They are not entitled to old age security, Guaranteed Income Supplement and/or financial assistance (GAIN) for this length of time. The sponsoring children sign an enforceable agreement to take care of their parents for ten years. Many seniors and a large section of the Punjabi community are now lobbying to reduce that wait period to three years so that they can become naturalized Canadian citizens after three years, thus becoming eligible for old age benefits. But, another section of the Punjabi community (and the mainstream) is of the opinion that those sponsored elderly, who have not worked in Canada and have made no contribution in taxes and pension funds, should not get any OAS and GIS.

The general consensus is that all immigrant seniors should get a free bus pass (after three months permanent residency) so that they may become more independent in their own mobility and visit community centres, seniors centres, Gurdwaras, Mandirs, libraries and relatives or friends. Generally, social security's guarantee of a retirement income and related benefits releases the family of many caring responsibilities (Cole, Achenbaum, Jacobi & Kastenbaum, 1993).

Punjabi elderly have faith in their religion (and spirituality) and pray for their own and humankind's good health. An elderly man said, "With luck and by God's blessing, I will stay healthy. I really do feel that you could wish for your old age to be in a certain mould; but it does not mean it will occur." He further said, "Evidently, the ultimate worry and fear is to be in a vegetative state and to be totally helpless, and have some one look after you. That I would utterly dread and hate." Another person stated, "You know we have become the invisible majority because the people just don't notice you. They will overlook you" (Sanghera,1991). But grey power is increasing and politicians are taking note. These seniors are active in Gurdwaras as well as municipal, provincial and federal elections. As such, they are not as "overlooked" as the preceding quote might suggest.

The Punjabi community has identified family, community relation and spirituality as key factors in healthy aging. Its seniors rate family support and care giving as the most important factor in healthy aging. But, some seniors experience isolation and marginalization as they are not receiving traditionally expected deferential treatment. There are rumors of abuse and there are unreported incidences of elder abuse (physical, mental and financial), but, none have been verified (Hansson & Carpenter, 1994). Barriers to identification are: lack of awareness of rights, shame, embarrassment and betrayal, feeling they deserve it, not wanting to hurt the culprit, confidentiality issues, religious values, inability to express due to impairment, fear of powerlessness and having limited social support per se.

Though some traditions are gradually disappearing, substantial assistance and care giving in a variety of forms is still given to the Punjabi elderly. They do live in a community and community culture strongly values caregiving and support (Sokolovsky, 1990). Many Punjabi seniors maintain ties with relatives and friends in India, visit Punjab regularly, place prominent value on religious and ethnic traditions, (Tran, Kaddatz & Allard, 2005) and consider Sri Harimandir Sahib (Golden Temple, Amritsar) as the epitome of virtue, piety and sanctum sanctorum of the Sikhs.

Punjabi families will try to keep the elderly with disabilities and mobility difficulties at home and request homecare. They will not place the elderly in a long term care home due to inherent feelings of guilt, which arises from conflicting values of filial piety versus shame (Koehn, 2004). Long term care homes need to employ more ethnic minority workers who speak residents' languages such as Punjabi, Cantonese, and Mandarin to serve their unique needs. Some Punjabi community agencies have now established long term care Punjabi homes, employing Punjabi speaking workers and serving Punjabi food. A 54 one bed room unit has been established by the Rainbow Community Health Co-operative with provincial grants. Progressive Intercultural

Community Services Society (PICS) manages this facility and also runs subsidized housing for the independent Punjabi seniors. Punjabi community families have placed extended care elders in this facility. People are now realizing that, at some stage, Punjabi elderly may have to be permanently placed in a nursing home. But to facilitate this, long-term care must develop lists of such facilities and also arrange for enhanced culturally and religiously sensitive services.

It is imperative for health care services and health care professionals to be creative, open, non-judgmental, friendly and culturally sensitive. They must implement elder and ethnic friendly systems and arrange geriatric consultation services via a team approach to determine and address high risk situations. Mental health issues are often stigmatized in the Punjabi community so service providers must take the lead to transmit information that mental illness is a disease which requires treatment. Health care professionals and service providers should be aware that the Punjabi elderly consult bio-medical doctors first but that they also use alternative traditional (Desi-Indian's) medicine (Ayurvedic) and popular medicine (Granny's Recipe) as an adjunct. Many Punjabi elderly parents, if confronted by their general practitioner, will be hesitant to admit or deny the use of alternative medicine (Ghosh & Khan, 2005). Many Punjabi families and elderly are dissatisfied with services of hospitals and the attitudes, conduct and management in the emergency department. Management must explain procedures and take these communities into their confidence.

The Punjabi elderly are still not aware of many available services and some are not fully utilized, such as, transportation services and meals services. Red Cross services such as loaning walkers, toilet seats and crutches are now being used by some. Some Punjabi seniors and families are aware of the importance of guardianship issues and wills. It is essential to have further information disseminated about such issues. Seniors organizations and lawyers can be consulted to deal with the practicalities of guardianship without violating the rights and autonomy of the elderly.

Punjabi seniors' organizations receive grants for mutual help projects and even for buildings and renovations. They invite professionals to provide information about various services. They also assist in applications to seek those services. But, these seniors are generally not included in consultations and decision making. They and their families do not seem to be fully aware of adult day care programs which "provide non-institutional support for those unable to remain in the community without it" (Chappell, Strain & Blandford, 1986, p. 121). The primary goal of these programs is to meet the needs of those who require help in social and physical functioning and/or whose families need some respite or relief from their responsibility.

The Punjabi elderly and their families may have heard about certain services but, may have no understanding how these services work. Some are not easily accessible due to procedures, language (English/French) barriers and answering machines blurt-

00000000000000000000

0000000000

ing out impersonal and long complicated instructions. Many Punjabi elderly and their families still feel that racism exists in various services and service agencies and that it is "practiced" subtly and covertly.

It is vitally important that community services be culturally sensitive, easily and equitably accessible and inclusive: meaning Punjabi and other communities must be involved in decision making processes and policies which implement action. Enhanced and easily comprehensible information about these services must be publicly available. Ethnic media, religious and cultural centres along with liaisons, community centres, mainstream media, community schools, post offices and parliamentary offices can be utilized to disseminate knowledge. The information services need to be provided through a warm, respectful and supportive human relationship model to make the elderly feel wanted and to find meaning in their lives. Through a process of mutual respect, understanding and compassion, the goals of minority elderly service providers and their intended clients can be harmonized, realized and furthered.

References

Aad Guru Granth Sahib Ji (Holy Book). *Amritsar: Shironmani Gurdwara Parbandhak* Committee.

Basran. G. & Bolaria, B. (2003). *The Sikhs in Canada; Migration, race, class and gender.* New Delhi: Oxford University Press.

Bergston, V. (1973). *The social psychology of aging.* Indianapolis, Indiana: Bobbs-Merrill.

Bhai Gurdass. (1982). *41 Vaaraan. Amritsar:* Jawahar Singh, Kirpal Singh & Co.

Chappell, N.L., Strain, A. & Blandford, A. (1986). *Aging and health care: A social perspective.* Toronto: Holt, Rinehart and Winston of Canada.

Cole, T., Achenbaum, A., Jacobi, P. & Kastenbaum, R. (1993). *Voices and visions of aging: Toward a critical gerontology.* New York: Springer Publishing Company.

Cottrell, L. (1942). The adjustment of the individual to his age and sex roles. American *Sociological Review, 7,* 617-620.

Cowgill, O.D. (1972). *Aging and Modernization. New York:* Appleton, Century, Crofts & Homes.

Ghost, P. & Khan, S. (2005). *Transcultural geriatrics: Caring for the elderly of Indo-Asian origin.* London: Radcliffe Publishing.

Hagestad, G. (1990). Social Perspectives on Life course. In Binstock, H.R., George, L.K. & Shanes, E. et al (Ed), *Handbook of aging and the social sciences* (pp. 151-168). San Diego CA: Academic Press.

Hansson, R. & Carpenter, B. (1994). *Relationships in old age: Coping with the challenge of transition.* New York: The Guildford Press.

Hsu, F.L.K. (1970). *American Chinese reflections on two cultures and their people.* New York: Doubleday.

Koehn, S. (2005). Community - based research seeks to address barriers to access to care for ethnic minority seniors. *GRC News, 24*(2), 4-6.

Marshall, V. (1987). *Aging in Canada: Social perspectives.* Markham, Ontario: Fitzheny & White Side.

Neugarten, B. (1976). *The psychology of aging: An overview.* Washington, D.C.:American Psychological Association.

Pathak, J.D. (1978). *Our elderly.* Bombay: Bombay Medical Research Centre.

Riley, M. & Riley, J. (1986). Longevity and social structure; The potential of added Years. In A. Pifer & L. Bronte (Eds.), *Our aging society: Paradox and promise.* (pp. 53-78).. New York: W.W. Norton.

Sanghera, G.S. (1991). *The male Punjabi elderly of Vancouver: Their background, health beliefs and access to health care services.* Vancouver: University of British Columbia (unpublished major paper for MSW).

Sokolovsky, J. (ed.) (1990). *The cultural context of aging* – Worldwide perspectives. New York: Bergin & Garvey Publishers.

Tran, K., Kaddatz, J. & Allard, P. (2005). South Asian in Canada: Unity through Diversity. *Canadian Social Trends, Autumn, 2005,* 20-25.

22

Concluding Thoughts: "All bets are off"

Douglas Durst and Michael MacLean, (University of Regina)

A favorite expression of my mother's was: "All bets are off," meaning that with new information old ideas or assumptions were probably false and therefore, the "bet" must be withdrawn. This book brings new ideas and challenges numerous assumptions and beliefs that many of us have regarding aging and immigrants. So, when the topic comes to immigrant seniors and aging: all bets are off!

There is sometimes a tendency to view elderly immigrants as some kind of victim. All immigrants are poor, marginalized and lack empowerment. Their weak language skills marginalize and create barriers to accessing services and programs. They are left on the fringes of Canadian society. For some groups, this may be true but it is wrong to generalize. Many senior immigrants are healthy and active in a variety of sectors in Canadian society. They may be working or volunteering in numerous capacities. Other immigrants aged in Canada and have as much knowledge of the Canadian way of life and are actively involved in the same way as many native-born Canadians.

It is an assumption that most elderly immigrants who came under the Family Class wanted to come to Canada. Koehn, Spencer and Hwang tell the reader that this belief is in fact false, and that most elderly immigrants would have preferred to age in their homeland with familiar surroundings, language, culture and friends. For these senior immigrants, the experience is a huge leap into the unknown and unfamiliar. There are assumptions that families want to care for their elders and that the elders want to live in their adult child's home. Filial piety remains strong in many cultures but there are dramatic changes in assumptions about preferences for living and housing arrangements. How filial piety is expressed has changed in their new homeland. Both Kim and Sanghera explore how various expectations undergo cultural transformation through the adjustment process.

Accessing health care services remains a problem for some groups. Services such as long-term care remain a source of discontent and frustration for some groups but new trends in ethno-cultural homecare, special care homes and long-term care facilities have created a new industry aimed at aging immigrants.

Assumptions about multiculturalism have been challenged as well. Some argue that Canada's version of multiculturalism is a model for the world. Others argue that multiculturalism is dead and a failure at ensuring a reasonable acculturation while maintaining cultural identity. The myth of the cultural mosaic is perpetuated. Community cultural festivals are nothing more than superficial demonstrations of the four "Ds": dance, diet, dress and dialect. In fact, people live in separate enclaves. Kuo shows us how individuals maintain their homeland identity while creating a new identity in their new country that does not conflict with the old.

The world of immigrant seniors is much more complicated and complex than many would like to believe. For example, for many westerners there is a tendency to understand all "Asian" immigration as if they were one group. The Japanese immigrants overwhelming aged in Canada and are in a very different situation than the more recent Chinese immigrants who are almost all under family reunification. The Korean immigrants are aging in Canada but many with poor language and acculturation skills; still many remain active in their small businesses. Among the Chinese elders are diverse groups of recent mainland immigrants, long-time immigrants from Hong Kong and a host of Chinese who have come to Canada by way of Indonesia, Vietnam, Philippines, and other Pacific nations. Even among the Indians, there are those who aged in Canada, those who aged in India and those who came via the United Kingdom, South Africa and other global communities. The picture is complex and confusing making assumptions and generalizations risky.

In recent years, Canada has experienced a change in source countries. Dramaticaly the senior immigrants, under family class, are arriving from China. Yet the dynamics of the young adult immigrants have shifted from Eastern Asia to the Middle East and Africa. This will have impacts in the senior population in some years to come. Strangely, the numbers of immigrants from Central and South America have been proportionately decreasing.

This complexity offers challenges to researchers, policy developers and service providers alike. Researchers need to be careful not to construct false categories with false and mis-leading generalization. Assumptions about preferences for services and programs can be untrue. Policy makers and service providers need to re-examine their assumptions and beliefs. There is a new need for research that recognizes the complexities and accounts for them in the generation of new knowledge. It is like looking through a prism. If the angle of light is changed, ever so slightly, the hue changes. If the angle is changed slightly more, the color changes. This book attempts to demonstrate the complexities and provide an opportunity to learn from each other. Each chapter keeps changing the angle and providing new light.

There are a number of critical issues that need to be addressed or accommodated in future research. Some researchers have been careless in lumping immigrants with refugees and making assumptions about both groups. There are important differences between immigrants and refugees in education, health, income and other variables. Refugees are generally at much greater disadvantage in all categories. In addition, refugees may have experienced severe trauma that influences and shapes their immigrant experience. There are differences between those who age in their homelands and those who aged in their new country. Those who aged in Canada are much richer, healthier and better skilled at accessing services and programs.

In Canada, there are subtle and not so subtle forms of racism, discrimination and agism. There is a need for research to cut to a deeper level and move beyond superficial and sweeping assumptions. For example, the experiences of Black Africans are different than Asians so their perceptions about services and programs are shaped by these experiences. As Canada continues in its trends of diversification, it would be useful to understand how groups view each other. Most of the research on racism examines attitudes and behaviors of "mainstream Canadians." Every year, "mainstream" becomes less and less "white, Anglo/Francophone, middle class male." For example, little is know about how Chinese Canadians view other minorities. Little is known about the attitudes within so-called groups. For example, most of the Vietnamese in Canada arrived, after 30 years of war, as refugees. It would be interesting to know how established Vietnamese refugees view northern Vietnamese who were former "enemies." It has taken a long time for the animosity between politically left versus right refugees from El Salvador to diminish. Similar political divisions and attitudes prevail among Ukrainian, Chinese and other immigrants. In Regina, for many years, each group hosted its own pavilion during its annual cultural mosaic; there were two "Ukrainian" and two "Chinese" pavilions separated politically. Ironically the festival was an event to sponsor awareness and harmony. Generally the young have little interest in harboring old feelings of distrust and sometimes hate as it is the seniors/elders who hold on to old grudges. It is also the seniors/elders who volunteer their time to coordinate and operate these cultural events for the community within and beyond.

An interesting demographic trend has appeared in the United States but not in Canada. The Hispanic population has been growing rapidly and is now greater than the African American population. Similar trends are not appearing in Canada and immigration from Latin American nations remains low; yet, African immigration has been increasing. These differences and shifts in immigration will impact on our senior population. It is worth exploring some of these changes and differences.

Research is needed to understand the senior clients who are not receiving services and benefits and those who are. Federal and provincial health and social services provide an array of pamphlets, books, advertising and web pages to share the information but it is not clear who is accessing services and programs. Information could influence policies about health and social programs and provide opportunities for prevention. Diabetes is rapidly growing amongst populations where it was almost non-existent a decade ago. With diet and lifestyle change, rates of diabetes are rapidly rising amongst all Asian groups including Chinese and Indian. Knowledge about what programs and services are successful, where they work, and why they work is urgently needed.

Similar research about housing and home care supports are needed as well. Assumptions about independent living and the cultural meaning of independence need to be explored. There are differences in individuals but little is understood about the cultural meanings of independence, support from informal and formal caregivers, and institutional care.

Another interesting field of study is the relationship between adult children and their aging parents. There is considerable research and discussion about the "sandwich generation" who have responsibilities for young children and aging parents. Little is known about immigrant adults who are trying to support elderly and failing parents in far-away lands. These efforts to help with elderly parents who are on the other side of the globe create emotional stress, guilt and perhaps shame for failing to meet filial responsibility. Issues around end-of-life care are especially difficult and guilt ridden.

As this volume has demonstrated, Canada's population has changing faces and greying temples. The goal is healthy and active aging. There is much to do and much to understand. However, it must be viewed as a partnership with all "stakeholders" equal in responsibility. Immigrant communities of all ages need to participate in empowering their aging and elderly seniors. Researchers need to explore these topics from new angles and approaches to generate new knowledge. Practitioners need to challenge themselves to explore new ways to deliver services and programs. The world of immigrant seniors will benefit from the contribution of all of these stakeholders. This book is part of this contribution. Keep well.

Douglas Durst and Michael MacLean

October, 2010.

Canadian Research Centres on Aging

Centre on Aging, University of Victoria
P.O. Box 1700 Stn CSC
Office: Sedgewick A104
Victoria, British Columbia V8W 2Y2
Tel: 250-721-6369
Fax: 250-721-6499

Dr. ElainGallagher (Director)
E-mail: egallagh@uvic.ca
E-mail: senage@uvic.ca
Web site: www.coag.uvic.ca

The Gerontology Research Centre, Simon Fraser University at Harbour Centre
2800 - 515 West Hastings
Vancouver, British Columbia V6B 5K3
Tel: 604-291-5062
Fax: 604-291-5066
E-mail: gero@sfu.ca

Dr. Andrew Sixsmith (Director)
E-mail: sixsmith@sfu.ca
Dr. Andre Wister (Assoc. Director)
E-mail wister@sfu.ca
Web site: www.harbour.sfu.ca/gero

Alberta Centre on Aging, University of Alberta
305 Campus Tower
Edmonton, Alberta T6G 1K8
Tel: 780-492-3207
Fax: 780-492-3190

Dr. Laurel A. Strain (Director)
E-mail: laurel.strain@ualberta.ca
E-mail: aging@ualberta.ca
Web: uofaweb.uablerta.ca/aging

Centre on Aging and Health, University of Regina
University of Regina
Regina, Saskatchewan S4S 0A2
Tel: 306-337-2537
Fax: 306-337-2321

Dr. Thomas Hadjistavropoulos (Director)
E-mail: thomas.hadjistavropoulos@
uregina.ca
E-mail: cah@uregina.ca
Web site:www.uregina.ca/hadjistt/centre.index.htm

Centre on Aging, University of Manitoba
338 Isbister Building
Winnipeg, Manitoba R3T 2N2
Tel: 204-474-8754
Fax: 204-474-7576

Dr. Verena Menec (Director)
E-mail: menec@cc.umanitoba.ca
E-mail: aging @umanitoba.ca
Web site: www.umanitoba.ca/centres/aging/

Centre for Educfation & Research on Aging and Health, Lakehead University
Health Services North
955 Oliver Road
Thunder Bay, Ontario P7B 5E1
Tel: 807-766-7299
Fax: 807-343-2104

Dr. Mary Lou Kelly (Director)
E-mail: mlkelley@lakeheardu.ca
E-mail: cerah@lakeheardu.ca
Web site: www.lakeheadu.ca/~necahwww

R. Samuel McLaughlin Centre for Research and Education in Aging and Health, McMaster University

1280 MainStreet West, Rm 330   Dr. Parminder Raina (Co-Director)
Hamilton, Ontario L8S 4L8   E-mail praina@mcmaster.ca
Tel: 905-525-9140 ext. 22547   Dr. Alexandra Papaioannau (Co-Director)
Fax: 905-522-7681   Mary Gauld (Senior Research Coordinator)
E-mail: gauld@mcmaster.ca
Web site: www.fhs.mcmaster.ca/mcah

McMaster Centre for Gerontological Studies, McMaster University

Kenneth Taylor Hall, Room 226   Dr. Margaret Denton (Director)
Hamilton, Ontario L8S 4M4   E-mail: mdenton@mcmaster.ca
Tel: 905-525-9140, ext. 24449   E-mail: gercntr@mcmaster.ca
Fax: 905-525-4198   Web: www.socsci.mcmaster.ca/gerontology/

Sheridan Elder Research Centre, Sheridan Institute of Technology and Advanced Learning

1430 Trafalger Road   Pat Spadafora (Director)
Oakville, Ontario L6H 2L1   E-mail: pat.spadafora@sheridanc.on.ca
tel: 905-845-9430, ext. 8615   Web site: www.sheridanc.on.ca/serc/
Fax: 905-815-4233

Elizabeth Bruyere Research Institute, University of Ottawa

43 Bruyere Stree   Dr. Larry W. Chambers (Chair & President)
Ottawa, Ontario K1N 5C8   E-mail: lchamber@scohs.on.ca
Tel: 613-562-6045   Linda Plante (Adminstrative Assistant)
Fax: 613-562-4266   E-mai: lplante@scohs.on.ca
Web site: www.scohs.on.ca/bins/index.asp

Institute for Human Development, Life Course and Aging, University of Toronto

222 College Street, suite 106   Dr. Lynn McDonald (Director)
Toronto, Ontarkio M5T 3J1   E-mail: lynn.mcdonald@utotonto.ca
Tel: 416-978-0377   Susan Murphy (Administration)
Fax: 416-978-4771   E-mail: susan.murphy@utoronto.ca
Web site: www.utoronto.ca/lifecourse/

Rotman Research Institute – Baycrest Centre for Geriatric Care

3560 Bathurst Street   Dr. Donald T. Stuss (Director)
Toronto, Ontario M6A 2E1   E-mail: dstuss@rotman-baycrest.on.ca
Tel: 416-785-2500, exst. 3550   E-mail: sng@rotman-baycrest.on.ca
Fax: 416-785-9999   Web site: www.rotman-baycrest.on.ca/

Cetnre for Studies in Aging, Sunnybrook & Women's College Health Sciences Centre (SWCHSC)

2075 Bayview Avenu
Toronto, Ontario M4N 3M5
Tel: 416-480-5858
Fax: 416-480-5856

Dr. Brian Maki (Dirctor)
E-mail: brian.maki@sri.utoronto.ca
Web: www.sunnybrook.utoronto.ca/~csia/index.htm

Canadian Centre for Activity and Aging, University of Western Ontario

1490 Richmond Street
London, Ontario N6G 2M3
Tel: 519-661-1603
Fax: 519-661-1612

Clara Fitzgerald (Director)
E-mail: cfitzge4@uwo.ca
Web site: www.uwo.ca/actage

Aging & Health Research Centre, University of Western Ontario

Room 3205, Social Sciences Centre
Longon, Ontario N6A 5C2
Tel: 519-661-2111, X84713 or X8471

Dr. William R. Avison (Dircector)
E-mail: wavison@uwo.ca
E-mail: ahrc@uwo.ca
Web: www.ssc.uwo.ca/sociology/aging/health

R.B. Schlegel – University of Waterloo Research Institute for Aging

325 Max Beck Drive, Suite 202
Kitchener, Ontario N2E 4H5
Tel: 519-688-4567, ext. 3150
Fax: 519-746-6776

Dr. Mike Sharratt (Director)
E-mail: sharratt@healthy.uwaterloo.ca
E-mail: btaylor@rbjschlegel.com
Web site: www.ahs.uwaterloo.ca/research.ria

McGill Centre for Studies in Aging (MCSA), Douglas Hospital

6825 La Salle Bopulevard
Verdun, Quebec H4H 1R3
Tel: 514-766-2010
Fax: 514-888-4050

Dr. Judes Poirier (Director)
E-mail: judes.poirier@mcgill.ca
E-mail: info.mncsa@mcgill.ca
Web site: www.aging.mcgill.ca

Centre d recherche de institut universitarie de geriatrie de Montreal
The Institut universitarie de geriatrie de Montreal (UGM)

Head Office
4565 Queen-Mary Road
Montral, Quebec H3W 1W5
Tel: 514-340-2800
Fax: 514-340-2802

Dr. Yves Joanette (Director ofResearch)
E-mail: yves.joanette@umontreal.ca
Pierrette Boivin (Communications)
E-mail: pierrette.boivin.iugm@ssss.gouv.qc.ca
Web site: www.iugm.qc.ca

PavillonAlfre-DesRochers
5325 avenue Victoria
Montreal, Quebec K3W 2P2
Tel: 514-340-2800
Fax: 514-731-2136

Centre de recherche sur le vieillissement/Research Centre on Aging, Universite de Sherbrooke

Pavilon d'Youville
1036, rue Belvedere Sud
Sherbrooke, Quebec J1H 4C4
Tel: 819-829-7131
Fax: 819-829-7141

Dr. StephenCunnane (Director)
E-mail: Stephen.Cunnane@USherbrooke.ca
Web site: www.cdrv.ca

Institut sur le vieillissement et la partiiation sociale des aires (IVPSA), Univerite Laval

Local 2472-C
Pavilon De Koninck
Universite Laval
Quebec, Quebec G1K 7P4
Tel: 418-656-2131, #11555
Fax: 418-656-3567

Dr. Rene Verreauit (Co-Director)
E-mail: Reve.Verreault@msp.ulaval.ca
Dr. Aline Vezina (Co-Director)
E-mail: Aline.Vezina@svs.ulaval.ca
Web site: www.ivpsa.ulaval.ca

Centre de recherche et d'expertise en gerontologie sociale

5800 Boulevard Cavendish, Suite 500
Cote St-Luc, Quebec HWw 2T5
Tel: 514-488-9163
Fax: 514-488-2822

Professor Nancy Guberman
E-mail: guberman.nancy@uqam.ca

Third Age Centre, St. Thomas University

Brian Mulroney Hall, Room 101
Fredericton, New Brunswick E3B 5G3
Tel: 506-452-0526
Fax: 506-452-0611
E-mail: 3rdage@stu.ca
Web site: www.stu.ca/research/3rdage/

The Fredericton 80+ Study
c/o Department of Gerontology
Fredericton, New Brunswick E3B 5G3
Tel: 506-452-0516
Fax: 506-452-0611
William L. Randall (Project Director)
E-mail: randall@stu.ca
Web site: www.stu.ca/research/80plus/index.htm

Nova Sotia Centre on Aging, Mount Saint Vincent University

166 Bedford Highway
Halifax, Nova Scotia B3M 2J6
Tel: 902-457-6546
Fax: 902-457-6508

Dr. Janice Keefe (Director)
E-mail: janice.keefe@msvu.ca
Web site: www.msvu.ca/campus-information/caging

Maritime Data Centre for Aging Research & Policy Analysis, Mounst Saint Vincent University

66 Bedford Highway
Halifax, Nova Scotia B3M 2J6
Tel: 902-457-6780
Fax: 902-457-6226

Dr. Janice Keele (Associate Professor & Canada Research Chair in Aging & Caregiving Policy)
E-mail: janice.keefe@msvu.ca
E-mail: mdc.aging@msvu.ca
Web site: www.msvu.ca/mdcaging/index.asp

Prince Edward Island Centre on Health & Aging
Charlottetown, Prince Edward Island   Olive Bryanton (Director)
Tel: 902-368-9008 / 902-566-0737   E-mail: obryanton@upei.ca
Fax: 902-368-9006